T0344424

Complex Disorders in Pediatric Psychiatry: A Clinician's Guide

Complex Disorders in Pediatric Psychiatry: A Clinician's Guide

DAVID DRIVER, MD
Director
Psychiatry
Healthy Foundations Group
Bethesda, MD, United States
Child, Adolescent and Adult Psychiatrist
Healthy Foundations Group
Bethesda, MD, United States

SHARI S. THOMAS, MD
Child and Adolescent Psychiatry
Healthy Foundations Group
Bethesda, MD, United States

ELSEVIER

ELSEVIER

3251 Riverport Lane
St. Louis, Missouri 63043

Content Strategist: Kayla Wolfe
Content Development Manager: Lucia Gunzel
Content Development Specialist: Casey Potter
Publishing Services Manager: Deepthi Unni
Project Manager: Janish Ashwin Paul
Designer: Gopalakrishnan Venkatraman

Working together
to grow libraries in
developing countries

Printed in United States of America

Last digit is the print number: 9   8   7   6   5   4   3   2   1

www.elsevier.com • www.bookaid.org

List of Contributors

Editors

David Driver, MD
Director
Psychiatry
Healthy Foundations Group
Bethesda, MD, United States
Child, Adolescent and Adult Psychiatrist
Healthy Foundations Group
Bethesda, MD, United States

Shari S. Thomas, MD
Child and Adolescent Psychiatry
Healthy Foundations Group
Bethesda, MD, United States

Authors

Maxine Ames, MD
Sidney Kimmel Medical College
Thomas Jefferson University
Department of Pediatrics
Nemours, A. I. DuPont Hospital for Children
Wilmington, DE, United States

Afsoon Anvari, BS
Medical Student
2d Lieutenant of USAF
Uniformed Services University of the Health Sciences
Bethesda, MD, United States

Victoria Bacon, MPS
The Center for Anxiety and Behavioral Change
Rockville, MD, United States

Rebecca Begtrup, DO, MPH
Clinical Instructor
Department of Psychiatry and Behavioral Sciences at
   the Children's National Health Systems
Washington, DC, United States

Steven J. Berkowitz, MD
Associate Professor of Psychiatry
University of Pennsylvania
Perelman School of Medicine
Director
Penn Center for Youth and Family Trauma Response
   and Recovery
Philadelphia, PA, United States

Lawrence W. Brown, MD
Director, Pediatric Neuropsychiatry Program
Associate Professor of Neurology and Pediatrics
Division of Neurology
Children's Hospital of Philadelphia
Philadelphia, PA, United States

Brenda Bursch, PhD
Professor
Department of Psychiatry and Biobehavioral Sciences
David Geffen School of Medicine At UCLA
Los Angeles, CA, United States

Samantha Busa, PsyD
Clinical Assistant Professor
Hassenfeld Children's Hospital at NYU Langone
Department of Child and Adolescent Psychiatry
Child Study Center
New York, NY, United States

Irene Chatoor, MD
Professor of Psychiatry and Pediatrics
The George Washington University School of
   Medicine
Vice Chair
Department of Psychiatry and Behavioral Sciences
Director of the Infant and Toddler Mental Health
   Program at the Children's National Health
   Systems
Washington, DC, United States

Jessica Crawford, MD
Stanford University School of Medicine
Stanford, CA, United States

Russell C. Dale, MD
Professor of Paediatric Neurology
Department of Clinical Neuroimmunology
Institute for Neuroscience and Muscle Research
Children's Hospital at Westmead
University of Sydney
Sydney, New South Wales, Australia

Jonathan Dalton, PhD
Director
Psychology
The Center for Anxiety and Behavioral Change
Rockville, MD, United States

Mary L. Dell, MD
Departments of Psychiatry and Pediatrics
Nationwide Children's Hospital
The Ohio State University College of Medicine
Columbus, OH, United States

Stephen DiDonato, PhD, LPC
Assistant Professor
Community & Trauma Counseling Program
Jefferson: Philadelphia University + Thomas Jefferson
    University
Philadelphia, PA, United States

David Driver, MD
Director
Psychiatry
Healthy Foundations Group
Bethesda, MD, United States
Child, Adolescent and Adult Psychiatrist
Healthy Foundations Group
Bethesda, MD, United States

Josephine Elia, MD
Sidney Kimmel Medical College
Thomas Jefferson University
Department of Pediatrics and Psychiatry
Nemours, A. I. DuPont Hospital for Children
Wilmington, DE, United States

Jennifer Frankovich, MD, MS
Clinical Associate Professor
Department of Pediatrics
Division of Allergy, Immunology & Rheumatology
Stanford University
Stanford, CA, United States

Michelle Goldsmith, MD, MA
Stanford University School of Medicine
Stanford, CA, United States

Alexander J. Gordon, BA
Doctoral Fellow
Department of Psychology
St. John's University
Queens, NY, United States

Elora Hilmas, Pharm D
Nemours, A. I. DuPont Hospital for Children
Wilmington, DE, United States

Geeta Ilipilla, MD
Departments of Psychiatry and Pediatrics
Nationwide Children's Hospital
The Ohio State University College of Medicine
Columbus, OH, United States

Aron Janssen, MD
Associate Professor, Child and Adolescent Psychiatry
Clinical Director, Gender and Sexuality Service
Co-Director, Pediatric Psychiatry Consultation-Liaison
    Service
Hassenfeld Children's Hospital at NYU Langone
Department of Child and Adolescent Psychiatry
Child Study Center
New York, NY, United States

Grace Unsal, DO
C/O Drexel Department of Psychiatry
Philadelphia, PA, United States

Michael Kelly, MD
Clinical Assistant Professor
Stanford University
Department of Psychiatry and Behavioral Sciences
Stanford, CA, United States

Francis Loeb, BS
Intramural Research Training
Awardee (IRTA)
National Institute of Mental Health
Bethesda, MD, United States

Anne McHugh, MD
Pediatric Rheumatology
Fellow
Department of Pediatrics
Division of Allergy, Immunology & Rheumatology
Stanford University
Stanford, CA, United States

Gaurav Mishra, MD
Child & Adolescent Psychiatrist
Imperial County Behavioral Health Services
El Centro, CA, United States

Noga Or-Geva, PhD
Postdoctoral Research Fellow
Interdepartmental Program in Immunology
Department of Neurology and Neurological Sciences
Stanford University School of Medicine
Stanford, CA, United States

Temitayo O. Oyegbile, MD, PhD
Assistant Professor
Departments of Pediatrics and Neurology
Division of Pediatric Neurology
MedStar Georgetown University Hospital
Washington DC, United States

Zachariah D. Pranckun, DO
Child & Adolescent Psychiatrist
Department of Psychiatry & Human Behavior
Sidney Kimmel Medical College
Thomas Jefferson University
Philadelphia, PA, United States

Judy Rapoport, MD
Principle Investigator
National Institute of Mental Health
Bethesda, MD, United States

Adelaide S. Robb, MD
Professor
Psychiatry and Pediatrics
George Washington University School of Medicine
Washington, DC, United States
Children's National Medical Center
Washington, DC, United States

Jay Salpekar, MD
Director
Neuropsychiatry in Epilepsy Program
Kennedy Krieger Institute
Johns Hopkins University School of Medicine
Baltimore, MD, United States

Stefanie Sequeira, BS
Department of Psychology
Clinical/Developmental Program
University of Pittsburgh
Pittsburgh, PA, United States

Richard Shaw, MD
Stanford University School of Medicine
Stanford, CA, United States

Meghan Starner, MD
Department of Psychiatry
Sidney Kimmel Medical College
Thomas Jefferson University
Philadelphia, PA, United States

Margo Thienemann, MD
Clinical Professor
Department of Psychiatry and Behavioral Sciences
Division of Child and Adolescent Psychiatry
Stanford University
Stanford, CA, United States

Shari S. Thomas, MD
Child and Adolescent Psychiatry
Healthy Foundations Group
Bethesda, MD, United States

Alix Timko, PhD
Assistant Professor of Psychology in Psychiatry
Department of Child and Adolescent Psychiatry and
    Behavioral Sciences
Children's Hospital of Philadelphia
Perelman School of Medicine at The University of
    Pennsylvania
Philadelphia, PA, United States

Paula Tran, MD
Assistant Professor of Clinical Psychiatry and
    Pediatrics
Children's Hospital Los Angeles - University of
    Southern California
Los Angeles, CA, United States

Heather Van Mater, MD, MS
Associate Professor
Department of Pediatrics
Division of Rheumatology
Duke University
Durham, NC, United States

Laurel Weaver, MD, PhD
Assistant Professor of Psychiatry
Department of Child and Adolescent Psychiatry and
    Behavioral Sciences
Children's Hospital of Philadelphia
Perelman School of Medicine at The University of
    Pennsylvania
Philadelphia, PA, United States

Hunter Wernick, MD
Nemours, A. I. DuPont Hospital for Children
Wilmington, DE, United States

Joshua Wortzel, MSc
Stanford University School of Medicine
Stanford, CA, United States

Nassim Zecavati, MD, MPH
Associate Professor
Department of Pediatrics
Pediatric Neurology
MedStar Georgetown University Hospital
Washington, DC, United States

Dale Zhou, BS
Child Psychiatry Branch
National Institute of Mental Health
National Institutes of Health
Bethesda, MD, United States

Preface

In the demanding world of patient care, we can easily become inundated and overwhelmed by both volume and diversity. Additionally, the landscape of pediatric psychiatry is expanding at a dizzying pace. For our patients, this means that we now have an improved ability to understand their suffering and offer evidence-based interventions. For providers, a more assorted group of individuals are seeking care, putting pressure on our ability to quickly identify needs and develop evidence-based treatment plans.

In this book, we hope to shorten the journey to understanding recent advances by compiling the expertise of leaders from around the country. The authors in this book pioneer research, coin nomenclature, write criteria, and develop novel treatments. They are clinicians, educators, and scientists. As such, there is in-depth discussion of the pathophysiology, diagnosis, and treatment of some of the most complex illnesses in pediatric psychiatry.

The frontlines of pediatric psychiatry are in pediatricians' offices, urgent care clinics, and pediatric emergency rooms. Our hope for this volume is that providers will find it both useful as an in-clinic resource and as a starting point for the pursuit of a more thorough understanding of the various in-office presentations.

We would like to express our sincere gratitude for the authors who took time to share their expertise. Their contributions have allowed this book to have a breadth and depth that ensure clinicians can incorporate vital information into their daily practice of medicine. The editorial staff at Elsevier have been patient and supportive as this project evolved, and we would like to thank them for their commitment to this book. Lastly, we would like to thank our patients who inspire us to continuously strive to provide excellent care.

David Driver, MD
Healthy Foundations Group
Bethesda, MD, United States
Shari S. Thomas, MD
Healthy Foundations Group
Bethesda, MD, United States

Contents

List of Tables and Boxes

CHAPTER 1

Gender Dysphoria in Childhood and Adolescence

ARON JANSSEN, MD • SAMANTHA BUSA, PSYD

The concept of gender may appear to be simple for those who have never thought about the fact that their biologic sex is congruent with their gender identity; however, it is a complex term with complex meanings. It can morph and change over time and can be expressed in an infinite number of ways. For children and adolescents, gender identity can be especially confusing. Historically, the assumption was that a child is born with a set of chromosomes that defined gender identity: XY for boys and XX for girls. These chromosomes were thought to be typically associated with the assigned gender marker, a congruent gender identity, congruent gender role/expression, and an attraction to the opposite sex. But there have always been individuals who have not had fit so neatly into this paradigm. With the recent increase in coverage of gender variance within the media, more children are exposed to the idea that gender is more complex than just boy or girl. For mental health professionals, an understanding of gender development is crucial in treating youth, particularly among those who present with gender dysphoria.

We first aim to help providers have a sense of the difference between assigned sex, gender identity, and gender role and how gender dysphoria affects children and adolescents. It is important to have a common language to discuss the differences and relationships between sex, gender identity, and gender expression. Biologic sex is defined as the set of anatomic and hormonal differences that have historically defined male and female. These are affected by the individual's genetic makeup. This is different from an individual's gender identity, which is an individual's subjective sense of his/her own gender as male, female, or another gender identification. Gender variance is encompassed within gender identity, as it describes any variability in gender identity or gender role. Gender role is the behaviors and roles learned by an individual as determined by the cultural norms. Gender expression is how an individual presents his/her gender through his/her actions, dress, and demeanor, and how those presentations are based on gender norms.

Gender dysphoria is a term created by the *Diagnostic and Statistical Manual of Mental Disorders, Fifth Edition* (*DSM-5*) to describe the distress that might be present in the context of incongruence between sex assigned at birth and gender identity. There is some controversy around the inclusion of gender dysphoria within the diagnostic manuals, as it may inadvertently pathologize gender variance through its inclusion in this manual. Gender variance is a healthy exploration of the gender spectrum. Although we do not believe that gender variance is pathologic, we know that individuals who experience incongruence between biologic sex and gender identity are forced to face intense minority stress, overtly and covertly, and it is unsurprising that transgender adolescents often have alarmingly high rates of mental health issues, including increased suicidal ideation and suicide attempts.[1] Minority stress is seen systemically through the chronic violence toward transgender and gender nonconforming individuals, high rates of homelessness, underemployment, and poor medical care for these individuals.[2–4] An individual presenting with gender dysphoria might have symptoms that stem from minority stress or might be independent of minority stress; however, the dysphoria is not the result of the individual's gender identity itself.[5] In this chapter, we seek to discuss gender variance and how gender identity develops within childhood and also to describe gender dysphoria and treatment associated with it. We will also discuss the important role of parental support as a mediator of outcomes for transgender youth with gender dysphoria.

DEVELOPMENT OF GENDER IDENTITY

The development of gender identity is complex and not the same for every individual. Kohlberg defined developmental stages of gender identity development and posited that children move through these stages and see things as more complex as they age.[6] Through his work he identified that around 2–3 years of age, the construct *gender identity* becomes apparent. Children in this age have a sense of who they are, but it is not stable. Children aged 4–5 years understand the concept of *gender stability* that their own gender is stable. Between ages 5–7 years, children begin to understand *gender constancy*, the concept that everyone's gender is stable. For some children, this period where gender constancy solidifies is when we begin to see an increase in gender dysphoria, as there is less fluidity in gender cognitively at this period. When children enter puberty, there is also an increase in questioning around gender identity. Because the body begins to change, many children are more aware of the discrepancy between their sex assigned at birth and their gender identity.

DIAGNOSTIC CRITERIA FOR GENDER DYSPHORIA IN CHILDHOOD AND IN ADOLESCENCE

The diagnosis of gender dysphoria has a history that is controversial in nature. Distress related to gender identity was first acknowledged in *DSM-II*[7] in 1968 as sexual deviation, and in children this distress was not addressed until *DSM-III*.[8] Since then, the diagnosis has morphed in its naming to gender dysphoria rather than gender identity disorder. Although the diagnosis does not fully encapsulate the concept of minority stress, it is important to give this diagnosis when appropriate. *DSM-5*[9] defines gender dysphoria in children as incongruence between assigned sex and gender identity and expression that occurs for at least 6 months. It must be accompanied by at least six symptoms (see Table 1.1).[9] In adolescents, the criteria for gender dysphoria are the same as for adults and include incongruence between assigned sex and gender identity that occurs for at least 6 months and two accompanying symptoms (see Table 1.1).[9]

EPIDEMIOLOGY AND ETIOLOGY

There are a number of challenges associated with identifying the prevalence of gender nonconforming and transgender youth. Some of these methodological

TABLE 1.1
DSM-5 Criteria for Gender Dysphoria in Children and Adolescents

Gender Dysphoria in Children	Gender Dysphoria in Adolescents and Adults
A. A marked incongruence between one's experienced/expressed gender and assigned gender, of at least 6 months duration, as manifested by at least six of the following (one of which must be Criterion A1): 1. A strong desire to be of the other gender or an insistence that one is the other gender (or some alternative gender different from one's assigned gender) 2. In boys (assigned gender), a strong preference for cross-dressing or simulating female attire; or in girls (assigned gender), a strong preference for wearing only typical masculine clothing and a strong resistance to the wearing of typical feminine clothing 3. A strong preference for cross-gender roles in make-believe play or fantasy play 4. A strong preference for the toys, games, or activities stereotypically used or engaged in by the other gender 5. A strong preference for playmates of the other gender 6. In boys (assigned gender), a strong rejection of typically masculine toys, games, and activities and a strong avoidance of rough-and-tumble play; or in girls (assigned gender), a strong rejection of typically feminine toys, games, and activities 7. A strong dislike of one's sexual anatomy 8. A strong desire for the primary and/or secondary sex characteristics B. The condition is associated with clinically significant distress or impairment in social, school, or other important areas of functioning	A. A marked incongruence between one's experienced/expressed gender and assigned gender, of at least 6 months duration, as manifested by at least two of the following: 1. A marked incongruence between one's experienced/expressed gender and primary and/or secondary sex characteristics 2. A strong desire to be rid of one's primary and/or secondary sex characteristics, or a desire to prevent the development of the anticipated secondary sex characteristics 3. A strong desire for the primary and secondary sex characteristics of the other gender 4. A strong desire to be of the other gender (or some alternative gender different from one's assigned gender) 5. A strong desire to be treated as the other gender 6. A strong conviction that one has the typical feelings and reactions of the other gender B. The condition is associated with clinically significant distress or impairment in social, occupational, or other important areas of functioning

challenges include changes in diagnostic criteria, differences in defining constructs, measurement differences, and the fact that gender identity can be fluid. In Amsterdam, there have been two studies looking at older adolescents and adults identifying that approximately 3%–4.5% report an "ambivalent gender identity" and approximately 1% report an "incongruent gender identity."[10] In a study specifically assessing children and adolescents rated by their parents using the Child Behavior Checklist (CBCL), approximately 2.5%–5% children were identified as behaving like the other sex and 1%–2% reported "identifying as the other sex."[11] For adolescents in this sample, approximately 1.1%–3.1% reported an ambivalent gender identity, and 0.2%–0.4% reported a transgender identity. In the most recent samples, approximately 0.7% of adolescents aged 13–17 years identify as transgender.[12] Although these data give us a picture about transgender youth, they do not capture the rates of gender nonconforming youth. The etiologic process of gender identity development is even less clear, and there is not enough literature at this time to understand the biologic and genetic components of gender identity clearly. Gender identity is separate from sex, gender role, and gender expression; therefore it is difficult to understand gender identity's etiologic mechanisms fully at this time.

When addressing whether these symptoms persist into adulthood, there are a number of prospective studies that report predictors of persistence of a transgender or gender nonconforming identity into adulthood, including intensity of the incongruence between natal sex and gender identity, cognitive identification, age of presentation, and having made a social role transition.[13,14] Children who persist through puberty are more likely to persist into adulthood, although it is impossible to predict with full certainty the future gender identity for an individual. Children who persist into adulthood might be more likely to say they are the other gender, rather than saying they have a wish to be the other gender, although this is not universally predictive. In addition, adolescents who identify as transgender are more likely to persist in their identity than those who identify as transgender earlier.[13] Further research is needed to be able to determine how to better predict persistent transgender identity to tailor interventions.

SCREENING/DIAGNOSIS

One of the primary tasks of health professionals providing services to youth experiencing gender dysphoria is to evaluate the extent to which the patient and his/her

family understand the short- and long-term consequences of gender-affirming medical interventions.[15] Mental health professionals specifically conduct comprehensive evaluations to assess for concurrent mental health vulnerabilities, treatment adherence concerns, familial attitudes and beliefs about gender identity, and a reasonable capacity for informed consent.[16] Referrals for gender dysphoria have increased over the past few years, and it is important for providers to have a sound assessment process. Within this process, families seeking care are looking for a multidisciplinary team where primary care providers are able to collaborate with mental health providers. Although there is no standardized assessment process for transgender youth within the mental health setting for these youth, there are a number of screening instruments and suggestions for a sound clinical interview. Starting with a phone screen and intake documents, it is important to be sure to have registration and intake forms, as well as staff who are trained to be welcoming and inclusive. Access to care is hindered by minority stress; therefore awareness of these challenges can help families know your team will be welcoming and inclusive. This chapter will not address these issues specifically; however, the Fenway Institute has guidelines on how to create a welcoming environment and examples of inclusive forms.[17]

When scheduling an assessment, it is imperative to have time to meet with both the child and his/her parents individually and together when assessing for gender dysphoria, as a developmental history can guide treatment recommendations. It is also important to gather information from the child's school and other collaborating providers. The sociocultural context of an individual is also important, and the fact that treatment might depend on the support of others, safety, finances, and access to care should be recognized. When meeting a family for the first time, it is important to not make assumptions regarding an individual's identity or preferred pronouns. At the beginning of each new evaluation, asking a child his/her preferred name and pronoun is a way to establish a validating environment within the office. It is also important to separate assessment of gender from assessment of sexual history and preferences, as these are separate constructs.

For clinics that are not specifically addressing gender dysphoria, there are ways to screen if gender identity is a source of stress for a child. Many clinics use the Achenbach Scales to broadly assess psychiatric conditions.[18] For providers who use the Achenbach CBCL, parents are able to report if their child "behaves like the opposite sex" and "wishes to be the other sex." In addition to these universal screening items, there are

TABLE 1.2
Screening Instruments for Gender Dysphoria

Scale	Number of Items	Focus
Body Image Scale[1]	30 items to rate on a Likert-type scale	Current self-report of dysphoria related to body and image
Gender Identity Interview for Children[2]	12 items to rate on a Likert-type scale	Current self-report of gender identity development
Gender Identity Question-naire for Children[3]	16 items to rate on a Likert-type scale	Parent report of gender identity development
Recalled Childhood Gender Identity Scale[4]	22 items to rate on a Likert-type scale	Retrospective self-report of gender role
Utrecht Gender Dysphoria Scale[5]	12 statements to rate on a Likert-type scale Male and female version	Current self-report of dysphoria related to gender

Data from

1. Lindgren TW, Pauly IB. A body image scale for evaluating transsexuals. *Arch Sex Behav*. 1975;4(6):639–656.
2. Zucker KJ, Bradley SJ, Sullivan CBL, Kuksis M, Birkenfeld-Adams A, Mitchell JN. A gender identity interview for children. *J Pers Assess*. 1993;61(3):443–456.
3. Johnson LL, Bradley SJ, Birkenfeld-Adams AS, et al. A parent-report gender identity questionnaire for children. *Arch Sex Behav*. 2004;33(2):105–116.
4. Zucker KJ, Mitchell JN, Bradley SJ, Tkachuk J, Cantor JM, Allin SM. The recalled childhood gender identity/gender role questionnaire: psychometric properties. *Sex Roles*. 2006;54(7–8):469–483.
5. Schneider C, Cerwenka S, Nieder TO, et al. Measuring gender dysphoria: a multicenter examination and comparison of the Utrecht gender dysphoria scale and the gender identity/gender dysphoria questionnaire for adolescents and adults. *Arch Sex Behav*. 2016; 45(3):551–558.

a number of screening instruments validated through research and specifically created to address gender dysphoria, including the Recalled Childhood Gender Identity Scale,[19] Utrecht Gender Dysphoria Scale,[20] the Gender Identity Interview for Children,[21] the Gender Identity Questionnaire for Children,[22] and the Body Image Scale[23] (see Table 1.2 for detailed information about these scales). Although these screening measures can be helpful in understanding an individual's thoughts and feelings around his/her gender identity, they are not enough to make a diagnosis of gender dysphoria and should be accompanied by a thorough clinical interview.

To thoroughly assess gender-related concerns, it is necessary to address gender identity, gender role and expression, and discomfort in an individual's body. To assess gender identity, we look for statements either reported or spontaneously offered in the assessment of "I wish I was a girl" or "I want to grow up to be a mom" for natal males and vice versa for natal females. For younger children, they might draw themselves as a gender other than their sex assigned at birth, might have dreams about being a gender other than their sex assigned at birth, and might have confusion when asked to participate in gendered activities. Children are able to answer questions regarding play and preferences directly, and parents can also be an invaluable source of information. For older children and adolescents, there is better articulation of these wishes. Questioning of gender and sexuality is common and normative at this age; however, for those who have a persistent distress related to exploration of identity for at least 6 months, gender dysphoria could be a possible diagnosis.

Assessment of gender role and expression is focused on dress, play, and playmates through parent and child report. Natal males with gender dysphoria would be likely to report or be described by their parents as insisting on growing out their hair and wearing more stereo-typically female clothing such as skirts and leggings. Natal females with gender dysphoria might report or be described by their parents as wanting short hair and to wear more stereotypic masculine clothing. As adolescents have more independence from their parents, they might bind their breasts and shop in the men's section. For all children, assessing play and playmates is complicated, as with some families gendered toys and friends who are the opposite sex are strongly discouraged within families. In these cases, collateral information from school is important, allowing the provider to see what the individual prefers at home versus in school.

In assessing discomfort related to the body, assessing the position a child urinates can provide clues around distress related to his/her genitals. More specifically, children who are very young might attempt to remove genitalia or ask to "have different parts." Children who are young might look toward getting older and worry about changes that occur when he/she "is an adult," such as development of breasts or having a beard. Older adolescents might attempt to not allow their body to make changes, possibly restricting food to avoid breasts. Across childhood and adolescence, it is important to ask both parents and children about the frequency and comfort level of masturbation. It is also important to assess romantic and sexual attraction, as well as feelings about sex. All of these factors are to be assessed and in concert and then discussed with the family during a thorough feedback session. Feedback should include resources, impressions, and recommendations for treatment, which will be discussed next.

PSYCHOTHERAPY

There are a number of interventions that are recommended for children and teenagers with gender dysphoria through both psychotherapy and medical approaches. The guidelines for care have been created by the World Professional Association for Transgender Health.[24] Psychotherapeutic approaches focus on a gender-affirming model, allowing the child or teen to explore his/her gender identity, help the family to come to terms with the child's exploration and identity, and seek social and medical transition if he/she is interested. Therapy also aims to provide a space to address comorbid conditions. Social transition is often another focus of psychotherapy. Social transition has been identified as a protective factor for many transgender and gender nonconforming youth. Therapy can look to define gender and gender development; identify diversity in gender expression; navigate family relationship to gender identity; find ways to advocate, find support, and address challenges in school and in the community; find ways to communicate with friends and peers about gender; process sexual and romantic identities; balance multiple areas of diversity (i.e., race, ethnicity, sexual orientation); and manage stressful challenges.

Social transition includes interventions such as name and gender marker change, change in name and gender markers on identity documents, breast binding or padding, hair removal, and voice and communication therapy. These interventions allow a child to feel as though he/she can "pass" more effectively. A longitudinal study assessed transgender youth between the ages of 9–14 years matched to control subjects or siblings to determine depression and anxiety symptom differences. In this study, transgender youth who have socially transitioned report no differences in depression and slightly higher levels of anxiety,[25] which is in contrast to mental health data for youth who have not socially transitioned. In addition to social transition, support from parents is crucial to mental health outcomes and has also been seen as protective against a variety of risk factors for gender nonconforming youth.[26–32] However, it is clear that there is a correlation between perceived support across settings and long-term psychologic adjustment.[29]

For parents, the experience of a child identifying as gender nonconforming or transgender might be accompanied by fear, guilt, shame, embarrassment, concern, sadness, grief, and acceptance. Many parents experience distress following a child's coming out.[33] Parents may feel anxiety over the potential stigma gender nonconforming youth might experience.[34,35] Parents may also feel anxious about whether the child will persist in his/her identity.[36] Providing parental support and gender-affirming care can occur at the same time but may need to occur separately. It is essential to assess the entire family system for their experiences throughout the therapeutic process. Within this, providers might help families develop a script to talk about a child in their extended families or within schools. Providers might also be involved in helping families advocate within less supportive environments. Providers can also validate a parent's experience while encouraging him/her to process his/her feelings outside of his/her relationship with his/her child. Although psychotherapy can be helpful, it is not necessary for all youth who identify as gender nonconforming or transgender to attend therapy services. Many individuals will socially transition without the help of a mental health professional. In addition, therapy does not need to focus solely on the child or adolescent but also on the parents and family. Individuals can participate in parent and child support groups, in person or online.

MEDICAL INTERVENTIONS

Medical interventions for gender dysphoria are meant to delay or reverse the physiologic and visible changes that emerge in puberty. Although mental health providers do not prescribe these medical interventions, it is essential that psychiatrists and psychologists have a clear understanding of the process related to referring individuals for treatment and the impact that they have on gender dysphoria symptoms. Having a network of gender-affirming multidisciplinary providers that include adolescent medicine, plastic and reconstructive surgery, endocrinology, gynecology, urology, and vocal surgery and therapy is very important when working with transgender youth and adults. Another role of mental health providers is that they can provide letters of support for medical interventions and have the ability to assess readiness for intervention guided by the WPATH Standards of Care.[24]

The criteria related to beginning these types of intervention require that individuals must be able to demonstrate capacity to consent to the medication and that psychologic/mental health challenges are "reasonably well controlled."[24] Another important aspect to this type of intervention is the idea that some individuals solely want to transition socially and may never want to take hormones or have surgery to affirm their gender identity. Some may require these procedures to experience relief in their experiences of gender dysphoria. The three classes of medical interventions are puberty suppression medications, gender-affirming hormones, and gender-affirming surgery. Referrals for these interventions can be made by any mental health professional with at least a master's degree, familiarity with using the *DSM*, training in gender dysphoria and gender nonconforming identities, and continuing education in the treatment of gender dysphoria.[37]

Puberty suppression medications limit the development of secondary sex characteristics and are given to individuals at the beginning of puberty. These medications include GnRH analogues, spironolactone, and oral contraceptive pills. This form of intervention is reversible. Puberty suppression is meant to alleviate some dysphoria related to the development of secondary sex characteristics that are not in line with an individual's gender identity. This allows children entering puberty to have more time to explore their gender, as puberty suppression medications are meant to put a pause button on development of distressing sex characteristics in puberty. Puberty suppression drugs are thought to allow patients to also feel as though they can pass more effectively. Previous research has shown that this feeling is significantly related to prosocial outcomes.[38] Puberty suppression hormones are fully reversible and allow the adolescent to explore his/her gender nonconformity further while preventing the development of sex characteristics that are more difficult to reverse if the adolescent decides to pursue sex reassignment.

WPATH[24] and the Endocrine Society[39,40] guidelines recommend that the use of hormone-suppressing therapy is indicated when (1) there is a persistent and pervasive history of gender nonconformity or gender dysphoria; (2) the gender dysphoria emerged or worsened with the onset of puberty; (3) any cooccurring psychologic, medical, or social difficulties that might interfere with treatment are addressed; and (4) the adolescent and family have given informed consent. The informed consent process includes education regarding the use of the treatment and a full understanding of risks and benefits of the intervention itself. It is encouraged that parents and children participate in this process together.

Puberty suppression medications have been studied in a number of contexts. The Amsterdam Gender Clinic in the Netherlands has been a leader in medical interventions for children and adolescents with gender dysphoria, by publishing a protocol for use in treatment.[41] In this protocol, puberty-suppressing medications were first recommended at 12 years of age, after a child enters Tanner Stage II of sexual development. Puberty suppression has been documented to have a number of advantages to treatment through a number of studies, specifically related to transgender youth who have mental health outcomes being comparable to cisgender youth.[1,42–44]

Gender-affirming hormones are used to allow an individual to develop secondary sex characteristics congruent with his/her gender identity. These include testosterone for natal females and estrogen for natal males. If estrogen is used in natal males, breasts will develop, hair will soften, hips will widen, and the face will take on a more feminine appearance. The use of testosterone in natal females will allow for increases in muscle mass, changes in the voice, and development of an Adam's apple. The use of both estrogen and testosterone will affect an individual's emotions, as he/she is essentially going through a second puberty if hormone blockers were not used or going through puberty for the first time if blockers were used. The Endocrine Society notes that these changes can begin within 3 months but can take up to 3 years to show full effects. WPATH[24] guidelines recommend that the use of hormone-suppressing therapy can be initiated when an individual is 16 years old; however, more recent guidelines note that these guidelines are flexible and can begin earlier in adolescence.[40,45] An informed consent process is essential to this process that involves an expert team of multidisciplinary professionals.

Finally, irreversible interventions include a number of different types of gender-affirming surgery, which are categorized as top and bottom surgeries. Top surgery includes breast augmentation or reconstructive chest surgery to create a more male-contoured chest. Bottom surgeries include orchiectomy (removal of the testicles), penectomy (removal of the penis), vaginoplasty (creation of a vagina), metoidioplasty (increasing the size of the clitoris), scrotoplasty (creation of a scrotum), and phalloplasty (creation of a penis). For some individuals, additional plastic surgeries are used to change the cosmetic appearance of the face, neck, or other regions the body. As discussed previously, an individual may want some, none, a few, or many of these interventions, and it is important to have open and accepting conversations with the individual about these interventions. WPATH and the Endocrine Society recommend that surgery is not considered until a child is the age of majority in his/her respective country (18 years in the United States); however, there is an increasing number of adolescents who have top surgeries before the age of 18 years.[24,40] Some recommendations state that individuals should live continuously in the gender role congruent with his/her gender identity, and transgender male patients seeking chest surgery should wait until at least 1 year of testosterone treatment is completed. Overall, these guidelines are less clear and require more targeted research to see the cost and benefit. Regardless, one letter for chest surgery and two letters for genital surgery are required for these interventions. In adults, gender-affirming surgeries can increase sexual satisfaction[46] and psychologic outcomes.[47] Unfortunately, the cost of these procedures is high, and although there has been an increase in coverage by health insurance companies, access to care continues to be a crucial challenge.[48]

COOCCURRING MENTAL ILLNESS

As discussed previously, minority stress places transgender and gender nonconforming youth at risk for mental health concerns. Rates of mental health conditions in transgender adults vary greatly in the literature, although diagnoses span mood, anxiety, and psychotic disorders.[47] Importantly, most children and teens who meet criteria for gender dysphoria do not have a cooccurring mental health issue.[1] In clinic-referred youth, there is a high proportion of individuals with gender dysphoria seeking mental health services, although only 32.4% have at least one cooccurring mental health concern.[1] When we compare transgender and cisgender youth, we see high rates of mental health concerns across the spectrum of disorders and elevated probability of diagnosis of a number of mental health issues, including depression, suicidal ideation, suicide attempt, and inpatient and outpatient hospitalization.[49] Approximately 45%

of transgender youth report outpatient mental health treatment and 22.8% report inpatient psychiatric hospitalization. When looking specifically at symptoms, between 6% and 42% of transgender and gender nonconforming youth endorse depressive symptoms, and between 10% and 45% of transgender youth endorse suicide attempts.[49,50] Nonsuicidal self-injurious behavior is also a concern, where between 14% and 39% of youth endorse self-harm thoughts and actions.[51,52] For anxiety, approximately 26% of children report symptoms.[1,13,49,50] Many transgender and gender nonconforming youth also have an attention deficit hyperactivity disorder diagnosis.[1,13,50] There is also a significant amount of youth who identify as gender nonconforming or transgender with an autism spectrum disorder diagnosis.[53-58] Specifically, some studies have identified that restricted interests related to gender could be an indicator of the link between autism spectrum disorders and gender dysphoria.[59] Other studies have seen a higher representation of natal females presenting with gender dysphoria, autism, and other developmental delays.[60] There are many potential reasons for these high rates, and many studies suggest that the elevated rates of mental health concerns stem from the social stress associated with being transgender or gender nonconforming.

PROTECTIVE FACTORS AND CLINICAL IMPLICATIONS

Transgender and gender nonconforming youth are extremely vulnerable; these vulnerabilities are a consequence of environmental factors.[1,61,62] Many factors are societal in nature and require time for broad changes both politically and within communities. One malleable protective factor for these youth is parental support. Parental support has been shown to be related to lower the levels of anxiety, posttraumatic stress, suicidal ideation, and suicide attempts.[26,27,63,64] Restriction of social and medical transition for youth who present with gender dysphoria is related to an increase in anxiety and depression.[16,65] Youth who perceive parental support report greater life satisfaction overall,[26,27,63] report "good" mental health, and are significantly at less risk for homelessness.[66] Therefore, mental health providers can make significant impacts through facilitating and encouraging parental support. This can ameliorate the impact of gender dysphoria and promote positive outcomes.

As a field, it is important to assess gender identity, role, and expression routinely. At a minimum, changing practices to ask for the preferred name and pronouns is a way to create a more welcoming environment within your clinical setting. The literature surrounding treatment for this population is continually emerging, although there are a number of guidelines for assessment and treatment. First, assessment must be comprehensive and involve both parents and children. Providers need to be aware of the guidelines for treatment in the WPATH Standards of Care and use them to guide treatment planning.[24] Providing support to youth and their families can be protective to these youth. Finally, it is important to not assume an individual's gender identity, gender role, or gender expression, as gender is a continuum rather than a binary concept. Assessing gender dysphoria can be a complex process, and a multidisciplinary team is essential in working with these youth.

CLINICAL RECOMMENDATIONS WHEN MEETING WITH TRANSGENDER AND GENDER NONCONFORMING YOUTH

1. Do not assume an individual's gender identity and pronouns. Ask at the beginning of the visit. Also remember that gender identity is separate from sexual and romantic identity.
2. Do not assume these identities exist on a binary.
3. Affirm the child or teen's gender identity. Be an ally.
4. Remember that it is difficult to talk about these topics, do not push.
5. Work with a multidisciplinary team and seek supervision.
6. Medical examinations can be uncomfortable. Be sure to provide space to discuss these issues.
7. Be sure to train staff and clinicians with whom you work (including front desk staff, intake staff, and clinicians).
8. Do not assume what someone wants regarding transition. Ask open-ended questions and explore.
9. Assess for cooccurring mental health conditions. Remember that these conditions are likely due to minority stress and not due to an individual's gender identity.
10. Provide space for the family members to process their own thoughts/feelings about their child while educating them about the profound impact of family support.

PATIENT REFERENCES

World Professional Association for Transgender Health: www.wpath.org.
PFLAG: www.pflag.org.
Gender Spectrum: www.genderspectrum.org.

REFERENCES

1. de Vries AL, Doreleijers TA, Steensma TD, Cohen-Kettenis PT. Psychiatric comorbidity in gender dysphoric adolescents. *J Child Psychol Psychiatry.* 2011;52(11):1195–1202.
2. Russell ST, Ryan C, Toomey RB, Diaz RM, Sanchez J. Lesbian, gay, bisexual, and transgender adolescent school victimization: implications for young adult health and adjustment. *J Sch Health.* 2011;81(5):223–230.
3. Toomey RB, Ryan C, Diaz RM, Card NA, Russell ST. Gender-nonconforming lesbian, gay, bisexual, and transgender youth: school victimization and young adult psychosocial adjustment. *Dev Psychol.* 2010;46(6):1580.
4. Roberts AL, Rosario M, Slopen N, Calzo JP, Austin SB. Childhood gender nonconformity, bullying victimization, and depressive symptoms across adolescence and early adulthood: an 11-year longitudinal study. *J Am Acad Child Adolesc Psychiatry.* 2013;52(2):143–152.
5. Grant JM, Mottet LA, Tanis J, Herman JL, Harrison J, Keisling M. *National Transgender Discrimination Survey Report on Health and Health Care.* Washington, DC: National Center for Transgender Equality and the National Gay and Lesbian Task Force; 2010.
6. Kohlberg LA. *Cognitive-Developmental Analysis of Children\'s Sex-role Concepts and Attitudes;* 1966.
7. Association AP, Nomenclature Co, Statistics. *DSM-II: Diagnostic and Statistical Manual of Mental Disorders* The Association; 1975.
8. Association AP. *Diagnostic and Statistical Manual (DSM-III).* Washington, DC: American Psychiatric Association; 1980.
9. Association AP. *Diagnostic and Statistical Manual of Mental Disorders (DSM-5®).* American Psychiatric Pub; 2013.
10. Kuyper L, Wijsen C. Gender identities and gender dysphoria in The Netherlands. *Arch Sex Behav.* 2014;43(2):377–385.
11. Cohen-Kettenis PT, Pfäfflin F. *Transgenderism and Intersexuality in Childhood and Adolescence: Making Choices.* vol. 46. Sage; 2003.
12. Herman J, Flores A, Brown T, Wilson B, Conron K. *Age of Individuals Who Identify as Transgender in the United States.* Los Angeles: Williams Institute; 2017.
13. Wallien MS, Swaab H, Cohen-Kettenis PT. Psychiatric comorbidity among children with gender identity disorder. *J Am Acad Child Adolesc Psychiatry.* 2007;46(10):1307–1314.
14. Steensma TD, Biemond R, de Boer F, Cohen-Kettenis PT. Desisting and persisting gender dysphoria after childhood: a qualitative follow-up study. *Clin Child Psychol Psychiatry.* 2011;16(4):499–516.
15. Levin SB. Ethical concerns about emerging treatment paradigms for gender dysphoria. *J Sex Marital Ther.* 2017. https://doi.org/10.1080/0092623X.2017.
16. Byne W, Bradley SJ, Coleman E, et al. Report of the American Psychiatric Association Task Force on treatment of gender identity disorder. *Arch Sex Behav.* 2012;41(4):759–796.

17. Makadon HJ, Mayer KH, Potter J, Goldhammer H. *The Fenway Guide to Lesbian, Gay, Bisexual and Transgender Health*. ACP Press; 2015.

18. Achenbach TM. *Child Behavior Checklist/4-18*. University of Vermont, psychiatry; 1991.

19. Zucker KJ, Mitchell JN, Bradley SJ, Tkachuk J, Cantor JM, Allin SM. The recalled childhood gender identity/gender role questionnaire: psychometric properties. *Sex Roles*. 2006;54(7–8):469–483.

20. Schneider C, Cerwenka S, Nieder TO, et al. Measuring gender dysphoria: a multicenter examination and comparison of the Utrecht gender dysphoria scale and the gender identity/gender dysphoria questionnaire for adolescents and adults. *Arch Sex Behav*. 2016;45(3):551–558.

21. Zucker KJ, Bradley SJ, Sullivan CBL, Kuksis M, Birkenfeld-Adams A, Mitchell JN. A gender identity interview for children. *J Pers Assess*. 1993;61(3):443–456.

22. Johnson LL, Bradley SJ, Birkenfeld-Adams AS, et al. A parent-report gender identity questionnaire for children. *Arch Sex Behav*. 2004;33(2):105–116.

23. Lindgren TW, Pauly IB. A body image scale for evaluating transsexuals. *Arch Sex Behav*. 1975;4(6):639–656.

24. WPATH TWPAfTH. *Standards of Care for the Health of Transsexual, Transgender, and Gender Nonconforming People, Seventh Version*. vol. 2017. World Professional Association for Transgender Health; 2011.

25. Durwood L, McLaughlin KA, Olson KR. Mental health and self-worth in socially transitioned transgender youth. *J Am Acad Child Adolesc Psychiatry*. 2017;56(2):116–123. e112.

26. Bauer GR, Scheim AI, Pyne J, Travers R, Hammond R. Intervenable factors associated with suicide risk in transgender persons: a respondent driven sampling study in Ontario, Canada. *BMC Public Health*. 2015;15:525.

27. Davey A, Bouman WP, Arcelus J, Meyer C. Social support and psychological well-being in gender dysphoria: a comparison of patients with matched controls. *J Sex Med*. 2014;11(12):2976–2985.

28. Darby-Mullins P, Murdock TB. The influence of family environment factors on self-acceptance and emotional adjustment among gay, lesbian, and bisexual adolescents. *J GLBT Fam Stud*. 2007;3(1):75–91.

29. Espelage D, Aragon S, Birkett M. Homophobic teasing, psychological outcomes, and sexual orientation among high school students: what influence do parents and schools have? *Sch Psychol Rev*. 2008;37(2):202–216.

30. Friedman MS, Koeske GF, Silvestre AJ, Korr WS, Sites EW. The impact of gender-role nonconforming behavior, bullying, and social support on suicidality among gay male youth. *J Adolesc Health*. 2006;38(5):621–623.

31. Ryan C, Huebner D, Diaz RM, Sanchez J. Family rejection as a predictor of negative health outcomes in white and Latino lesbian, gay, and bisexual young adults. *Pediatrics*. 2009;123(1):346–352.

32. Stanton B, Cole M, Galbraith J, et al. Randomize trial of a parent intervention: parents can make a difference in long-term adolescent risk behaviors, perceptions, and knowledge. *Arch Pediatr Adolesc Med*. 2004;158:947–955.

33. Grossman AH, D'augelli AR, Salter NP. Male-to-female transgender youth: gender expression milestones, gender atypicality, victimization, and parents' responses. *J GLBT Fam Stud*. 2006;2(1):71–92.

34. Johnson SL, Benson KE. "It's always the mother's fault": secondary stigma of mothering a transgender child. *J GLBT Fam Stud*. 2014;10(1–2):124–144.

35. Hill DB, Menvielle E. "You have to give them a place where they feel protected and safe and loved": the views of parents who have gender-variant children and adolescents. *J LGBT Youth*. 2009;6(2–3):243–271.

36. Edwards-Leeper L, Spack NP. Psychological evaluation and medical treatment of transgender youth in an interdisciplinary "Gender Management Service"(GeMS) in a major pediatric center. *J Homosex*. 2012;59(3):321–336.

37. Coleman E, Bockting W, Botzer M, et al. Standards of care for the health of transsexual, transgender, and gender-nonconforming people, version 7. *Int J Transgend*. 2012;13(4):165–232.

38. Lawrence AA. Factors associated with satisfaction or regret following male-to-female sex reassignment surgery. *Arch Sex Behav*. 2003;32(4):299–315.

39. Hembree WC, Cohen-Kettenis P, Delemarre-van de Waal HA, et al. Endocrine treatment of transsexual persons: an Endocrine Society clinical practice guideline. *J Clin Endocrinol Metabol*. 2009;94(9):3132–3154.

40. Hembree WC, Cohen-Kettenis PT, Gooren L, et al. Endocrine treatment of gender-dysphoric/gender-incongruent persons: an endocrine society* clinical practice guideline. *J Clin Endocrinol Metabol*. 2017;102(11):3869–3903.

41. Delemarre-van de Waal HA, Cohen-Kettenis PT. Clinical management of gender identity disorder in adolescents: a protocol on psychological and paediatric endocrinology aspects. *Eur J Endocrinol*. 2006;155(suppl 1):S131–S137.

42. Cohen-Kettenis PT, Schagen SEE, Steensma TD, de Vries AL, Delemarre-van de Waal HA. Puberty suppression in a gender-dysphoric adolescent: a 22-year follow-up. *Arch Sex Behav*. 2011;40:843–847.

43. Wren B. Early physical intervention for young people with atypical gender identity development. *Clin Child Psychol Psychiatry*. 2000;5(2):220–231.

44. de Vries AL, McGuire JK, Steensma TD, Wagenaar EC, Doreleijers TA, Cohen-Kettenis PT. Young adult psychological outcome after puberty suppression and gender reassignment. *Pediatrics*. 2014;134(4):696–704.

45. Steever J. Cross-gender hormone therapy in adolescents. *Pediatr Ann*. 2014;43(6):e138–e144.

46. Klein C, Gorzalka BB. Continuing medical education: sexual functioning in transsexuals following hormone therapy and genital surgery: a review (CME). *J Sex Med*. 2009;6(11):2922–2939.

47. Gijs L, van der Putten-Bierman E, De Cuypere G. Psychiatric comorbidity in adults with gender identity problems. In: Kreukels BP, Steensma TD, de Vries AL, eds. *Gender Dysphoria and Disorders of Sex Development: Progress in Care and Knowledge*. Springer; 2014:255–276.

48. Baker KE. The future of transgender coverage. *N Engl J Med*. 2017;376(19):1801–1804.

49. Reisner SL, Vetters R, Leclerc M, et al. Mental health of transgender youth in care at an adolescent urban community health center: a matched retrospective cohort study. *J Adolesc Health.* 2015;56(3):274–279.

50. Mustanski BS, Garofalo R, Emerson EM. Mental health disorders, psychological distress, and suicidality in a diverse sample of lesbian, gay, bisexual, and transgender youths. *Am J Public Health.* 2010;100(12).

51. Skagerberg E, Parkinson R, Carmichael P. Self-harming thoughts and behaviors in a group of children and adolescents with gender dysphoria. *Int J Transgend.* 2013; 14(2):86–92.

52. Holt V, Skagerberg E, Dunsford M. Young people with features of gender dysphoria: demographics and associated difficulties. *Clin Child Psychol Psychiatry.* 2016;21(1): 108–118.

53. Strang JF, Meagher H, Kenworthy L, et al. Initial clinical guidelines for co-occurring autism spectrum disorder and gender dysphoria or incongruence in adolescents. *J Clin Child Adolesc Psychol.* 2016:1–11.

54. Strang JF, Kenworthy L, Dominska A, et al. Increased gender variance in autism spectrum disorders and attention deficit hyperactivity disorder. *Arch Sex Behav.* 2014; 43(8):1525–1533.

55. Jacobs LA, Rachlin K, Erickson-Schroth L, Janssen A. Gender dysphoria and co-occurring autism spectrum disorders: review, case examples, and treatment considerations. *LGBT Health.* 2014;1(4):277–282.

56. Janssen A, Huang H, Duncan C. Gender variance among youth with autism spectrum disorders: a retrospective chart review. *Transgend Health.* 2016;1(1):63–68.

57. de Vries AL, Noens IL, Cohen-Kettenis PT, van Berckelaer-Onnes IA, Doreleijers TA. Autism spectrum disorders in gender dysphoric children and adolescents. *J Autism Dev Disord.* 2010;40(8):930–936.

58. May T, Pang K, Williams KJ. Gender variance in children and adolescents with autism spectrum disorder from the National Database for Autism Research. *Int J Transgend.* 2016;18(1):7–15.

59. VanderLaan DP, Postema L, Wood H, et al. Do children with gender dysphoria have intense/obsessional interests? *J Sex Res.* 2015;52(2):213–219.

60. Kaltiala-Heino R, Sumia M, Tyolajarvi M, Lindberg N. Two years of gender identity service for minors: overrepresentation of natal girls with severe problems in adolescent development. *Child Adolesc Psychiatry Ment Health.* 2015;9:9.

61. D'Augelli AR, Grossman AH, Starks MT. Childhood gender atypicality, victimization, and PTSD among lesbian, gay, and bisexual youth. *J Interpers Violence.* 2006;21(11):1462–1482.

62. Simon L, Zsolt U, Fogd D, Czobor P. Dysfunctional core beliefs, perceived parenting behavior and psychopathology in gender identity disorder: a comparison of male-to-female, female-to-male transsexual and non-transsexual control subjects. *J Behav Ther Exp Psychiatry.* 2011;42(1):38–45.

63. Bouris A, Guilamo-Ramos V, Pickard A, et al. A systematic review of parental influences on the health and well-being of lesbian, gay, and bisexual youth: time for a new public health research and practice agenda. *J Prim Prev.* 2010;31(5–6):273–309.

64. Simons L, Schrager SM, Clark LF, Belzer M, Olson J. Parental support and mental health among transgender adolescents. *J Adolesc Health.* 2013;53(6):791–793.

65. Drescher J, Byne W. Gender dysphoric/gender variant (GD/GV) children and adolescents: summarizing what we know and what we have yet to learn. *J Homosex.* 2012; 59(3):501–510.

66. Travers R, Bauer G, Pyne J, Bradley K, Gale L, Papadimitriou M. Impacts of strong parental support for trans youth: a report prepared for Children's Aid Society of Toronto and Delisle Youth Services. *Trans Pulse.* 2012:1–5.

CHAPTER 2

School Refusal

JONATHAN DALTON, PHD • VICTORIA BACON, MPS

INTRODUCTION

School attendance is the foundation of a student's ability to receive education and the benefits that such education provides. However, this most basic ability of attending school consistently proves elusive for many students. There are myriad proximal and distal factors that contribute to school absenteeism, which include physical health, mental disorders, and family, school, and community variables. For practitioners, when a patient presents with problematic absenteeism, it can be difficult to formulate a case conceptualization and a treatment plan, particularly because this problem exists as a behavior rather than a diagnosis. Despite the varied complexities involved, treatment for patients who struggle to attend school can be successful in enabling them to resume sustained school attendance. For the sake of brevity, we will use the term children to include both children and adolescents unless otherwise noted.

It is important to begin with defining the many terms commonly used to describe missing school, which are not necessarily interchangeable. Broadly, *absenteeism* refers to any excusable or inexcusable absence from school, planned or unplanned.[1] As absenteeism by nature is not always considered a concern, and in certain cases may be normative, there are further terms to delineate problematic and nonproblematic absenteeism. To combat disparities in terminology, the proposed standard definition of problematic school absenteeism in the literature includes (1) missing at least 25% of total school time for at least 2 weeks, (2) severe difficulty attending classes for at least 2 weeks with significant interference in the child or family's daily routine, and/or (3) absences for at least 10 days of school during any 15-week period while school is in session (with absence defined as 25% or more of the school day missed).[1] *Truancy* is a legal definition, which varies state to state but is generally considered an amount of 20% or more school days missed within a 6-week period.[2] Although not mutually exclusive with school refusal, in the literature, truancy is generally separated by a lack of anxiety or fear base.[3] *School refusal*, also previously referred to as school phobia, generally refers to school absenteeism related to anxiety-based reasons.[4]

Furthermore, *school refusal behavior*, which can be associated with school refusal or truancy, broadly refers to behaviors such as missing full days of school, tardiness, reluctance to go to school in the morning, or difficulty remaining in classes.[4,5] Although definitions vary from country to country, school refusal is an issue that has been identified and studied across the globe and is a focus of the Global Program of Child Mental Health.[6–9]

There are disparities in the literature regarding the prevalence of school refusal, likely in part due to differences in definitions of truancy, school refusal, and absenteeism. Additionally, it can be hard to quantify, as not all school refusal behaviors result in missed days of school. From the results of various studies on school refusal and analyses of the national educational data, school refusal prevalence rates can be estimated as somewhere between 1% and 28%.[10–13] Although some studies suggest insignificant differences in prevalence between gender, race, and income level, others suggest that rates may be higher in lower-income rural or urban areas.[11,12] School refusal behaviors most commonly begin in children aged 10–13 years;[14] however, some studies suggest that rates are higher among older children.[14]

It is important to stress that school refusal is not a disorder as defined by the *Diagnostic and Statistical Manual of Mental Disorders, Fifth Edition* (*DSM-5*). For the anxiety-based school refusal that we focus on in this chapter, missing school is, in essence, a symptom of the underlying anxiety disorder(s). School refusal is heterogeneous in nature and has a multitude of family and environmental factors to consider in its treatment, for those with and without underlying psychiatric disorders. There are various risk factors that have been linked to school refusal, and when conceptualizing a school refusal case, it is important to consider all the child-, family-, parent-, peer-, school-, and community-based factors.[1]

It is suggested that school refusal be conceptualized based on the functionality of the school refusal behaviors, which fall into one of the four major categories.[15] These categories are divided into students who refuse school to (1) avoid school-related stimuli that provoke a general sense of negative affectivity (i.e., anxiety and depression); (2) escape school-related aversive social and/or evaluative situations; (3) gain attention from significant others (e.g., parents); and/or (4) pursue tangible reinforcement outside of school (e.g., shopping, playing with friends, or drug use).[15] School refusal to avoid negative affectivity or to gain attention tends to be found more in younger children, whereas school refusal to avoid aversive social/evaluative situations or to pursue tangible reinforcement tends to be found more in older children.[15] One study suggests that the majority of children fall into the two categories that include pursuit of positive reinforcement (i.e., attention or tangible reinforcement).[16]

There are many reasons why a child may not attend school, with medical reasons cited as one contributor to missed school days. Absenteeism has been linked to students who experience high levels of pain, have unmet dental needs, experience chronic headaches, and/or are overweight/obese.[17-20] Absenteeism has also been linked to students with frequent somatic complaints[21] and sleep difficulties, particularly insomnias, parasomnias, and daytime sleepiness.[22] Interestingly, one sample showed no significant differences in chronic health problems for students with high rates of absenteeism but did show differences in perceived health by the students.[23]

Children with increased behavioral problems and greater severity of psychiatric symptoms tend to have higher rates of absenteeism.[23] Some studies suggest that although students with both internalizing and externalizing problems exhibit school absenteeism, the relationship between absenteeism and internalizing problems was not linked, whereas the relationship between absenteeism and externalizing problems was.[24] Interestingly, although school refusal has been linked to anxiety disorders, students with higher rates of absenteeism tend to report lower levels of fear, which could suggest that, although anxiety disorders may be a risk factor, there are other variables indicated to result in a student refusing school.[14]

Higher rates of school absenteeism have been noted among children from single-parent families, low-income families, and families with low parental education.[25] Children from families with less emphasis on personal development and recreational activities outside of the home also show greater rates of absenteeism.[14] Additional familial risk factors for school refusal include physical punishment by parent, parental or child physical illness, and parental mental illness.[26] Studies have also looked at the link between school refusal and parental self-efficacy (PSE), a parent's

appraisal of their competence to parent a child refusing school.[27] PSE was linked to parental anxiety and depression, as well as higher levels of family dysfunction.[27] PSE was found to be lower in parents of students refusing school,[27] which could in part explain why it has been suggested that parents may have difficulty forcing their child to attend school, particularly when the child is expressing fear.[28]

As noted previously, students may refuse to attend school to avoid aversive social and/or evaluative situations. Being bullied has been linked to higher rates of absenteeism,[23] and for students who refuse school, poor peer relationships in general are linked to future nonattendance.[28] Students may even stay home from school when they do not feel safe either at school or on their way to/from school.[29]

Absenteeism has been linked to school environment particularly for older children, which can include variables such as sharing of resources, order and discipline, parental involvement, student interpersonal relationships, and student-teacher relationships.[30] Teachers' classroom management has been specifically linked to school refusal as a predictive risk factor or a reductive risk factor, especially in relation to a teacher's ability to influence relationships among peers.[28] For example, children who missed school with comorbid medical diagnoses associated with high levels of pain were less likely to miss school when they perceived their teachers as highly supportive of competence and autonomy.[17]

Because of the heterogeneity of school refusal, the risks associated are also varied; however, the consequence of school refusal, which is arguably most notable, is school dropout. As of 2015, 88% of adults have at least a high-school diploma, with lower rates of graduation among Hispanics and foreign-born adults.[31] Although not all dropouts are related to school refusal, absences from school even as early as the elementary years are a significant predictor of eventual school dropout.[10,32] Additionally, absenteeism is also linked to increased levels of anxiety and depression, increases in conduct problems, suicide attempts, risky sexual behavior, teen pregnancy, and substance use.[25,33] School refusal has also been linked to continued social, economic, and occupational problems into adulthood,[33] which can include continued psychiatric care as an adult and continuing to live at home with parents.[34]

DIAGNOSTIC ASSESSMENT

School refusal is a cluster of behaviors that are related to mental disorders that often interact in complex manners with the youths' environment. Consequently, assessment of youth exhibiting school refusal must be multifaceted and comprehensive. Specifically, this assessment should examine diagnostic, dimensional, and functional characteristics of the child and of the school refusal behavior.

With regard to diagnostic evaluation, it is important to consider a broad range of disorders and the absence of a diagnosable mental disorder. Kearney and Albano[15] found that among the children refusing school, 22.4% met criteria for separation anxiety disorder, 10.5% for generalized anxiety disorder, 8.4% for oppositional defiant disorder, and 4.9% for depression. Interestingly, approximately one-third of the children (32.9%) did not meet criteria for any mental disorder.

In addition to mental disorders, school-refusing children often report a range of somatic complaints. The rates of problematic somatic complaints among children refusing school range from 36.5%[35] to 79.4%.[36] Somatic complaints are myriad and wide-ranging and have been found to include headache, stomachache, nausea or vomiting, fatigue, sweating, light-headedness, abdominal pain, heart palpitations, diarrhea, shortness of breath, and menstruation symptoms.[4] Clearly, these symptoms overlap considerably with the symptoms of anxiety disorders, mood disorders, and somatic symptom disorders. However, these symptoms can obviously also be indicative of an underlying general medical condition, which themselves are often related to the onset of school refusal. For this reason, it is important that medical rule-outs be performed by qualified medical professionals.

Commonly used assessment measures used to assist in the evaluation of children exhibiting school refusal include the Screen Child Anxiety Related Disorders,[37] Anxiety Disorders Inventory Schedule,[38] School Refusal Assessment Scale–Revised (SRAS-R),[39] Self-Efficacy questionnaire for School Situations,[40] Child Behavior Checklist,[41] Multidimensional Anxiety Scale for Children,[42] and the Child Depression Inventory.[43]

It is recommended that in addition to the use of a clinical interview and psychometrically sound measures listed earlier, it is also important to include a behavior avoidance task (BAT) during the assessment. The BAT should include measuring the avoidance of interoceptive cues (e.g., dyspnea, light-headedness, tachycardia) and external stimuli (e.g., perceived social evaluation, separation from parents, phobic item). In addition to allowing the clinician to directly observe both the intensity and the topography of the avoidant behavior in response to various cues and thus obtain convergent or discriminatory diagnostic information,

the BAT is believed to be particularly sensitive to treatment outcome[44] and may be used to assess progress during and after treatment.

DIMENSIONAL ASSESSMENT

However, the particularly complex interactions observed between the child, his/her family, and school while treating school refusal behavior speak to the importance of a dimensional assessment of the phenomenological experience of the affected child to properly design an effective treatment. For example, the polythetic nature of the *DSM-5* produces 715 unique combinations of symptoms possible within a single panic attack.

To that end, it is recommended that each child's constellation of avoided and/or feared situations be examined in depth. These feared and/or avoided situations that form this constellation are not randomly distributed and serve as "branches on a tree," while the core fear serves as the "tree trunk," from which the avoidance of specific stimuli emerges. For example, a teen with social anxiety disorder who completes the sentence "I'm afraid that people will think of me as …" with "weird" will have a different constellation of avoidance and fear than a teen who completes that sentence with "stupid."

Specifically, the teen whose core fear centers around being seen as "weird" will be more likely to avoid unstructured social situations such as lunch or time between classes when there is no clear social rubric to follow and in which he/she will be more likely to say or do something that might be interpreted as socially inappropriate or weird. However, this same teen may feel much lower levels of anxiety while giving a well-rehearsed class presentation or answering a question from a teacher because these situations provide less of an opportunity to be judged as "weird." However, a teen who fears being seen as "stupid" may exhibit the opposite pattern of fear and avoidance and primarily attempt to avoid a situation during which his/her intellectual abilities may be scrutinized.

In addition, assessment of the manner of a child's anxiety acquisition directly informs the treatment design. For example, some children will display a marked aversion to cognitions associated with feared catastrophic outcomes that are exceptionally unlikely to be experienced at school, such as severe illness resulting in death, natural disasters, and school shootings, which are often acquired through information transfer. These children are clearly experiencing overvalued ideation and struggling to contextualize the probability of risk and are likely to exhibit a marked intolerance of uncertainty. The low-frequency and high-intensity nature of the feared outcome means that habituation following exposure to a school setting will be slow because the children will not likely attribute the absence of feared events to the absence of danger, but rather to luck, in a manner similar to someone who survived a game of Russian roulette.

On the contrary, some children have experienced events at school, which have produced a learning history that has resulted in a conditioned fear response to school, which has in turn become a conditioned stimulus. Such events can include bullying, sexual assault, and even panic attacks while at school. These individuals will likely experience consistently high levels of anxious arousal when presented with school-related stimuli (including entering the school building) while not engaging in safety behaviors. Thankfully, these individuals will likely experience a more rapid habituation while remaining in the presence of the school-related stimuli. However, the level of anxiety and the topography of the observed avoidant behavior can appear indistinguishable, regardless of the process of fear acquisition. Nonetheless, it is critical to understand the nature of this acquisition, as it will determine the extent to which the treatment design will need to incorporate extinction learning in the school itself versus training in metacognitive skills related to intrusive and overvalued ideation.

In addition, it is helpful to assess the child's level of distress tolerance. For some children, avoidance can be reflexive and can occur very early within the escalation in anxious arousal. In fact, these children's avoidance can be so effective that the child may not experience even moderate levels of anxiety unless avoidance is unavailable as a coping response. These children tend to exhibit lower levels of self-efficacy and more reliance on proximity to caregivers as a method of emotional regulation. These children often escalate their behavior quickly upon parental insistence of the child entering into an anxiety-provoking situation, which is often negatively reinforced by rapid parental acquiescence. Distress tolerance can be assessed in a variety of ways, but we favor direct observation of a parent-involved behavioral avoidance task (BAT), which also allows us to examine the interaction between the child and the parent as the child is asked to confront an anxiety-inducing stimuli. When such a pattern of poor distress tolerance and parental negative reinforcement of anxiety-based behavior are encountered, parent management training (PMT) will often be the focus of the treatment design.

Finally, it is critical for the clinician to assess ecologic and contextual variables related to the school refusal behavior. These variables include parental psychopathology, family system, and school resources. For example, some children have a history of learning disorders (e.g., executive functioning disorder, processing speed disorder) but have not exhibited school refusal behavior (or other problematic avoidant coping behaviors) until attempting to reintegrate back into school following a prolonged absence due to illness, injury, bereavement, etc. Learning disabilities in these children were manageable in earlier grades without accommodations because of a lighter workload or lower demands for higher-order cognitive skills. These children often experience marked distress when they can no longer complete the work at a level commensurate with internal or external expectation and struggle to accommodate this new information about themselves and thus begin to avoid school entirely as a means of coping. For these children, treatment will often have an early focus on academic remediation, attaining appropriate school accommodations regarding missed work, and assistance in planning and organizing an effective approach to completing missed work while also completing current assignments.

On the other hand, many assessments of a youth exhibiting school refusal behavior will reveal very problematic family systems. For example, a child with a prior diagnosis of an anxiety disorder who begins to exhibit high levels of hostility toward a custodial parent following his/her parents' divorce and who is himself/herself currently struggling with tolerating distress may prompt that parent to avoid conflict with the child through an increase in permissive parenting, which ultimately results in parental complicity in the child's anxious avoidance of school. In situations such as these, the parent(s) will be referred for individual treatment, parent training focused on authoritative parenting strategies will likely need to occur concurrently with the child's treatment, and family therapy itself may be recommended.

Unfortunately, many children present with an insidious onset of school refusal behavior that began early as intermittent refusal and gradually increased over the course of several academic years until complete refusal to attend school is observed. These children often present with a complex interaction of mental disorders, family system pathology, learning challenges, and problematic interactions between the family and school. These children, we find, will benefit from aggressive and comprehensive treatment that consists of four major treatment components.

FUNCTIONAL ASSESSMENT

Treatment for school refusal behavior is directly informed by the functions that underlie the behavior. Therefore, it is critical that a comprehensive assessment of the child who is refusing school include a functional assessment. As outlined earlier, Kearney and Albano[15] found that, in students, the categories of functions underlying the school refusal behavior include (1) avoidance of school-related stimuli that provoke a general sense of negative affectivity (i.e., anxiety and depression); (2) escape from school-related aversive social and/or evaluative situations; (3) obtainment of attention from significant others (e.g., parents); and/or (4) pursuit of tangible reinforcement outside of school (e.g., shopping, playing with friends, or drug use).

This assessment may include standardized instruments (i.e., SRAS-R), an observational functional analysis performed by the clinician as a parent attempts to gain a child's compliance in attending school, ABC (Antecedent, Behavior, Consequence) data collection sheets completed by parents, or a history obtained from the family and/or school. The results of this functional assessment directly inform the focus of the clinical intervention. More specifically, a child who is primarily positively reinforced through parent attention will benefit from a treatment emphasis on training parents on extinction and differential reinforcement through modeling and role-playing active ignoring, lowered level of parental expressed emotion, and psychoeducation on the extinction burst and the coercive parent-child cycle. On the other hand, the treatment of a child whose school refusal behavior is negatively reinforced by avoidance of negative affect will emphasize appropriate cognitive behavior therapy (CBT) techniques (as outlined below) such as psychoeducation regarding anxiety acquisition, maintenance, and extinction; exposure therapy; cognitive reappraisal strategies; and distress tolerance techniques.

COGNITIVE BEHAVIORAL TREATMENT

School refusal behavior is a multifaceted phenomenon that results from a complex interaction between mental disorders, family systems, school environment, and coping history. As a result of these complex interactions, school refusal behavior is often an entrenched and very difficult-to-treat presenting problem. Thankfully, CBT for school refusal has been shown to produce clinically significant results.[45–48] Interestingly, a recent metaanalysis indicated that treatment for school refusal was significant for an increase in school attendance but not for a reduction in anxiety.[49]

PHARMACOTHERAPY

The current literature regarding the effectiveness of pharmacotherapy in the treatment of school refusal has produced mixed results. For example, Bernstein et al.[50] investigated whether supplementing an 8-week CBT protocol with imipramine produced a superior outcome as measured by hours in school. Specifically, Bernstein et al.[50] utilized a randomized, double-blind placebo in which 63 school-refusing adolescents with either anxiety disorders or mood disorders were given imipramine versus placebo. They found that among youth who were refusing school, 54% of patients receiving imipramine were able to achieve attendance on 75% of school days, while this was only true of 17% of patients who received the placebo.

On the other hand, Melvin et al.[48] compared CBT, CBT + fluoxetine, and CBT + placebo in adolescents with anxiety disorders. They found that adding fluoxetine to CBT did not affect outcomes at either the 6-month or 1-year follow-up in the treatment of school refusal but did lead to greater adolescent-reported satisfaction with treatment as compared with CBT alone or CBT + placebo.

COMPREHENSIVE TREATMENT DESIGN

As school refusal is a complicated behavior that involves the interaction of individual, family, and school variables, it is reasonable to conclude that effective treatment will need to be comprehensive in nature and systematically target individual, family, and school variables. To that end, four specific treatment components have been identified: (1) individual exposure-based CBT, (2) group therapy for youth exhibiting school refusal behavior, (3) PMT, and (4) school consultation and collaboration. Each of these components will be outlined in the following.

Although individual child-focused treatment must be individualized based on the comprehensive assessment outlined earlier, a basic treatment template can be delineated. The essential first component of child-focused treatment is psychoeducation. The aim for the child and family is to become "curious, but informed, observers" of the anxiety response, beginning with the urge to avoid or escape. Mowrer[51] described the reinforcing nature of escape and avoidance and their role in anxiety maintenance. Because school refusal is often associated with the reinforcing nature of escape and avoidance,[39] it is critical that the children and their family understand how avoidance supports the continuation of the anxiety over time. This avoidance is normalized by describing how evolution has primed humans to quickly avoid things that make us sick, hurt, or scared. The problematic role of avoidance in anxiety disorders can be explained in a developmentally appropriate manner such as "anxiety and avoidance are teammates" or "we don't treat anxiety, we treat avoidance." This can be further explained by discussing how avoidance prevents further corrective feedback and learning regarding their inaccurate appraisal of danger, or "it prevents you from learning that while the anxiety was real, the danger never was."

The psychoeducation phase continues with information regarding the physiologic, cognitive, and emotional aspects of the anxiety. The goal for the child and family is to be able to adopt an informed perspective that allows them to accurately contextualize the phenomenological experience of anxiety or distress. To that end, information regarding (1) the function of consequences of hypervigilance and threat bias, (2) the body's sympathetic nervous system and the various sensations that may be produced by its activation, and (3) the role of emotions in directing and prioritizing our attention is described. To help the child understand and process this information, a hypothetical fire alarm in a high-rise building is used as an example, in which he/she is asked to list the likely thoughts, sensations, and emotions he/she would feel in this hypothetical situation.

Furthermore, it is discussed that it is not the alarm but rather the appraisal of the hypothetical alarm as an indication of danger that produces the symptoms he/she described. In other words, it is what he/she thinks the alarm means that produces the reaction. This is used as a bridge to beginning training in cognitive reappraisal of anxious arousal. Specifically, the child is asked what his/her reaction would be to a likely false alarm in this situation, and how the only difference in the scenarios is what he/she thinks the alarm means. Finally, the child is educated that "their anxiety alarm cannot be stopped from going off, at least in the beginning of treatment. But he/she can be helped to think in a different way about what this anxious alarm means but more importantly about what it doesn't mean."

As the cognitive portion of treatment commences, it is recommended that coping self-statements are created. Examples of self-statements are presented in Box 2.1.

The children are taught that these statements are not self-reassurance regarding reasons why they should not be anxious but rather how they can and why they should persist in the presence of anxiety. It is stressed that it is this confrontation with the anxiety rather than the avoidance of the anxiety, which is the mechanism of change during extinction learning. To communicate this information in a developmentally appropriate

---

BOX 2.1
Self-statement Examples

Courage is what I do, not what I feel.
Just because it's hard doesn't mean I can't do it.
I am stronger than my fear.
Anxiety is temporary and harmless.
I can do it while I am anxious.
It's okay to be scared.
I can choose how I think about my anxiety.
I know I can do it because I've done hard things before.
Scary thoughts are not dangerous to have.
I don't have to be certain about how it will go.
Thoughts are not evidence, and feelings are not facts.
Right now I am noticing that I'm having a scary thought about_____.

---

manner, children are asked why we would not simply "arm" a child with a fear of butterflies with bug spray and fly swatters if he/she is somewhere where butterflies are present. Children usually are able to understand that this approach would be problematic because the child would only feel less anxious when he/she was properly "armed," and more importantly, the child would never learn that butterflies are not dangerous. This analogy is extended to the child's own anxiety, and they are encouraged to stop "swatting butterflies" as a means of coping with the feared situation of stimulus.

Once children and their families are provided this psychoeducation and trained in skills related to cognitive reappraisal of anxious arousal, it is highly recommended that exposure therapy commences. Exposure therapy enjoys broad empirical support and has been identified as an empirically supported treatment[52] that has been shown to be both effective and efficacious in treating posttraumatic stress disorder, obsessive-compulsive disorder, panic disorder, generalized anxiety disorder, social anxiety disorder, and specific phobia.

As exposure therapy commences, children and their families are taught that school refusal is like an allergic reaction to a casserole, and it is important that treatment specifically targets the right "ingredient" that results in disordered anxiety and avoidance, and not simply "school." The exposure hierarchy may certainly include school stimuli such as completing schoolwork, being in the parking lot, or being in the school building; the hierarchy should be constructed around the core fear that fuels the urge to avoid school as a means of emotional regulation. To better elucidate the exposure therapy process, a sample hierarchy for a teen

> ### BOX 2.2
> #### Social Anxiety Hierarchy Example
>
> Reading tongue twisters aloud in front of clinician
>
> Reading age appropriate text aloud in front of clinician
>
> Reading a text well above age level in front of clinician
>
> Calling stores and asking when they close
>
> Calling stores and asking for the store's phone number
>
> Reading a book in public that is written for much younger child
>
> Giving an extemporaneous speech in front of clinician
>
> Defining SAT level vocabulary words
>
> Reciting the alphabet backward under timed condition
>
> Asking stranger for directions to an obvious location (e.g., asking where a store is while standing in front of store)
>
> Meeting teacher at school to review missed classwork
>
> Sitting in an empty classroom with clinician and repeating earlier exposure
>
> Attending a single class in "audit" fashion
>
> Adding additional classes in "audit" fashion
>
> Completing classwork for one class
>
> Completing classwork in additional classes
>
> Raising hand in one class
>
> Raising hand in additional classes
>
> Raising hand in class and intentionally giving wrong answer

with social anxiety disorder with a core fear of being appraised as "stupid" who is exhibiting school refusal behavior, is listed in Box 2.2.

This hierarchy is constructed in a collaborative manner with children who will play a major role in determining the order of the exposure items. However, it is common that this hierarchy and its order need to be modified as the exposure begins. For example, children may initially rate an exposure as a "2" on a 1–10 scale but find that it is much higher once they begin to do the exposure task. For that reason, children are instructed in advance that the hierarchy will likely be altered throughout treatment because their ratings are only informed guesses.

During the exposure, children are asked to practice using their coping cards as a means of sustaining nonavoidant coping in the presence of anxiety. They are also given frequent specific praise and tangible rewards that have been developed in conjunction with PMT. In addition, they are reminded that feeling anxiety while engaging in exposure therapy is the equivalent of becoming sweaty while working out; it simply means

that they are getting a good workout and is not an indication that they are doing anything wrong. As exposure therapy continues, focus is placed on the development of self-efficacy or in the children's belief in their ability to cope effectively with an anxiety-inducing situation. The emerging research appears to support the mediating effect of self-efficacy in outcome for school refusal treatment.[53]

CHILD GROUP THERAPY FOR SCHOOL REFUSAL

Not surprisingly, youth who refuse school tend to be socially isolated from their peers,[47] resulting in fewer opportunities for social learning and social support from peers. This lack of opportunities may lead to the development of or calcification of poor social skills, which may, in turn, become an obstacle to school reentry. In addition, research has shown that perceived social support among adolescents serves as a protective factor and a source of psychologic resilience.[54]

Consequently, using adjunctive group therapy for youth who are refusing school appears particularly well suited in that it provides opportunity for social learning, including participant modeling, social support, corrective feedback from peers, and destigmatization of their current difficulty.[55-58] The group model developed by our center is based on this facilitation of social learning and support. Specifically, included group members are intentionally drawn from various stages of school reentry, ranging from prolonged (multiyear) continuous refusal through maintenance of school attendance following reentry. This mixed composition provides opportunity for coping models, instillation of hope, and opportunities for leadership roles for group members more advanced in their progress. However, it is likely that adolescents with long histories of avoidant coping will require individual treatment before being able to take part in the group format, which they may initially see as more uncertain and aversive than individual therapy, resulting in a stronger urge to avoid the group.

The group is ongoing in nature, with members graduating as they are able to sustain school attendance or leave for college or work. Each group consists of 8–11 group members, with a high number intentionally included because of the high rate of absenteeism that may be observed. Group members are expected to attend a minimum of 75% of sessions to keep their slot in the group, and group refusal is treated like school refusal with regard to exigent contingencies. Group members who are not able to attend 75% of sessions are asked to engage in more intensive individual treatment before being allowed to rejoin the group at a later point.

Each session involves a review of each member's goals from the previous week and obstacles and successes in his/her ability to meet his/her own goals. Group members also review other sources of stress and receive feedback in the form of both support and being challenged by other group members. At the conclusion of group, each member states his/her goals for the following week, which must be appropriate, measurable, and achievable before the next group session.

PARENT MANAGEMENT TRAINING

PMT is recognized as an important component of the treatment of youth refusing school.[59] However, the research supporting the added benefit for this training to child-focused treatment of school refusal is mixed. For example, Heyne et al.[60] found that the addition of a parent training program for children between 7 and 14 years of age did not produce added benefits to the child treatment program.

However, the wealth of support for PMT as a clinical intervention in modifying the problematic behavior of children appears to suggest its appropriateness for the treatment of school refusal. Specifically, PMT's basic tenets of teaching parents basic behavioral concepts, such as positive and negative reinforcement, positive and negative punishment, and contingency management, are directly relevant to the skills parents utilize to improve their child's school attendance. However, PMT was developed and directed toward youth having primary externalizing behavioral disorders, such as oppositional defiance disorder and conduct disorder. Supplementing traditional PMT with information regarding information directly relevant to anxiety disorders, such as habituation, extinction, escape, avoidance, unconditioned versus conditioned stimuli, and spontaneous recovery of fear, is theoretically consistent and likely beneficial, although published research answering this question is not available.

It is recommended that PMT for school-refusing youth be conducted when possible in a group format with other parents of school-refusing youth. This modality facilitates interpersonal learning, support, and accountability to complete weekly therapeutic homework assignments while allowing more families to receive concurrent treatment. The model of parent training comprises eight 90-min sessions that are largely didactic in nature.

Topics covered in PMT include the importance of removing competition for school attendance (i.e., children are not allowed to do activities during school hours that are not allowed at school), authoritative parenting (labeled "loving firmness"), positive reinforcement, negative reinforcement, the parent-child coercive cycle, extinction learning and the extinction burst, the process of habituation, differential reinforcement (both differential reinforcement of incompatible behavior and differential reinforcement of other behavior), contingency management, positive and negative punishment (used for circumscribed circumstances, such as aggression destruction, or threats of either), token economies, coping skills for parents (including obtaining appropriate social support), the protection trap,[61] and appropriate assertiveness with school personnel. In addition, information on relapse prevention and the importance of continued consistency of implementation of parenting principles outlined during the sessions are stressed.

In addition to the didactic topics covered during the PMT session, parents take turns reviewing their child's progress at the beginning of the session with other group members, discuss obstacles that may have arisen during the week, share any data collected that week (e.g., ABC data collection sheets, list of incompatible positive behaviors to reinforce), and offer support and modeling for one another.

SCHOOL CONSULTATION

Because school reentry directly involves school personnel (e.g., teachers, counselors, social workers, school psychologists, administrators), it is essential for school personnel be involved in the plan for reintegration back into the classroom. It has proven successful to arrange a multidisciplinary meeting with the treating clinician, parents, school-refusing children (if possible), teachers, administrators, and other educational professionals in the room. The goal of this meeting, broadly defined, is to remove uncertainty about what to expect from the reentry process for the child, from large issues such as missed work completion to more logistical concerns such as current seating arrangements.

Specifically, this meeting is individually tailored to each child's needs but may address issues such as information of the child's mental disorder if he/she has been diagnosed with one, the extent to which schoolwork that has been missed is required to be completed and how much can be excused, the design of a plan for missed work completion and missed content remediation, the responsibility of the student for current assignments while missed content is being remediated, the process of completing group projects if any exist, the development of an appropriate "cover story" for peers that may inquire about the child's absences, the differences between appropriate accommodation versus enabling avoidance on behalf of educators, and whether seating arrangements have changed. Furthermore, it is usually recommended that students during the initial phase of reentry are allowed to be in "auditing mode" during which time (usually 3–5 days) the student will not be responsible for classwork or homework of any variety and will not be called upon unless he/she raised his/her hand. Finally, the teachers are instructed to not draw attention to the newly returning student in the classroom.

More broadly, it is recommended that one representative from the school serves as the contact with the student's family and that this person should work to project a nonjudgmental stance while communicating with the family.[1] The authorization for the child to use "flash passes" to leave the classroom and visit a counselor is allowed, but it is recommended that these passes be limited to no more than once per day and any "unused" passes at the end of the week can be traded in for points or other items of value. This arrangement provides an ability to escape a situation at school (designed to elicit compliance to go to school while having intrusive thoughts about needing to leave a classroom) while providing an incentive to use nonavoidant coping in the moment of heightened distress.

Additionally, many school personnel inquire about referring the child to a variant of Home and Hospital Teaching. Home and Hospital offers many drawbacks including the fact that it negatively reinforces avoidant behavior, it allows for continued social isolation, it removes urgency for treatment and does not address avoidant coping, and it is often seen by the student as a valid alternative to school attendance. For these reasons, it is recommended that home-based education be limited to children who cannot safely be returned to school because of suicidality, aggression, or other dangerous behavior during an extinction burst or who are suffering from comorbid medical conditions that preclude school attendance.

CONCLUSION

School refusal is a complex phenomenon with myriad proximal and distal antecedents, including child, family, school, and community variables, which interact to produce entrenched behavior patterns that are quite difficult to treat effectively. In addition, school refusal results in short- and long-term sequela that often place the affected child on a different developmental trajectory that includes poor academic functioning, impaired social functioning, and lowered self-efficacy, as well as challenges as adults including higher rates of unemployment, marital discord, and the presence of persistent mental disorders.[33]

These long-term consequences of school refusal have less to do with the absence of specific academic skills such as correctly conjugating a verb or using the Pythagorean Theorem but rather are more related to the child's reliance on avoidant coping as a method of regulating emotions in the presence of distress. Because the stakes are so high and the behavior so complex, effective treatment must be comprehensive in nature and address the multiple variables involved in the refusal behavior with the targeted goal of providing the child the knowledge and skills required to use nonavoidant coping and the encouragement and motivation to use it effectively and consistently.

REFERENCES

1. Kearney C. An interdisciplinary model of school absenteeism in youth to inform professional practice and public policy. *Educ Psychol Rev.* 2008;20(3):257–282. Available from: PsycINFO, Ipswich, MA.
2. Gentle-Genitty C, Karikari I, Chen H, Wilka E, Kim J. Truancy: a look at definitions in the USA and other territories. *Educ Stud.* 2015;41(1–2):62–90. Available from: PsycINFO, Ipswich, MA.
3. Fremont W. School refusal in children and adolescents. *Am Fam Phys.* 2003;68(8):1555–1561.
4. Kearney C. School absenteeism and school refusal behavior in youth: a contemporary review. *Clin Psychol Rev.* 2008;28(3):451–471. Available from: PsycINFO, Ipswich, MA.
5. Kearney C, Silverman W. The evolution and reconciliation of taxonomic strategies for school refusal behavior. *Clin Psychol Sci Pract.* 1996;3(4):339–354. Available from: PsycINFO, Ipswich, MA.
6. Remschmidt H. How can we prevent school avoidance and behavior problems in preschool children? *Dtsch Ärzteblatt Int.* 2015;112(39):645–646. Available from: PsycINFO, Ipswich, MA.
7. Knollmann M, Knoll S, Reissner V, Metzelaars J, Hebebrand J. School avoidance from the point of view of child and adolescent psychiatry: symptomatology, development, course, and treatment. *Dtsch Ärzteblatt Int.* 2010;107(4):43–49. Available from: PsycINFO, Ipswich, MA.
8. Inoue K, Tanii H, Ono Y, et al. Current state of refusal to attend school in Japan. *Psychiatry Clin Neurosci.* 2008;62(5):622. Available from: PsycINFO, Ipswich, MA.

9. Inglés C, Gonzálvez-Maciá C, García-Fernández J, Vicent M, Martínez-Monteagudo M. Current status of research on school refusal. *Eur J Edu Psychol.* 2015;8(1):37–52. Available from: PsycINFO, Ipswich, MA.

10. Epstein J, Sheldon S. Present and accounted for: improving student attendance through family and community involvement. *Educ Res.* 2002;95(5):308–318. Available from: PsycINFO, Ipswich, MA.

11. Kearney C. *School Refusal Behavior in Youth: A Functional Approach to Assessment and Treatment* [e-book]. Washington, DC, US: American Psychological Association; 2001. Available from: PsycINFO, Ipswich, MA.

12. Balfanz R, Byrnes V. *Chronic Absenteeism: Summarizing what We Know from Nationally Available Data.* Baltimore: Johns Hopkins University Center for Social Organization of Schools; 2012.

13. Sheldon S, Epstein J. Getting students to school: using family and community involvement to reduce chronic absenteeism. *Sch Comm J.* 2004;14(2):39–56. Available from: PsycINFO, Ipswich, MA.

14. Hansen C, Sanders S, Massaro S, Last C. Predictors of severity of absenteeism in children with anxiety-based school refusal. *J Clin Child Psychol.* 1998;27(3):246–254. Available from: PsycINFO, Ipswich, MA.

15. Kearney C, Albano A. The functional profiles of school refusal behavior: diagnostic aspects. *Behav Modif.* 2004;28(1):147–161. Available from: PsycINFO, Ipswich, MA.

16. Dube S, Orpinas P. Understanding excessive school absenteeism as school refusal behavior. *Child Sch.* 2009;31(2):87–95. Available from: PsycINFO, Ipswich, MA.

17. Vervoort T, Logan D, Goubert L, De Clercq B, Hublet A. Severity of pediatric pain in relation to school-related functioning and teacher support: an epidemiological study among school-aged children and adolescents. *Pain.* 2014;155(6):1118–1127. Available from: PsycINFO, Ipswich, MA.

18. Agaku I, Olutola B, Adisa A, Obadan E, Vardavas C. Association between unmet dental needs and school absenteeism because of illness or injury among U.S. school children and adolescents aged 6–17 years, 2011–2012. *Prev Med.* 2015;72:83–88. Available from: PsycINFO, Ipswich, MA.

19. Rousseau-Salvador C, Amouroux R, Annequin D, Salvador A, Tourniaire B, Rusinek S. Anxiety, depression and school absenteeism in youth with chronic or episodic headache. *Pain Res Manag.* 2014;19(5):235–240. Available from: PsycINFO, Ipswich, MA.

20. Echeverría S, Vélez-Valle E, Janevic T, Prystowsky A. The role of poverty status and obesity on school attendance in the United States. *J Adolesc Health.* 2014;55(3):402–407. Available from: PsycINFO, Ipswich, MA.

21. Zolog T, Ballabriga M, Domenech-llaberia E, et al. Somatic complaints and symptoms of anxiety and depression in a school-based sample of preadolescents and early adolescents. Functional impairment and implications for treatment. *J Cogn Behav Psychother.* 2011;11(2):191–208. Available from: PsycINFO, Ipswich, MA.

22. Hochadel J, Frölich J, Wiater A, Lehmkuhl G, Fricke-Oerkermann L. Prevalence of sleep problems and relationship between sleep problems and school refusal behavior in school-aged children in children's and parents' ratings. *Psychopathol.* 2014;47(2):119–126. Available from: PsycINFO, Ipswich, MA.

23. Ingul J, Nordahl H. Anxiety as a risk factor for school absenteeism: what differentiates anxious school attenders from non-attenders? *Ann Gen Psychiatry.* 2013;12. Available from: PsycINFO, Ipswich, MA.

24. Ingul J, Klöckner C, Silverman W, Nordahl H. Adolescent school absenteeism: modelling social and individual risk factors. *Child Adolesc Ment Health.* 2012;17(2):93–100. Available from: PsycINFO, Ipswich, MA.

25. Wood J, Lynne-Landsman S, Ialongo N, et al. School attendance problems and youth psychopathology: structural cross-lagged regression models in three longitudinal data sets. *Child Dev.* 2012;83(1):351–366. Available from: PsycINFO, Ipswich, MA.

26. Bahali K, Tahiroglu A, Avci A, Seydaoglu G. Parental psychological symptoms and familial risk factors of children and adolescents who exhibit school refusal. *East Asian Arch Psychiatry.* 2011;21(4):164–169. Available from: PsycINFO, Ipswich, MA.

27. Carless B, Melvin G, Tonge B, Newman L. The role of parental self-efficacy in adolescent school-refusal. *J Fam Psychol.* 2015;29(2):162–170. Available from: PsycINFO, Ipswich, MA.

28. Havik T, Bru E, Ertesvåg S. School factors associated with school refusal- and truancy-related reasons for school non-attendance. *Soc Psychol Educ.* 2015;18(2):221–240. Available from: PsycINFO, Ipswich, MA.

29. Eaton D, Kann L, Kinchen S, et al. Youth risk behavior surveillance-United States, 2009. *Surveill Summ MMWR.* 2010:59.

30. Hendron M, Kearney C. School climate and student absenteeism and internalizing and externalizing behavioral problems. *Child Sch.* 2016;38(2):109–116. Available from: PsycINFO, Ipswich, MA.

31. Ryan C, Bauman K. Educational attainment in the United States: 2015. *Curr Popul Rep.* 2016:20–578.

32. Lehr C, Sinclair M, Christenson S. Addressing student engagement and truancy prevention during the elementary school years: a replication study of the check & connect model. *J Educ Students Placed Risk.* 2004;9(3):279–301. Available from: PsycINFO, Ipswich, MA.

33. Kearney C, Spear M, Mihalas S. *School Refusal Behavior. Translating Psychological Research into Practice* [e-book]. New York, NY, US: Springer Publishing Co; 2014:83–88. Available from: PsycINFO, Ipswich, MA.

34. Flakierska-Praquin N, Lindström M, Gillberg C. School phobia with separation anxiety disorder: a comparative 20- to 29-year follow-up study of 35 school refusers. *Compr Psychiatry.* 1997;38(1):17–22. Available from: PsycINFO, Ipswich, MA.

35. Egger H, Costello E, Angold A. School refusal and psychiatric disorders: a community study. *J Am Acad Child Adolesc Psychiatry.* 2003;42(7):797–807. Available from: PsycINFO, Ipswich, MA.

36. Honjo S, Nishide T, Nishide Y, et al. School refusal and depression with school attendance in children and adolescents: comparative assessment between the Children's Depression Inventory and somatic complaints. *Psychiatry Clin Neurosci.* 2001;55(6):629–634. Available from: PsycINFO, Ipswich, MA.

37. Birmaher B, Brent D, Chiappetta L, Bridge J, Monga S, Baugher M. Psychometric properties of the screen for child anxiety related emotional disorders (scared): a replication study. *J Am Acad Child Adolesc Psychiatry.* 1999;38(10):1230–1236. Available from: PsycINFO, Ipswich, MA.

38. Silverman W, Abano A. *Anxiety Disorders Interview Schedule (ADIS-IV)*; 2004.

39. Kearney C. Identifying the function of school refusal behavior: a revision of the school refusal assessment scale. *J Psychopathol Behav Assess.* 2002;24(4):235–245. Available from: PsycINFO, Ipswich, MA.

40. Heyne D, King N, Myerson N, et al. The self-efficacy Questionnaire for school situations: development and psychometric evaluation. *Behav Change.* 1998;15(1):31–40. Available from: PsycINFO, Ipswich, MA.

41. Achenbach T, Rescorla L. *Manual for the ASEBA School-age Forms & Profiles*; 2001.

42. March J, Parker J, Sullivan K, Stallings P, Conners C. The multidimensional anxiety scale for children (MASC): factor structure, reliability, and validity. *J Am Acad Child Adolesc Psychiatry.* 1997;36(4):554–565. Available from: PsycINFO, Ipswich, MA.

43. Kovacs M. *Child Depression Inventory 2 (CDI 2)*; 2010.

44. Castagna P, Davis T, Lilly M. The behavioral avoidance task with anxious youth: a review of procedures, properties, and criticisms. *Clin Child Fam Psychol Rev.* 2016. Available from: PsycINFO, Ipswich, MA.

45. King N, Tonge B, Ollendick T, et al. Cognitive-behavioral treatment of school-refusing children: a controlled evaluation. *J Am Acad Child Adolesc Psychiatry.* 1998;37(4):395–403. Available from: PsycINFO, Ipswich, MA.

46. Heyne D, Sauter F, Van Widenfelt B, Vermeiren R, Westenberg P. School refusal and anxiety in adolescence: non-randomized trial of a developmentally sensitive cognitive behavioral therapy. *J Anxiety Disord.* 2011;25(7):870–878. Available from: PsycINFO, Ipswich, MA.

47. Pina A, Zerr A, Gonzales N, Ortiz C. Psychosocial interventions for school refusal behavior in children and adolescents. *Child Dev Perspect.* 2009;3(1):11–20. Available from: PsycINFO, Ipswich, MA.

48. Melvin G, Dudley A, Tonge B, et al. Augmenting cognitive behavior therapy for school refusal with fluoxetine: a randomized controlled trial. *Child Psychiatry Hum Dev.* 2017;48(3):485–497. Available from: PsycINFO, Ipswich, MA.

49. Maynard B, Heyne D, Esposito Brendel K, Bulanda J, Thompson A, Pigott T. Treatment for school refusal among children and adolescents. *Res Social Work Pract.* 2015. https://doi.org/10.1177/1049731515598619.

50. Bernstein G, Borchardt C, Last C, et al. Imipramine plus cognitive-behavioral therapy in the treatment of school refusal. *J Am Acad Child Adolesc Psychiatry.* 2000;39(3):276–283. Available from: PsycINFO, Ipswich, MA.

51. Mowrer O. On the dual nature of learning—a re-interpretation of 'conditioning' and 'problem-solving.' *Harv Educ Rev.* 1947;17:102–148. Available from: PsycINFO, Ipswich, MA.

52. Kaczkurkin AN, Foa EB. Cognitive-behavioral therapy for anxiety disorders: an update on the empirical evidence. *Dialogues Clin Neurosci.* 2015;17(3):337–346.

53. Maric M, Heyne D, MacKinnon D, van Widenfelt B, Westenberg P. Cognitive mediation of cognitive-behavioural therapy outcomes for anxiety-based school refusal. *Behav Cogn Psychotherapy.* 2013;41(5):549–564. Available from: PsycINFO, Ipswich, MA.

54. Dumont M, Provost M. Resilience in adolescents: protective role of social support, coping strategies, self-esteem, and social activities on experience of stress and depression. *J Youth Adolesc.* 1999;28(3):343–363. Available from: PsycINFO, Ipswich, MA.

55. van Starrenburg ML, Kuijpers RC, Hutschemaekers GJ, Engels RC. Effectiveness and underlying mechanisms of a group-based cognitive behavioural therapy-based indicative prevention program for children with elevated anxiety levels. *BMC Psychiatry.* 2013. PMID:23827009.

56. Parenting an Anxious Child: A Proposed Model for Group-Administered Parent Training for Parents of Children With Anxiety Disorders. Presentation at: Anxiety Disorder Association of America Annual Conference, March 2011; Baltimore, MD.

57. When Anxiety Affects Education: Comprehensive Treatment of School Refusal. Oran Presentation at: Maryland Psychological Association; January 2015; Columbia, MD.

58. "I don't know Why, I just Can't go": Treating School Refusal and Teens with Complex Clinical Presentations Anxiety Disorder. Oral Presentation at: Association of America Annual Conference; April 2017; San Francisco, CA.

59. Kearney C, LaSota M, Lemos-Miller A, Vecchio J. *Parent Training in the Treatment of School Refusal Behavior. Handbook of Parent Training: Helping Parents Prevent and Solve Problem Behaviors* [e-book]. 3rd ed. Hoboken, NJ, US: John Wiley & Sons Inc; 2007:164–193. Available from: PsycINFO, Ipswich, MA.

60. Heyne D, King N, Ollendick T, et al. Evaluation of child therapy and caregiver training in the treatment of school refusal. *J Am Acad Child Adolesc Psychiatry.* 2002;41(6):687–695. Available from: PsycINFO, Ipswich, MA.

61. Silverman W, Kurtines W. *Anxiety and Phobic Disorders: A Pragmatic Approach* [e-book]. New York, NY, US: Plenum Press; 1996. Available from: PsycINFO, Ipswich, MA.

CHAPTER 3

Attention Deficit Hyperactivity Disorder and Anxiety

GEETA ILIPILLA, MD • ZACHARIAH D. PRANCKUN, DO • HUNTER WERNICK, MD • GRACE UNSAL, DO • JOSEPHINE ELIA, MD

INTRODUCTION

A high comorbidity for attention deficit hyperactivity disorder (ADHD) and anxiety has been reported in epidemiologic studies[1-3] and clinical psychiatric ADHD[4-13] and pediatric samples.[14]

This comorbidity is not innocuous but confers greater executive functional deficits,[10,15-18] greater social difficulties,[19] and poorer quality of life (QoL)[10] and precedes later substance use.[20] Despite the significant impairments, there is limited knowledge on the underlying neurobiology and treatment management for the combination.

BACKGROUND

The cooccurrence of ADHD and anxiety disorders is common in the pediatric population. Comorbid anxiety disorders are reported to occur in 30%–40% in clinical psychiatric samples of children with ADHD[4-13] and pediatric samples.[14] Epidemiologic studies also report high comorbid rates of 25% in the general population, suggesting that the comorbidity is not due to referral bias that might be expected in clinical samples. The comorbidity is bidirectional with high levels of ADHD (16%–24%) reported in children with anxiety.[1,21,22]

The comorbidity has significant impact because children with ADHD and comorbid anxiety disorders have greater attention, cognitive, and executive functioning difficulties than children with ADHD alone,[10,15-18] as well as greater social difficulties.[19] Sciberras and colleagues observed that children with multiple anxiety comorbidities (two or more) had poorer parent-reported QoL, more behavioral problems, poor peer interactions, and impaired daily functioning. Such poor functioning is not observed in children with single anxiety comorbidity, thus indicating that only the high and pervasive level of anxiety is associated with functional impairment. In addition, such high levels of anxiety may lead to avoidance and negative thought patterns that may negatively influence the functioning.[10] ADHD and anxiety disorders also precede later substance use.[20]

PREVALENCE

Data on the prevalence of comorbidity between ADHD and anxiety disorders are derived from both epidemiologic and clinical studies in children and adolescents. Clinical studies have limitations, as they recruit individuals from specialty treatment settings with more severe symptomatology and more impairment and those who come from families experiencing increased burden from their children's problems.

Summarized in Table 3.1 are the epidemiologic studies in children and adolescents that used standardized evaluations and reported the rate of comorbidities between ADHD and anxiety disorders to determine the joint odds ratio for the pairs of disorders.

Summarized in Table 3.2 are the representative clinical studies showing the prevalence of anxiety in children and adolescents with ADHD. Overall, results from both the epidemiologic and clinical studies indicate that the rates of comorbidity between ADHD and anxiety disorders occur at the rate of 25% with variations depending on age, gender, severity, and number of comorbidities.

The multimodal treatment ADHD (MTA) study found that the prevalence of anxiety disorders in a sample of 579 children with ADHD between the ages 7.0–9.9 years was 33.5%.[24] Studies have observed that a variety of anxiety disorders, including separation anxiety disorder, generalized anxiety disorder, overanxious disorder, posttraumatic stress disorder, panic disorder, and agoraphobia, occur in association with ADHD.[28] One study assessing the comorbidity in preschool-aged children with ADHD[13,29] found a similar rate of anxiety disorders in preschool children with a trend toward multiple comorbidities. The occurrence of one anxiety disorder should therefore merit careful screening for other anxiety disorders.

AGE AND DEVELOPMENT

Children with ADHD and anxiety are older in age at the time of presentation than children with ADHD alone.[4] Although comorbid anxiety disorders are seen in

TABLE 3.1
Epidemiologic Samples: Point Prevalence of Anxiety Disorders in Attention Deficit Hyperactivity Disorder (ADHD)

Study	N	Age (years)	Rate of ADHD Alone	Rate of Anxiety Alone	Rate of Anxiety in ADHD Group
Anderson et al.[1]	792	11	6.7	7.4	26.4
Bird et al.[21]	222	9–16	10	–	50.8
Smalley et al.[2]	9432	16–18	8.5	14.5	26.6%
Kessler et al.[3]	3195	18–44			PTSD 16.1 PD 5.5 GAD 7.2 SP 29.5 Soc. P 38.0 AP 4.0 OCD 1.4

AP, agoraphobia; *GAD*, generalized anxiety disorder; *OCD*, obsessive-compulsive disorder; *PD*, panic disorder; *PTSD*, posttraumatic stress disorder; *Soc. P*, social phobia; *SP*, specific phobia.

one-fourth (25%) of children with ADHD, they increase to one-third (33%) in adolescent age group and even higher in adults. In the National Comorbidity Survey Replication study (NCS-R), 47.7% of adults with ADHD had a comorbid anxiety disorder within the last 12 months.[3]

Increased rates of anxiety disorders have also been reported in clinical samples that were followed longitudinally as seen in Table 3.2. Biederman and colleagues also noted that the nature of these comorbid anxiety diagnoses in ADHD may change over time. Children with ADHD who progressed to have anxiety disorders in adulthood were more likely to present with simple phobias in their preschool years. They had high rates of separation anxiety and social anxiety disorders on entering school age and high rates of generalized anxiety disorder in adolescence. A 4-year follow-up study found that children with multiple anxiety disorders at baseline had significantly increased risk of agoraphobia, social phobia, and separation anxiety.[28] Studies in adults with ADHD have found high rates of comorbid generalized anxiety, social phobia, specific phobias, and posttraumatic stress disorders.[29] In part, the high rates in adults may be explained by increased help-seeking and self-referral for treatment in adults.

In a longitudinal twin study, Agnew-Blais and colleagues investigated childhood risk factors and young adult functioning of individuals with persistent, remitted, and late-onset ADHD. At age 18 years, individuals with persistent ADHD had more impairment at school or work, socially, higher levels of generalized anxiety disorder, marijuana dependence, and conduct disorder (CD) compared with those whose ADHD had remitted.[30]

GENDER

A review study from the Massachusetts General Hospital examining the gender effects on ADHD and comorbid anxiety found that girls with ADHD had greater prevalence of simple phobia, agoraphobia, and panic disorder compared with boys with ADHD. There also appears to be some gender difference in the rate of multiple comorbid anxiety disorders, which is about 33% in girls compared with 28% in boys.[25]

Pliszka has examined the nature of impulsivity in children with ADHD and comorbid anxiety and found that the group as a whole was inattentive but not impulsive on the continuous performance test (CPT).[4] Newcorn and colleagues reported high levels of impulsivity as rated by CPT that was irrespective of comorbidity except in ADHD girls who had lower levels.[15]

In a large-scale prospective longitudinal study that included 170 ADHD children compared with 88 non-ADHD controls, Smith and colleagues noted that preschool hyperactivity was a strong predictor of poor adolescent/adult outcomes for males and less for females.[31]

In one study using a dimensional measure of anxiety that examined the covariation of both of these symptoms cross-sectionally and over a 1-year follow-up the investigators noted that ADHD symptoms are associated with elevated physical anxiety symptoms and social and separation anxiety. These symptoms were linked with inattention and were pronounced in girls but not in boys. The study found no evidence that ADHD predicted the onset of anxiety symptoms or vice versa over a year of follow-up.[32]

TABLE 3.2
Clinical Samples: Comorbidity of Attention Deficit Hyperactivity Disorder (ADHD) and Anxiety Disorders

Study	N	Age (years)	Assessment	Prevalence of One or More Anxiety Disorders in ADHD	Other Findings
Pliszka[23]	79	–	Iowa-CTRS	27.8%	
Livingston et al.[8]			DISC	40%	
Woolston et al.[9]	35	4–14	DSM-IIIR CBCL	61%	
Pliszka[4]	107	6–12	DSM-IIIR Iowa-CTRS RCMAS SNAP-R	31.7%	
Jensen et al.[7] and MTA cooperative group[24]	579	7.0–9.9	DISC-P SNAP MASC CDI	33.5%	
Biederman et al.[5]	73	6–17	DICA-Parent	30%	AD 4% OCD 5% OA 19% SA 10% SP 16%
Biederman et al.[25]		6–17		33% versus 28% (girls vs. boys)	OCD 5% versus 4% OA 29% versus 30% SA 26% versus 29% SP 29% versus 19% Soc. P 14% versus 13% AP 16% versus 9% PD 5% versus 1% (girls vs. boys)
Wilens et al.[13]	165 / 381	4–6 / 7–9	K-SADS DSM-IIIR	28% / 33%	
Bedard and Tannock[26]	130	6–12	PICS TTI RCMAS	32%	
Elia et al.[6]	342	6–18	K-SADS	32.2%	GAD 15.2% SP 7.6% SA 7.0%
Sciberras[10]	392	5–13	ADIS-C	26%—one anxiety disorder 39% had more than two anxiety disorders	Soc. P—48% GAD 34% SA 32% OCD 8% PTSD 6%
Jarrett et al.[27]	134	6–17	ADIS-C/P CBCL MASC	23.1%	OCD 6.45% SP 35.48% PTSD 6.45% Soc. P 22.58% SA 22.58% GAD 54.8%

AD, avoidant disorder; *ADHD*, attention deficit hyperactivity disorder; *ADIS-CP*, Anxiety Interview Schedule for Child and Parent; *AP*, agoraphobia; *CBCL*, Child Behavior Checklist; *CD*, conduct disorder; *CDI*, Child Depression Inventory; *CTRS*, Conners' Teacher Rating Scale; *DICA*, Diagnostic Interview for Children and Adolescents; *DISC-P*, Diagnostic Interview Schedule for Children; *DSMIII-R*, *Diagnostic and Statistical Manual of Mental Disorders, Third Edition, Revised*; *GAD*, generalized anxiety disorder; *K-SADS*, Kiddie Schedule for Affective Disorders and Schizophrenia; *MASC*, Multidimensional Anxiety Scale for Children; *OA*, overanxious disorder; *OCD*, obsessive-compulsive disorder; *ODD*, oppositional defiant disorder; *PD*, panic disorder; *PICS*, Parent Interview for Child Symptoms; *PTSD*, posttraumatic stress disorder; *RCMAS*, Revised Children's Manifest Anxiety Scale; *SA*, separation anxiety; *SNAP*, Swanson, Nolan and Pelham; *Soc. P*, social phobia; *SP*, specific phobia; *TTI*, Teacher Telephone Interview.

SCREENING

There are several rating scales that are commonly used to screen for symptoms of ADHD and anxiety. The advantages of these tools include being economical, readily available, and easy to administer. The Vanderbilt ADHD Teacher (VADTRS) and Parent Rating Scales (VADPRS) are straightforward instruments that follow DSM-IV criteria for ADHD and include 12 criteria for Conduct Disorder and 7 criteria from the Pediatric Behavior Scale, which screen for anxiety and depression in children aged 6–12 years. Both versions of the Vanderbilt ADHD Rating Scale have been validated and shown to be statistically significant instruments.[33,34] The VADTRS and VADPRS are in the public domain and available widely free of charge.

ADHD measures can be generally grouped into broadband and narrowband instruments. Examples of broadband measures, which contain probes of both externalizing and internalizing disorders, include the Child Behavior Checklist (CBCL)[35,36] and the Devereux Scales of Mental Disorders (DSMD). Although helpful for identifying cooccurring conditions, they are lengthier making them perhaps clinically less useful over time.

ADHD-specific measures, or narrowband measures, include only questions related to ADHD. Examples include the Conners Rating Scale (CPRS)[37]; the Barkley's School Situations Questionnaire (SSQ-O-I); the Swanson, Nolan and Pelham Questionnaire (SNAP)[38]; the ADHD Rating Scale-IV[39]; and the ADHD Symptoms Rating Scale.[40]

In one review that sought to differentiate youth who had been referred for evaluation of ADHD from those who were not referred, using the CBCL (teacher and parent forms), DSMD, and CPRS (teacher and parent forms), Green and colleagues found an average effect size of 1.5 across broadband measures. In contrast, the ADHD-specific measures were found to be more beneficial in distinguishing youth with ADHD with the Conners' scale having the highest effect sizes (3.1–3.7) and the SSQ-O-I having the lowest (1.3).[41]

DIAGNOSIS

It is important for clinicians to assess for ADHD and anxiety as part of any comprehensive medical or mental health assessment.[42] A thorough clinical assessment includes separate interviews with the parent and child. Self-reporting should not be relied on for either ADHD or anxiety symptoms.[43] Also, Pliszka noted that about half of the children who met criteria for overanxious disorder by their own self-report are not rated as

anxious by their parents, indicating that parents may be unaware of their children's internalizing symptoms.[4] Children who met criteria for comorbid anxiety by self-report were also reported to have lower levels of self-confidence and more impairment in daily functioning compared with parent-reported anxiety.[16] Corroborating information from teachers is also very helpful.

The *Diagnostic and Statistical Manual of Mental Disorders, Fifth Edition* (*DSM-5*) can be helpful in delineating criteria that are helpful in arriving at a diagnosis.[44] For ADHD, one must establish a sufficient number of core symptoms and functional impairment in at least two settings. This is based on behavioral observations made by parents and teachers, which can be reported through behavior rating scales. It is important to note that parent and teacher reports of ADHD symptoms do not always align. In a study of 74 children, 55 youth met criteria for DSM-IV ADHD, based on either parent or teacher interviews; however, parents and teachers only agreed in 17 of these cases, with parents endorsing the diagnosis almost twice as often as teachers.[45] Furthermore, as elementary school teachers typically spend the majority of the day with children in one classroom, they may more accurately report symptoms of ADHD as compared with secondary school teachers who typically only see youth for one period a day. In fact, high-school teachers have shown little agreement with other raters on symptoms of ADHD.[36]

Observation of ADHD symptoms by the clinician in the office can be helpful but is not necessary for a diagnosis, as only 20% of patients show hyperactivity in novel settings, such as the clinic.[46] On the other hand, observation during the clinical interview is extremely helpful in identifying anxiety.

Structured interviews, such as the Diagnostic Interview Schedule for Children (http://www.columbia.edu/cu/csswp/journal/newsfall94/cdisc.html), the Diagnostic Interview for Children and Adolescents (DICA),[47,48] and the Kiddie Schedule for Affective Disorder and Schizophrenia (K-SADS),[49] are often not only used in research studies but can also be extremely useful in the clinical setting. Additionally, the Anxiety Disorders Interview Schedule for children, child, and parent versions (ADIS)[50] is a semistructured diagnostic interview that has been shown to be valid in assessing all DSM-IV anxiety disorders, as well as ADHD in children aged 6–17 years.[12] In a study examining interrater agreement on diagnoses using the ADIS, the level of agreement was determined to be excellent between raters for primary diagnosis ($\kappa = 0.92$) and individual anxiety disorders ($\kappa = 0.80$–1.0).[51]

> **TABLE 3.3**
> **Clinical Workup for Attention Deficit Hyperactivity Disorder (ADHD)/Anxiety**
>
> 1. Medical history
>   a. Review of systems
>   b. Medications (current and past)
>   c. Family history of ADHD, anxiety disorders
> 2. Physical examination
> 3. Height, weight, blood pressure, and heart rate
> 4. Electrocardiogram
> 5. Laboratory studies (CBC, CMP, ferritin)
> 6. Neuropsychologic testing (when indicated)

CLINICAL WORKUP

As summarized in Table 3.3, the clinical workup for the comorbid ADHD and anxiety disorders should include a medical history and physical examination. The medical history that includes a thorough review of systems is essential in ruling out visual, auditory, respiratory, cardiovascular, and neurologic factors. The history will also help identify medications (e.g., sympathomimetics used to treat asthma) that may contribute to the ADHD or anxiety symptoms, as well as substance use.

Although there are no specific physical or neurologic findings for either ADHD or anxiety disorder, listening for cardiac murmurs may be important for anxiety disorders such as panic disorder. Obtaining baseline measures of height and weight is important in identifying growth delays. Cardiovascular parameters such as blood pressure (BP) and heart rate (HR) and electrocardiogram are important especially if medications are considered. There are no laboratory studies specific for ADHD or anxiety; it is important to identify anemia, low serum ferritin and lead levels. A baseline comprehensive metabolic panel is important in checking blood glucose and calcium, as well as obtaining baseline liver function if medication treatment is considered. Although abnormalities in thyroid functioning can have effects on children's mood and behavior, studies do not support the regular evaluation of thyroid functioning when screening for ADHD.[52]

Assessing sleep is very important. Mayes and colleagues have noted that children with ADHD and comorbid anxiety or depression have significant sleep problems such as difficulty falling asleep, restlessness during sleep, waking during the night, nightmares, walking or talking in sleep, waking too early, and sleeping less than normal in the subgroups with anxiety/depression versus without anxiety or depression (e.g., ADHD-I plus anxiety/depression vs. ADHD-I alone).[53] These sleep difficulties are comparable to those in children with just anxiety or depressive disorders but are more prevalent in children with just ADHD. Polysomnography may need to be considered in children who snore and are restless during sleep.

When staring spells are present that are not attributed to inattention, an EEG may be necessary to investigate absence seizures and simple partial epilepsy.

NEUROPSYCHOLOGIC TESTS

Pliszka and colleagues used the Memory Scanning Test (MST) to differentiate cognitive functioning in children with ADHD with or without anxiety disorders. The children had to memorize four numbers and recognize when presented with computer displays of the number itself, the number within 4×4 matrix of letters, or the number within 4×4 matrix of numbers. The task becomes increasingly complex from single number displays to matrices with dissimilar distracters to similar distracters. The study found that as the display load became more difficult, children with ADHD and comorbid anxiety disorders became much slower to respond but had greater accuracy than the ADHD group without anxiety.[23] This indicates that there are information processing difficulties unique in children with ADHD and comorbid anxiety.

Livingston and colleagues reported that children with ADHD and comorbid anxiety disorders performed poorly on the coding subtest of the Wechsler Intelligence Scale for Children, Revised, and on the Trail making test. Such differences are particularly noted among boys with ADHD and anxiety disorders showing lower verbal IQ and arithmetic scores.[8]

PATHOPHYSIOLOGY/ETIOLOGY

Is Comorbidity Due to Overlapping Symptoms?

The cognitive symptoms of anxiety such as ruminating thoughts, vigilant apprehension, and catastrophic thinking about embarrassment and threat to life and the behavioral symptoms such as agitation, tantrums, attention-seeking behavior, increased dependence, and ritualistic behavior may be misinterpreted as ADHD symptoms.[54] This often leads to a question whether the high incidence of comorbidity is simply a product of overlapping symptoms. This issue is addressed by Milberger and colleagues[55] who used two approaches to examine the degree to which prevalence rates of both ADHD and comorbid disorders would be maintained after correcting for the symptomatic overlap. The first approach, named the subtraction method, involved subtraction of the symptoms common to both ADHD and the comorbid disorder, thus requiring a higher percentage of symptoms and making the diagnostic process more rigorous. The second approach, named the proportion method, required the percentage of observed symptoms after correction to be proportionately as large as it was before symptom deletion. Using both these approaches of correction, Milberger found that about 75% of cases maintained their diagnosis of generalized anxiety disorder, thus concluding that ADHD and the comorbid disorders are not simply artifacts of overlapping symptoms.

Does Anxiety Modulate Attention Deficit Hyperactivity Disorder Symptoms or Vice Versa?

Comorbid anxiety in ADHD subjects has been associated with poor performance on working memory tasks. Neural activity during a visual-spatial working memory task in 271 adolescents and young adults (average age of 17 years) showed that anxiety lowered neuronal activity in the cerebellum for working memory contrast and bilaterally in the striatum and thalamus for memory load contrast.[18]

Pliszka has examined the nature of impulsivity in children with ADHD and comorbid anxiety and found that the group as a whole was inattentive but not impulsive on the CPT.[4] Newcorn and colleagues reported high levels of impulsivity as rated by CPT that was irrespective of comorbidity except in ADHD girls who had lower levels.[15]

GENETICS

Biederman and colleagues investigated the familial relationship between ADHD and anxiety disorders. The study found that the risk of anxiety disorders was significantly higher in relatives of children with ADHD and anxiety disorders compared with relatives of children with ADHD without anxiety disorders.[5] The results indicate that ADHD and anxiety disorders are separate disorders, inherited independent of each other, or share familial etiologic factors.

Because ADHD and anxiety are both familial disorders, studying their association in families can help explain the nature of their association.[55a] Using familial risk analysis, Braaten and colleagues and Biederman and colleagues tested several hypotheses of transmission. They sought to determine whether ADHD and anxiety were transmitted independently, shared familial etiologic factors, or represented a distinct subtype. Braaten and colleagues looked at three subject groups,

which included ADHD only, ADHD and anxiety, and controls, and their relatives for ADHD and anxiety disorders. What they concluded was that the two disorders are transmitted independently because there were higher rates of ADHD in relatives of ADHD probands and higher rates of anxiety disorder only in relatives of probands with anxiety disorders.[56] Similarly, Biederman et al.[5] found that the risk for anxiety disorders was twice as high in relatives of ADHD probands with anxiety disorders compared with ADHD probands without anxiety disorders, supporting independent transmission as well.

Segenreich and colleagues conducted studies that took into account attempts to overcome assortative mating phenomenon and found that maternal ADHD, anxiety, and depression were more correlated with offspring variables than with paternal ones. Also maternal inattention but not hyperactivity was correlated with both inattention and hyperactivity in the offspring, and maternal anxiety was correlated with offspring inattention. Moreover, maternal inattention was correlated with anxiety in the offspring.[57]

Sonuga-Barke and colleagues investigated the interaction between positive maternal expressed emotion and genotype in children with ADHD and comorbid "conduct problems" and "emotional problems".[57a] Although "emotional problems" were not specific to anxiety disorders, the assessment included several questions related to anxiety. Results showed that those in the emotional problems group who had the 9R/10R and the 10R/10R allele of DAT1 were protected from the negative effects of low positive maternal expressed emotion, suggesting that genetic factors may alter sensitivity to positive or negative parenting. Although this study may point to variants in dopamine transporter genes in ADHD children with comorbidities, these results require replication specific to children with comorbid anxiety.

Gatt and colleagues investigated whether candidate genes associated with multiple disorders via pleiotropic mechanism and/or if other genes are specific to susceptibility for individual disorders. In this review of 1519 metaanalyses across 157 studies reporting multiple genes implicated in one or more of the five disorders (major depression, anxiety disorders, ADHD, schizophrenia, bipolar disorder), 134 genes were identified and 13 genetic variants were shared between two or more disorders (APOE e4, ACE Ins/Del, BDNF Val-66Met, COMT Val158Met, DAOA G72/G30 rs3918342, DAT1 40-bp, DRD4 48-bp, SLC6A4 5-HTTLPR, HTR1A C1019G, MTHR C677T, MTHR A1298C, SLC6A4 VNTR, and TPH1 218A/C). This suggests that pleiotropy (one gene influences two or more seemingly unrelated phenotypic traits) may be playing a role. Twelve metaanalyses of genome-wide association studies of the same disorders were identified, with no overlap in genetic variants reported.[58]

ADHD and anxiety disorders occur even more frequently in deaf impaired children compared with those without any hearing impairment. Antoine and colleagues have shown that in a mouse model, mutations in TBX1 or Slcl2a2 are responsible for both the hyperactivity and inner ear defects.[59]

Tryptophan hydroxylase (TPH) is the rate-limiting enzyme in the synthesis of serotonin, and the TPH2 polymorphism 703G/T is associated with aggressiveness and impulsivity. Laas and colleagues report that subjects, especially males, with TPH2 rs4570625 IT genotype had less aggression, had less impulsivity, and developed anxiety disorders less often by young adulthood, suggesting that this may be a protective variant.[60]

In a mouse model carrying a mutation of Pax 6, a gene with neurodevelopmental regulatory function, Yoshizaki and colleagues report differences in maternal separation–induced ultrasonic vocalizations in mice born from young father and in the level of hyperactivity in mice born from aged fathers in the open-field test compared with wild-type littermates. No differences in anxiety phenotypes were noted in aged versus young fathers, suggesting that paternal age may play a role in ADHD but not in anxiety.[61]

SIGNALING PATHWAYS

As reviewed by Keil and colleagues, the protein kinase A (PKA) signaling pathway is involved in the activation of the amygdala in mice leading to fear, learning, and memory impairments, and human studies of PKA signaling defects are also associated in humans with neuropsychiatric disorders such as anxiety, mood disorders, learning disorders, and ADHD.[62]

TREATMENTS

Behavioral Interventions

Nonpharmacologic treatments are important in the treatment of children with ADHD and anxiety given their safety, potential for no side effects or drug interactions, and effectiveness in combination with medications. Most of the studies in this age group implement psychosocial therapies in combination with pharmacotherapy. Cognitive behavior therapy (CBT) has the strongest evidence base in the treatment of childhood anxiety disorders. Major findings supporting the

benefits of psychosocial treatments come from the MTA study in which children with ADHD and anxiety comorbidity responded better to behavioral therapy alone than those with ADHD without anxiety. The children with ADHD, anxiety, oppositional defiant, and CDs responded well to a combination of medication and behavioral therapy.[7] The behavioral interventions in this study were aimed more toward ADHD than internalizing symptoms, and it can be surmised that some anxiety in children with ADHD is attributable to the core ADHD symptoms, and improvement in the core symptoms would lead to improvement in anxiety symptoms.

In a small pilot randomized trial of CBT for children with ADHD and anxiety, Sciberras and colleagues demonstrated the feasibility of using a standard anxiety program for children with anxiety, such as the Cool Kids CBT program. They made minor adaptations to the program to make it more acceptable for children with ADHD and their parents, including the use of an activity schedule and positive reinforcement to promote on-task behavior, 1-min "brain breaks" between activities, shortening and repetition of key concepts, and use of visual aids in the sessions and at home to promote skills practice. The CBT intervention group had marked improvements in child and parent well-being, including child anxiety, QoL, ADHD symptom severity and behavior, and improved parent mental health and parenting.[63]

Antshel and colleagues studied the efficacy of social skills training in children with ADHD and noted that children with ADHD and anxiety responded better to social skills training. They had improved parent-rated cooperation and assertiveness skills after social skills training.[64]

About 88% of youth with anxiety disorders show at least one sleep problem, with the most frequent ones being insomnia, nightmares, and fear of sleeping alone. Comorbid anxiety may explain the relationship between ADHD and sleep problems in children. Beriault and colleagues adapted the "Super Squirrel," which is a CBT treatment program designed for school-aged children with anxiety disorders in treatment of children with ADHD and anxiety and found it to be effective in decreasing anxiety. CBT was effective in reducing sleep onset latency and marginally decreased the total amount of sleep problems.[65]

PHARMACOTHERAPY

Stimulants: Effect on Attention Deficit Hyperactivity Disorder

Comorbid anxiety is considered as a moderator of treatment response in children with ADHD. Earlier short-term studies have observed that children with ADHD and comorbid anxiety show less robust response to stimulant treatment and experience more side effects than children with ADHD alone.[16,23] However, more recent long-term studies in ADHD children with or without anxiety treated with stimulants show concomitant improvement in internalizing symptoms and noted that they may be preferentially responsive to behavior therapy.[24,66]

Diamond et al.[66] observed that treatment with methylphenidate following a standard dose, titration, and duration schedule in children with ADHD and comorbid anxiety showed an equivalent response of ADHD symptoms regardless of their comorbidity.[66] Children with comorbid anxiety have higher physical anxiety symptoms at baseline, which may be mistaken for medication-related side effects.

Stimulants: Effect on Anxiety

Anxiety had been considered a side effect of stimulant treatment for ADHD. However, in a recent metaanalysis of 23 randomized controlled trials examining the likelihood of anxiety as a side effect of stimulant treatment in children with ADHD, Coughlin and colleagues demonstrated that the stimulant treatment significantly decreased the risk of anxiety when compared with placebo. They found no significant differences in the risk of anxiety based on the class of stimulants (methylphenidate vs. amphetamine derivatives), short-acting and long-acting formulations, dosage of stimulants, and duration of active treatment. Stimulants reduce anxiety symptoms indirectly by improving ADHD symptoms.

Successful treatment of ADHD would decrease the anxiogenic situations such as academic problems, peer and parental conflicts.[67] Therefore, comorbid anxiety is not a contraindication for stimulant treatment.

As summarized in Table 3.4, Pliszka observed that children with ADHD and comorbid anxiety disorders had only modest improvement in performance on working memory tasks on treatment with methylphenidate, which were not enhanced by higher doses.[23] Tannock and Schachar demonstrated that methylphenidate treatment improved auditory-verbal working memory only in nonanxious children with ADHD but not in those with comorbid anxiety.[16] A similar study by Bedard and Tannock looking at differential effects of methylphenidate on auditory-verbal versus visual-spatial modalities of storage and processing components of working memory found that stimulants selectively enhanced discrete processes such as auditory-verbal manipulation, visual-spatial storage, and manipulation only in children with ADHD without anxiety.[26] The cognitive aspect of anxiety, which is "worrying," is verbally mediated and therefore interferes selectively with auditory-verbal working memory. As anxious arousal is a function of the right prefrontal cortex, it is believed that anxious arousal competes with the cognitive operations of right prefrontal cortex, including visual-spatial working memory. Lower dose ranges of stimulants are observed to cause greater increase in HR in children with anxiety comorbidity.

The differences in anxiety outcomes among studies are likely due to methodological differences, as some

TABLE 3.4
Medications Treatments in Attention Deficit Hyperactivity Disorder (ADHD) + Anxiety

Coughlin[67]	Stimulants	Stimulants decreased risk of anxiety when compared with placebo
Pliszka[23]	MPH	Modest improvement on WM
Tannock and Schachar[16]	MPH	Improved WM only in nonanxious children and not in ADHD with comorbid anxiety
Bedard and Tannock[26]	MPH	Improved on WM only in ADHD without anxiety
Kratochvil et al.[68]	ATX + FLX versus ATX	Improved ADHD, anxiety, and depression
Abikoff et al.[69]	MPH + FLX versus FLX/PI	No greater reduction in anxiety for combination of SSRI + MPH than placebo
Weiss et al.[70]	D-AMPH + PX versus PX	No greater improvement in anxiety for combination of SSRI + D-AMPH

ATX, atomoxetine; *D-AMPH*, dextroamphetamine; *FLX*, fluoxetine; *MPH*, methylphenidate; *PX*, paroxetine; *SSRI*, selective serotonin reuptake inhibitor; *WM*, working memory.

studies used anxiety rating scales while others use diagnostic categories. It would be important to exclude common overlapping symptoms (for example, tension and restlessness) in preference of cognitive processes such as worrying, which could be more pathognomonic of anxiety in measuring outcomes.

The existing evidence strongly supports the use of stimulants as first-line agents in the treatment of ADHD symptoms even in children with comorbid anxiety, but use of caution is recommended. Expert consensus panels such as the Texas medical algorithmic panel recommend the initial treatment of stimulant monotherapy, followed by the addition of a selective serotonin reuptake inhibitor (SSRI) for children with ADHD and residual anxiety symptoms.

Multimodal Therapy + Stimulants

A study by van der Oord and colleagues, examining the benefits of adding 10-week intensive behavior therapy to children who were stable on methylphenidate, showed similar improvements on child-, parent-, and teacher-rated ADHD symptoms; anxiety; self-worth; and social skills, whether children received the combination or methylphenidate monotherapy.[71] Thus, the study found no evidence for the additive effect of multimodal behavior therapy next to optimally titrated methylphenidate.

The findings from the MTA study indicate that comorbid anxiety symptoms play a significant moderating role on the treatment outcomes of ADHD. Children with high parent-rated anxiety in the MTA study (33.5%) showed an enhanced response to behavioral therapy. Comorbid anxiety status conferred benefits to children as noted by greater effect sizes and robust responsiveness to all treatment modalities compared with children with ADHD alone or ADHD comorbid with oppositional defiant disorder (ODD) and CDs. In contrast, the dually comorbid children with ADHD, anxiety, and ODD/CD diagnoses showed a preferential response to combination interventions compared with either behavior therapy or medication management alone.[7]

ATOMOXETINE

Atomoxetine is a selective presynaptic norepinephrine reuptake inhibitor approved by the Food and Drug Administration (FDA) in the treatment of ADHD in children and adults. It is a nonstimulant medication recommended for use as a monotherapy for the treatment of ADHD for youth who are unresponsive to stimulants.

Even though the Cohen's effect size for atomoxetine for the treatment of ADHD is smaller (effect size: 0.6–0.7) compared with immediate-release (0.8–0.9) or long-acting stimulants (0.8–0.95), it is preferred in children with comorbid anxiety, as stimulants may increase symptoms such as tics, mania, aggression, anxiety, or suicidal ideation.

Evidence for the efficacy of atomoxetine in treatment of ADHD and comorbid anxiety has been demonstrated in several studies.[72,73] Geller and colleagues demonstrated that youth treated with atomoxetine at doses up to 1.8 mg/kg/day showed significantly greater improvement of ADHD Rating Scale-IV scores and anxiety scores compared with placebo.[73]

Adler and colleagues conducted a 14-week controlled trial of atomoxetine in adults with comorbid ADHD and social anxiety and noted a significant reduction in the Conners' adult ADHD rating scale scores compared with placebo. The scores on Liebowitz social anxiety scale also showed a similar significant reduction compared with placebo.[72] In a separate 12-week openlabeled study of 27 adults with ADHD and comorbid generalized anxiety disorders, atomoxetine was found to reduce ADHD symptoms and anxiety scores. Significant improvement was noted for both cognitive and somatic symptom subscales separately.[74]

Overall, there is positive evidence for effectiveness of atomoxetine on comorbid anxiety disorders in youth and adults with small to moderate effect sizes.

ATTENTION DEFICIT HYPERACTIVITY DISORDER MEDICATIONS + ANTIANXIETY MEDICATIONS

Stimulant + Selective Serotonin Reuptake Inhibitor

In clinical practice, children with ADHD and prominent anxiety comorbidity are often prescribed combination treatment for both ADHD and anxiety even though the evidence base supporting the use of combination medications is limited. The standard combination of stimulant medication for treatment of ADHD and SSRIs for the treatment of anxiety has no pharmacokinetic interactions and can be safely used. Two studies, which examined the combination of SSRIs and stimulants, have found no greater improvement of anxiety. The RUPP ADHD/anxiety study group reported data on treatment of residual anxiety symptoms in a group of 32 children, who were first treated with methylphenidate and then randomized to fluvoxamine or placebo. A minority of children (19%) had meaningful reduction of anxiety with stimulant monotherapy alone and did not need randomization. The combination of fluvoxamine and methylphenidate was well tolerated but did not cause greater reduction in anxiety scores compared with placebo.[69]

Weiss and colleagues conducted a similar study in adults using either monotherapy with problem-focused therapy or combination of dextroamphetamine and paroxetine with problem-focused therapy and found no greater improvement in anxiety with the combination compared with single treatment. The combination group had greater adverse effects and poorer tolerance compared with monotherapy.[70]

Atomoxetine + Selective Serotonin Reuptake Inhibitor

The combination of nonstimulant medicine atomoxetine and the SSRI antidepressants has challenges because of Cytochrome (Cyt) P450 2D6 interactions. Atomoxetine is metabolized by the Cyt-P450 2D6 enzyme, which is inhibited by the SSRIs, fluoxetine and paroxetine. The combination theoretically could increase plasma atomoxetine levels and result in better efficacy but poor tolerability. It is therefore recommended to maintain atomoxetine at the starting dose for 4 weeks and then increase to target dose only if there is lack of efficacy and if it is well tolerated.

Kratochvil and colleagues studied the combination of atomoxetine and fluoxetine (N = 127) compared with atomoxetine alone (N = 46) in children with ADHD and comorbid depressive and anxiety symptoms. The combination was well tolerated, and both the combination and monotherapy treatment groups had remarkable improvement in ADHD, anxiety, and depressive symptoms. The lack of a placebo comparison group limited the interpretation of the results in this study. The atomoxetine/fluoxetine combination group had greater elevations in the mean HR (change with A/F 11.9 beats/min vs. A/P 6.5 beats/min) and elevation in mean BP (mean [SD] change in diastolic BP mmHg, A/F 5.2 [9.4], A/P 0.3 [9.1], $P = .008$; mean [SD] change in systolic BP mm Hg, A/F 3.1 [8.9], A/P 0.14 [9.3]; $P = .070$), which did not reach statistical significance. However, the greater proportion of patients with sustained increases in diastolic BP on the combination (8.2% with A/F compared with 2.3% with A/P) indicates a greater need for BP monitoring when using the combination of atomoxetine and fluoxetine in treatment. Decreased appetite was the most common adverse effect in the combined treatment group (A/F 20% vs. A/P 6.8%, $P = .05$).[68] In summary, the available data suggest that atomoxetine monotherapy alone may be appropriate for youth with ADHD and anxiety

symptoms. However, if the use of a combination is clinically warranted, the data indicate that despite the higher plasma levels of atomoxetine, the combination with fluoxetine is well tolerated.

IMPLICATIONS FOR CLINICAL PEDIATRIC PRACTICE

Given that ADHD and anxiety disorders are highly comorbid, it is important to conduct a comprehensive assessment, including direct interviews of children and parents conducted separately, if possible. Parents are more reliable informants for externalizing disorders such as ADHD and children, and adolescents are more reliable informants for internalizing disorders such as anxiety (Table 3.5).

Comorbid anxiety has an important moderating role in treatment of ADHD. The anxiogenic potential of

---

TABLE 3.5
Implications for Clinical Pediatric Practice

1. Identify comorbid anxiety disorders in ADHD children
   Comprehensive assessment includes direct interview with the child and parent
   a. Clinical information needs to be obtained from both the parent and child
   b. If there is one anxiety disorder, it is important to evaluate for other anxiety disorders because multiple comorbidities confer more impairment
2. Comorbidity may modify the clinical presentation
   a. Anxious ADHD children may be less impulsive in the classroom
3. Treatments
   Behavioral therapy
       CBT effective with ADHD + anxiety
       CBT effective with ADHD + anxiety + ODD + CD
       CBT effective with high parent anxiety
   Stimulants
       Effective in ADHD with or without anxiety
       Effective in decreasing anxiety
   Atomoxetine
       Effective in ADHD
       Effective in ADHD + anxiety
   Stimulants + combination treatments
       Stimulants + multimodal therapy
           Effective in ADHD with anxiety, ODD, CD
           No additive effects of multimodal therapy when methylphenidate optimally titrated
   Stimulants + SSRI
       No benefit to combination

ADHD, attention deficit hyperactivity disorder; *CBT*, cognitive behavior therapy; *SSRI*, selective serotonin reuptake inhibitor.

stimulants has not been replicated in the recent studies, including the MTA study. The stimulants are still recommended as the first-line agents in treatment of ADHD in the presence of anxiety, but use of caution is recommended. Behavioral treatments need to be considered as first-line in children with anxiety comorbid with ADHD, as they have positive impact on academic and social functioning, as well as ADHD symptoms. The emerging evidence on treatment of residual anxiety symptoms using nonstimulant medication classes such as atomoxetine and stimulant and SSRI combinations is promising. A systematic assessment and treatment of anxiety in children with ADHD has the potential to improve functioning for these children.

SUMMARY

The comorbidity of ADHD and anxiety disorders is high throughout the developmental stages with increasing rates of anxiety with age. Assessing for comorbidity is important because children with ADHD and comorbid anxiety disorders have greater attention, cognitive, and executive functioning difficulties than children with ADHD alone. Studies have shown that multiple anxiety comorbidities are associated with poorer QoL and daily functioning, as well as more problematic behavior in children with ADHD.

The causes of this high comorbidity are not clearly understood. Genetic and genomic studies in psychiatric disorders, including ADHD and anxiety, indicate a complex picture. Although ADHD and anxiety disorders appear to be transmitted independently, they may share similar genetic variants that have pleiotropic effects. There may also be different risks depending on paternal and maternal risk genes. Epigenetic effects are less well known but are likely to play a major factor.

Data on treatment are also limited to CBT, stimulants, atomoxetine, and SSRIs. In general, multimodal treatments need to be considered when comorbidity is present. However, individualized treatment plans addressing the youngster's symptoms and impairments need to guide the choice of treatments and the time of implementation.

REFERENCES

1. Anderson JC, Williams S, McGee R, Silva PA. DSM-III disorders in preadolescent children. Prevalence in a large sample from the general population. *Arch Gen Psychiatry.* 1987;44(1):69–76.
2. Smalley SL, McGough JJ, Moilanen IK, et al. Prevalence and psychiatric comorbidity of attention-deficit/hyperactivity disorder in an adolescent Finnish population. *J Am Acad Child Adolesc Psychiatry.* 2007;46(12):1575–1583.
3. Kessler RC, Adler LA, Barkley R, et al. Patterns and predictors of attention-deficit/hyperactivity disorder persistence into adulthood: results from the national comorbidity survey replication. *Biol Psychiatry.* 2005;57(11):1442–1451.
4. Pliszka SR. Comorbidity of attention-deficit hyperactivity disorder and overanxious disorder. *J Am Acad Child Adolesc Psychiatry.* 1992;31(2):197–203.
5. Biederman J, Faraone SV, Keenan K, Steingard R, Tsuang MT. Familial association between attention deficit disorder and anxiety disorders. *Am J Psychiatry.* 1991;148(2):251–256.
6. Elia J, Ambrosini P, Berrettini W. ADHD characteristics: I. Concurrent co-morbidity patterns in children & adolescents. *Child Adolesc Psychiatry Ment Health.* 2008;2(1):15.
7. Jensen PS, Hinshaw SP, Kraemer HC, et al. ADHD comorbidity findings from the MTA study: comparing comorbid subgroups. *J Am Acad Child Adolesc Psychiatry.* 2001;40(2):147–158.
8. Livingston RL, Dykman RA, Ackerman PT. The frequency and significance of additional self-reported psychiatric diagnoses in children with attention deficit disorder. *J Abnorm Child Psychol.* 1990;18(5):465–478.
9. Woolston JL, Rosenthal SL, Riddle MA, Sparrow SS, Cicchetti D, Zimmerman LD. Childhood comorbidity of anxiety/affective disorders and behavior disorders. *J Am Acad Child Adolesc Psychiatry.* 1989;28(5):707–713.
10. Sciberras E, Lycett K, Efron D, Mensah F, Gerner B, Hiscock H. Anxiety in children with attention-deficit/hyperactivity disorder. *Pediatrics.* 2014;133(5):801–808.
11. Biederman J, Faraone SV, Keenan K, et al. Further evidence for family-genetic risk factors in attention deficit hyperactivity disorder. Patterns of comorbidity in probands and relatives psychiatrically and pediatrically referred samples. *Arch Gen Psychiatry.* 1992;49(9):728–738.
12. Jarrett MA, Wolff JC, Davis 3rd TE, Cowart MJ, Ollendick TH. Characteristics of children with ADHD and comorbid anxiety. *J Atten Disord.* 2016;20(7):636–644.
13. Wilens TE, Biederman J, Brown S, Monuteaux M, Prince J, Spencer TJ. Patterns of psychopathology and dysfunction in clinically referred preschoolers. *J Dev Behav Pediatr.* 2002;23(1 suppl):S31–S36.
14. Busch B, Biederman J, Cohen LG, et al. Correlates of ADHD among children in pediatric and psychiatric clinics. *Psychiatr Serv.* 2002;53(9):1103–1111.
15. Newcorn JH, Halperin JM, Jensen PS, et al. Symptom profiles in children with ADHD: effects of comorbidity and gender. *J Am Acad Child Adolesc Psychiatry.* 2001;40(2):137–146.
16. Tannock R, Ickowicz A, Schachar R. Differential effects of methylphenidate on working memory in ADHD children with and without comorbid anxiety. *J Am Acad Child Adolesc Psychiatry.* 1995;34(7):886–896.
17. Manassis K, Tannock R, Young A, Francis-John S. Cognition in anxious children with attention deficit hyperactivity disorder: a comparison with clinical and normal children. *Behav Brain Funct.* 2007;3:4.

18. van der Meer D, Hoekstra PJ, van Rooij D, et al. Anxiety modulates the relation between attention-deficit/hyperactivity disorder severity and working memory-related brain activity. *World J Biol Psychiatry*. 2017:1–11.

19. Biederman J, Faraone SV, Spencer T, et al. Patterns of psychiatric comorbidity, cognition, and psychosocial functioning in adults with attention deficit hyperactivity disorder. *Am J Psychiatry*. 1993;150(12):1792–1798.

20. Hahesy AL, Wilens TE, Biederman J, Van Patten SL, Spencer T. Temporal association between childhood psychopathology and substance use disorders: findings from a sample of adults with opioid or alcohol dependency. *Psychiatry Res*. 2002;109(3):245–253.

21. Bird HR, Gould MS, Staghezza BM. Patterns of diagnostic comorbidity in a community sample of children aged 9 through 16 years. *J Am Acad Child Adolesc Psychiatry*. 1993;32(2):361–368.

22. Last CG, Strauss CC, Francis G. Comorbidity among childhood anxiety disorders. *J Nerv Men Dis*. 1987;175(12):726–730.

23. Pliszka SR. Effect of anxiety on cognition, behavior, and stimulant response in ADHD. *J Am Acad Child Adolesc Psychiatry*. 1989;28(6):882–887.

24. A 14-month randomized clinical trial of treatment strategies for attention-deficit/hyperactivity disorder. The MTA Cooperative Group. Multimodal Treatment Study of Children with ADHD. *Arch Gen Psychiatry*. 1999;56(12):1073–1086.

25. Biederman J, Mick E, Faraone SV, et al. Influence of gender on attention deficit hyperactivity disorder in children referred to a psychiatric clinic. *Am J Psychiatry*. 2002;159(1):36–42.

26. Bedard AC, Tannock R. Anxiety, methylphenidate response, and working memory in children with ADHD. *J Atten Disord*. 2008;11(5):546–557.

27. Jarrett MA. Attention-deficit/hyperactivity disorder (ADHD) symptoms, anxiety symptoms, and executive functioning in emerging adults. *Psychol Assess*. 2016;28(2):245–250.

28. Biederman J, Monuteaux MC, Mick E, et al. Young adult outcome of attention deficit hyperactivity disorder: a controlled 10-year follow-up study. *Psychol Med*. 2006;36(2):167–179.

29. Wilens TE, Biederman J, Spencer TJ. Attention deficit/hyperactivity disorder across the lifespan. *Annu Rev Med*. 2002;53:113–131.

30. Agnew-Blais JC, Polanczyk GV, Danese A, Wertz J, Moffitt TE, Arseneault L. Evaluation of the persistence, remission, and emergence of attention-deficit/hyperactivity disorder in young adulthood. *JAMA Psychiatry*. 2016;73(7):713–720.

31. Smith E, Meyer BJ, Koerting J, et al. Preschool hyperactivity specifically elevates long-term mental health risks more strongly in males than females: a prospective longitudinal study through to young adulthood. *Eur Child Adolesc Psychiatry*. 2017;26(1):123–136.

32. Baldwin JS, Dadds MR. Examining alternative explanations of the covariation of ADHD and anxiety symptoms in children: a community study. *J Abnorm Child Psychol*. 2008;36(1):67–79.

33. Wolraich ML, Lambert W, Doffing MA, Bickman L, Simmons T, Worley K. Psychometric properties of the Vanderbilt ADHD diagnostic parent rating scale in a referred population. *J Pediatr Psychol*. 2003;28(8):559–567.

34. Wolraich ML, Feurer ID, Hannah JN, Baumgaertel A, Pinnock TY. Obtaining systematic teacher reports of disruptive behavior disorders utilizing DSM-IV. *J Abnorm Child Psychol*. 1998;26(2):141–152.

35. Papachristou E, Schulz K, Newcorn J, Bedard AC, Halperin JM, Frangou S. Comparative evaluation of child behavior checklist-derived scales in children clinically referred for emotional and behavioral dysregulation. *Front Psychiatry*. 2016;7:146.

36. Achenbach TM, Ruffle TM. The child behavior checklist and related forms for assessing behavioral/emotional problems and competencies. *Pediatr Rev*. 2000;21(8):265–271.

37. Conners CK, Sitarenios G, Parker JD, Epstein JN. The revised Conners' Parent Rating Scale (CPRS-R): factor structure, reliability, and criterion validity. *J Abnorm Child Psychol*. 1998;26(4):257–268.

38. Swanson JM, Schuck S, Porter MM, et al. Categorical and dimensional definitions and evaluations of symptoms of ADHD: history of the SNAP and the SWAN rating scales. *Int J Educ Psychol Assess*. 2012;10(1):51–70.

39. Reid R, DuPaul GJ, Power TJ, et al. Assessing culturally different students for attention deficit hyperactivity disorder using behavior rating scales. *J Abnorm Child Psychol*. 1998;26(3):187–198.

40. Holland ML, Merrell KW. Social-emotional characteristics of preschool-aged children referred for Child Find screening and assessment: a comparative study. *Res Dev Disabil*. 1998;19(2):167–179.

41. Green M, Wong M, Atkins D, Taylor J, Feinleib M. *Diagnosis of Attention-Deficit/Hyperactivity Disorder* Rockville, MD. ; 1999.

42. Pliszka S. Practice parameter for the assessment and treatment of children and adolescents with attention-deficit/hyperactivity disorder. *J Am Acad Child Adolesc Psychiatry*. 2007;46(7):894–921.

43. Barbosa J, Tannock R, Manassis K. Measuring anxiety: parent-child reporting differences in clinical samples. *Depress Anxiety*. 2002;15(2):61–65.

44. Association AP. *Diagnostic and Statistical Manual of Mental Disorders*. 5th ed. Washington, DC: American Psychiatric Publishing; 2013.

45. Mitsis EM, McKay KE, Schulz KP, Newcorn JH, Halperin JM. Parent-teacher concordance for DSM-IV attention-deficit/hyperactivity disorder in a clinic-referred sample. *J Am Acad Child Adolesc Psychiatry*. 2000;39(3):308–313.

46. Sleator EK, Ullmann RK. Can the physician diagnose hyperactivity in the office? *Pediatrics*. 1981;67(1):13–17.

47. Ezpeleta L, de la Osa N, Granero R, Domenech JM, Reich W. The diagnostic interview of children and adolescents for parents of preschool and young children: psychometric properties in the general population. *Psychiatry Res*. 2011;190(1):137–144.

48. Reich W. Diagnostic interview for children and adolescents (DICA). *J Am Acad Child Adolesc Psychiatry.* 2000;39(1):59–66.

49. Ambrosini PJ. Historical development and present status of the schedule for affective disorders and schizophrenia for school-age children (K-SADS). *J Am Acad Child Adolesc Psychiatry.* 2000;39(1):49–58.

50. Silverman WK, Saavedra LM, Pina AA. Test-retest reliability of anxiety symptoms and diagnoses with the Anxiety Disorders Interview Schedule for DSM-IV: child and parent versions. *J Am Acad Child Adolesc Psychiatry.* 2001;40(8):937–944.

51. Lyneham HJ, Abbott MJ, Rapee RM. Interrater reliability of the anxiety disorders interview schedule for DSM-IV: child and parent version. *J Am Acad Child Adolesc Psychiatry.* 2007;46(6):731–736.

52. Elia J, Gulotta C, Rose SR, Marin G, Rapoport JL. Thyroid function and attention-deficit hyperactivity disorder. *J Am Acad Child Adolesc Psychiatry.* 1994;33(2):169–172.

53. Mayes SD, Calhoun SL, Bixler EO, et al. ADHD subtypes and comorbid anxiety, depression, and oppositional-defiant disorder: differences in sleep problems. *J Pediatr Psychol.* 2009;34(3):328–337.

54. Spencer T, Biederman J, Wilens T. Attention-deficit/hyperactivity disorder and comorbidity. *Pediatr Clin N Am.* 1999;46(5):915–927. vii.

55. Milberger S, Biederman J, Faraone SV, Murphy J, Tsuang MT. Attention deficit hyperactivity disorder and comorbid disorders: issues of overlapping symptoms. *Am J Psychiatry.* 1995;152(12):1793–1799.

55a. Faraone SV, Perlis RH, Doyle AE, et al. Molecular Genetics of ADHD. *Biol Psychiatry.* 2005;57:1313–1323.

56. Braaten EB, Beiderman J, Monuteaux MC, et al. Revisiting the association between attention-deficit/hyperactivity disorder and anxiety disorders: a familial risk analysis. *Biol Psychiatry.* 2003;53(1):93–99.

57. Segenreich D, Paez MS, Regalla MA, et al. Multilevel analysis of ADHD, anxiety and depression symptoms aggregation in families. *Eur Child Adol Psychiatry.* 2015;24(5):525–536.

57a. Sonuga-Barke, Oades RD, Psychogiou L, et al. Dopamine and Serotonin transporter genotypes moderate sensitivity to maternal espressed emotion: the case of conduct and emotional problems in ADHD. *J Child Psychol Psychiatry.* 2009;50(9):1052–1063.

58. Gatt JM, Burton KL, Williams LM, Schofield PR. Specific and common genes implicated across major mental disorders: a review of meta-analysis studies. *J Psychiatr Res.* 2015;60:1–13.

59. Antoine MW, Vijayakumar S, McKeehan N, Jones SM, Hebert JM. The severity of vestibular dysfunction in deafness as a determinant of comorbid hyperactivity or anxiety. *J Neurosci.* 2017;37(20):5144–5154.

60. Laas K, Kiive E, Maestu J, Vaht M, Veidebaum T, Harro J. Nice guys: homozygocity for the TPH2 -703G/T (rs4570625) minor allele promotes low aggressiveness and low anxiety. *J Affect Disord.* 2017;215:230–236.

61. Yoshizaki K, Furuse T, Kimura R, et al. Paternal aging affects behavior in Pax6 mutant mice: a gene/environment interaction in understanding neurodevelopmental disorders. *PLoS One.* 2016;11(11):e0166665.

62. Keil MF, Briassoulis G, Stratakis CA, Wu TJ. Protein kinase a and anxiety-related behaviors: a mini-review. *Front Endocrinol.* 2016;7:83.

63. Sciberras E, Mulraney M, Anderson V, et al. Managing anxiety in children with ADHD using cognitive-behavioral therapy: a pilot randomized controlled trial. *J Atten Disord.* 2018;22(5):515–520.

64. Antshel KM, Remer R. Social skills training in children with attention deficit hyperactivity disorder: a randomized-controlled clinical trial. *J Clin Child Adol Psychol.* 2003;32(1):153–165.

65. Beriault M, Turgeon L, Labrosse M, et al. Comorbidity of ADHD and anxiety disorders in school-age children: impact on sleep and response to a cognitive-behavioral treatment. *J Atten Disord.* 2018;22(5):414–424.

66. Diamond IR, Tannock R, Schachar RJ. Response to methylphenidate in children with ADHD and comorbid anxiety. *J Am Acad Child Adolesc Psychiatry.* 1999;38(4):402–409.

67. Coughlin CG, Cohen SC, Mulqueen JM, Ferracioli-Oda E, Stuckelman ZD, Bloch MH. Meta-analysis: reduced risk of anxiety with psychostimulant treatment in children with attention-deficit/hyperactivity disorder. *J Child Adol Psychopharmacol.* 2015;25(8):611–617.

68. Kratochvil CJ, Newcorn JH, Arnold LE, et al. Atomoxetine alone or combined with fluoxetine for treating ADHD with comorbid depressive or anxiety symptoms. *J Am Acad Child Adolesc Psychiatry.* 2005;44(9):915–924.

69. Abikoff H, McGough J, Vitiello B, et al. Sequential pharmacotherapy for children with comorbid attention-deficit/hyperactivity and anxiety disorders. *J Am Acad Child Adolesc Psychiatry.* 2005;44(5):418–427.

70. Weiss M, Hechtman L. A randomized double-blind trial of paroxetine and/or dextroamphetamine and problem-focused therapy for attention-deficit/hyperactivity disorder in adults. *J Clin Psychiatry.* 2006;67(4):611–619.

71. van der Oord S, Prins PJ, Oosterlaan J, Emmelkamp PM. Does brief, clinically based, intensive multimodal behavior therapy enhance the effects of methylphenidate in children with ADHD? *Eur Child Adol Psychiatry.* 2007;16(1):48–57.

72. Adler LA, Liebowitz M, Kronenberger W, et al. Atomoxetine treatment in adults with attention-deficit/hyperactivity disorder and comorbid social anxiety disorder. *Depress Anxiety.* 2009;26(3):212–221.

73. Geller D, Donnelly C, Lopez F, et al. Atomoxetine treatment for pediatric patients with attention-deficit/hyperactivity disorder with comorbid anxiety disorder. *J Am Acad Child Adolesc Psychiatry.* 2007;46(9):1119–1127.

74. Gabriel A, Violato C. Adjunctive atomoxetine to SSRIs or SNRIs in the treatment of adult ADHD patients with comorbid partially responsive generalized anxiety (GA): an open-label study. *Atten Deficit Hyperact Disord.* 2011;3(4):319–326.

CHAPTER 4

Tourette Syndrome

LAWRENCE W. BROWN, MD

I look up and see nostrils flaring with black smoke as fiery red eyes glare into my own. The beast displays it enormous wings, eclipsing the light of the sun. Though I sit atop my steed the two-headed dragon towers over me. Their names are Obsessive Compulsive Disorder and Tourette Disorder. They speak no words, yet something in their gaze tells me that there's no hope, that I should simply drop my weapons and capitulate. In defiance I ignore their threats, unsheathe my sword, and charge headlong into the beast.

COLLEGE ESSAY BY PATIENT G.G, AGE 17.

INTRODUCTION

Tourette syndrome is a neuropsychiatric disorder beginning in childhood, which is characterized by chronic motor and verbal mannerisms with or without other features. Common coexisting challenges include attention deficit hyperactivity disorder (ADHD), obsessive-compulsive disorder (OCD), anxiety disorders, and other behavioral problems. Tourette syndrome is a relatively common, biologically based determined disorder with a strong genetic predisposition in most cases. It is not a functional disorder, although tics are often exacerbated by stress, disappear (for the most part) in sleep, and are usually suppressible (at least for brief periods). There is a wide spectrum of tics and behavioral symptoms that typically vary over time in a waxing and waning fashion. Although infection can precipitate or exacerbate tics, there is no evidence that Tourette syndrome is caused by a reaction to streptococcal infection, virus, or other autoimmune disorder.

A fundamental understanding of the pathophysiology of Tourette syndrome has been as elusive as the search for any underlying gene or genes. However, recent clinical advances have provided new directions in understanding genetic and basic neurobiologic mechanisms as well as new therapeutic options. Effective treatment is available for most affected individuals; this list no longer includes only medications, all of which have side effects that can limit otherwise effective intervention. Cognitive behavior therapy has been demonstrated to be effective and can also be synergistic with drug approaches. It is important to remember that pharmacologic treatment should be limited to symptoms with significant impact on daily functioning—in other words, when the tics cause pain, interfere with ability to concentrate, disrupt others in the classroom, or are otherwise socially disabling. It is often more important to first address coexisting neuropsychiatric problems such as ADHD, although one must always take into account the possibility that treatment of the comorbidity could further exacerbate the tic disorder.

BRIEF HISTORY

Tourette syndrome was first described in 1489 in a manuscript on witchcraft (*Malleus Maleficarum* or *Witch's Hammer*). The book described a priest with motor and vocal mannerisms believed to be the result of witchcraft, possession by the devil or exorcism. It was not until 1885 when George Gilles de la Tourette, at the time a medical student at the Salpetriere Hospital in Paris, described nine bizarre patients with a condition that he called "maladie des tics."[1] The characteristics included childhood onset, variability over time, and a variety of other symptoms, including phonic tics, premonitory urges, echolalia, and coprolalia. With remarkable foresight, Tourette noted a genetic tendency, but he unfortunately concluded that it was a weakened nervous system due to immorality of prior generations. For many decades, while psychoanalytic theory was the predominant treatment approach, Tourette syndrome was explained by severe, repressed childhood conflicts and difficulty with "ego synthesis" because of overprotective parents or repressed masturbatory thoughts.[2] It was not until the 1960s when treatment with first-generation neuroleptics proved to be effective in controlling tics that there was a shift to a more brain-based conceptualization of this disorder. Since then, there has been a veritable explosion in research, and Tourette syndrome is now understood as a heterogeneous neurodevelopmental disorder with strong genetic determinants.[3-6]

CLINICAL PRESENTATION

Tics are sudden, repetitive, nonrhythmic movements or sounds, which can be further broken down to simple or complex. Simple tics involve a single set of muscles and appear involuntary—motor mannerisms may be rapid like eye blinking and head jerking or slower (i.e., dystonic) like squinting or arm stretching; simple vocal tics include coughing, throat clearing, and sniffing. Complex tics imply more coordinated activity, which can sometimes appear to be intentional, including hopping or bending, repeating words or phrases (echolalia or palilalia), and unintentional vocal cursing (coprolalia) or gestures (copropraxia). In most cases there is a progression starting with simple motor tics followed by simple verbal and then complex motor and complex verbal tics, but there are many exceptions to the rule. Similarly, although 6–8 years is the most common age of onset of tics, some present as early as 2 or 3 years, whereas others present in adolescence. Interestingly, age of onset or initial complexity does not predict prognosis. Students of the natural history of tics have described a peak at approximately 10 years and a tendency to improve during adolescence with one large prospective clinical study finding that only 23% of 16-year-olds still having moderate or severe tics.[7,8]

Tourette syndrome is the accepted term given to the combination of waxing and waning motor tics plus at least one verbal mannerism beginning in childhood or adolescence over the course of at least 1 year (Box 4.1). Although the layperson's notion of Tourette syndrome includes coprolalia, it is actually present in a minority of patients.[9] There has been increasing awareness that the disorder is not simply a motor phenomenon

---

BOX 4.1
DSM-V Definitions of Tourette Syndrome and Tic Disorders

TOURETTE SYNDROME (TS)

- Two or more motor tics (for example, blinking or shrugging the shoulders) *and* at least one vocal tic (for example, humming, clearing the throat, or yelling out a word or phrase); however, they might not always happen at the same time.
- Presence of tics for at least a year. The tics can occur many times a day (usually in bouts) nearly every day, or off and on.
- Onset before 18 years of age.
- Symptoms that are not due to taking medicine or other drugs or due to having another medical condition (for example, seizures, Huntington disease, or postviral encephalitis).

PERSISTENT (CHRONIC) MOTOR OR VOCAL TIC DISORDER

- One or more motor tics (for example, blinking or shrugging the shoulders) or vocal tics (for example, humming, clearing the throat, or yelling out a word or phrase), but *not* both.
- Tics that occur many times a day nearly every day or on and off throughout a period of more than a year.
- Onset before 18 years of age.
- Symptoms that are not due to taking medicine or other drugs or due to having a medical condition that can cause tics (for example, seizures, Huntington disease, or postviral encephalitis).
- Not diagnosed with TS.

PROVISIONAL TIC DISORDER

- One or more motor tics (for example, blinking or shrugging the shoulders) or vocal tics (for example, humming, clearing the throat, or yelling out a word or phrase).
- Tics have been present for no longer than 12 months in a row.
- Onset before 18 years of age.
- Symptoms that are not due to taking medicine or other drugs or due to having a medical condition that can cause tics (for example, Huntington disease or postviral encephalitis).
- Not diagnosed with TS or persistent motor or vocal tic disorder.
  - Both multiple and one or more vocal tics that have been present at some time, although not necessarily concurrently.
  - Tics occur many times per day (usually in bouts) nearly on a daily basis or intermittently throughout a period of more than 1 year, during which there was never a tic-free period of more than 3 consecutive months.
  - Onset before 18 years of age.
  - The disturbance is not due to the direct physiologic effects of a substance (e.g., stimulants) or underlying medical conditions such as Huntington disease and postviral encephalitis.

From American Psychiatric Association. *Diagnostic and Statistical Manual of Mental Disorders*. 5th ed. 2013, with permission.

(verbal tics being a unique form of motor activity of the speech apparatus) but a response to a frequently ill-defined sensation ("premonitory urge") or tension that forms the basis of cognitive behavioral therapy for Tourette syndrome.[10] In that study of teens and young adults, more than 90% reported an impulse to tic ("had to do it") with intensification of premonitory sensations, if prevented from performing a motor tic.

Most often, tics first appear in the eyes or face; it is not uncommon for them to be treated as allergies or a persistent upper respiratory illness, and the initial symptoms may disappear for months or years before returning, sometimes with a suddenness that raises concern for an acute infectious or inflammatory condition. Over time, there is a cephalocaudal progression of motor mannerisms that can involve all parts of the body, in addition to repetitive vocal outbursts. Like motor tics, verbal mannerisms can be isolated and meaningless, or more complex. Tics are stereotyped—they occur in the same manner—but they typically evolve or morph over time, which helps to distinguish them from other similar phenomena such as stereotypies, chorea, and dyskinesia. They may be as mild and noninterfering as to be overlooked or overwhelming, continuous, and even medically serious as to cause significant pain, embarrassment, or injury.

There are common factors that can provoke tics such as stress, anxiety, and fatigue, but it is important to note that these issues are insufficient on their own to cause tics unless they help to manifest an underlying predisposition. Similarly, there is no evidence that ADHD medications directly cause tics, although the mechanism of action of stimulants can sometimes bring out or exacerbate tics in the genetically primed individual. It is also frequently reported that individuals with Tourette syndrome can suppress or temporarily control their tics, but this does not mean that the mannerisms are strictly functional and not brain-based. It is also a common feature that concentration and physical activity will reduce tics—many affected individuals will have tics as they wait in the batter's box but symptoms often disappear as soon as they walk up to the plate.

Although tics are generally not a life-threatening situation, there are times when they can be dangerous—in our own institution we have seen numerous individuals in the emergency department for cervical dislocations from neck whipping tics and one adolescent with vertebral artery dissection, leading to stroke similar to a patient already described in the literature.[11]

One of the challenging issues in understanding the epidemiology of Tourette syndrome is the variability of tics, which can be extremely severe and disabling as described above to so mild and infrequent that they never come to medical attention. Until recently, it was believed that tic disorders were extremely rare, but there have been several studies that changed the opinion. When research associates were sent to observe children in elementary schools several times in the course of a year, up to 1:5 had at least one tic on one occasion (and an even higher rate of 1:4 in special educational classes).[12] There have been population-based investigations that report a wide range of Tourette syndrome, which vary if the definition includes all tics or only those that interfere with daily life. This has led to marked variability with a prevalence range of 1–30 per 1000 children in population-based studies; however, other more recent epidemiologic studies indicate a prevalence rate as high as 1% if one eliminates the disabling criteria.[13] Data from the 2007 National Survey of Children's Health showed a prevalence rate of 0.3% among US children aged 6–17 years. This is likely an underestimate because data were gathered from a parent-reported survey who may not have well recognized those with fluctuating levels of symptoms or who have limited access to specialists.[14]

Patients have been identified in all countries and ethnic populations, with the lowest prevalence in African Americans and sub-Saharan black Africans.[15] The most common age of onset corresponds to early elementary school years (5–7 years), a peak in symptoms at ages 10–11 years, a gradual reduction during the teenage years, and a complete or near-complete remission by late adolescence. As discussed below, although tics form the defining features of the diagnosis, coexisting neuropsychiatric disorders are extremely common and one or more comorbidities can be seen in up to 90% of individuals. These comorbidities include ADHD, OCD, impulse control disorders, self-injurious behaviors, aggression, anxiety, depression, and oppositional defiant disorder. Even when tics disappear, other psychiatric features may persist.

As the field of genetics evolves, new technologies keep refining the role of heredity in leading to tics and Tourette syndrome.[16,17] In the past, family studies indicated a dramatic increase in the incidence of Tourette syndrome in first-degree relatives of index patients up to 20 times higher than in the general population. Twin studies also pointed to a strong genetic basis because concordance rates were much higher in monozygotic twins compared with dizygotic (50%–77% vs. 10%–23%). A different study with monozygotic twins showed 56% concordance for Tourette syndrome but 94% for all tic disorders. Twin studies also pointed to the impact of environment because it was typically the smaller and more medically complicated twin who had either the tic disorder or the greater degree of burden from the disorder, if both were symptomatic. Linkage analysis in sibling pairs and large pedigrees pointed to several associations of interest, but attempts to define candidate genes, particularly those involved in dopamine and other transmitters, could not be replicated. More recently, de novo copy number variants have been occasionally found on genome-wide arrays when triads (affected child with both unaffected parents), but none, are common in affected individuals or seem to point to common pathways. The latest "next gen" technology employing whole-exome sequencing is beginning to identify potentially important loci, especially now that multiple large well-defined research populations, which are studying both triads and large multigenerational families, are being combined to share data.

PATHOPHYSIOLOGY

The molecular, cellular, and biochemical basis for Tourette syndrome has not been fully explicated, but there has been increasing acceptance of the central role of structural and functional alterations in the basal ganglia and related neuronal networks both in the primary mechanism of tics and in related problems, including ADHD and OCD.[18] Normally, the basal ganglia provide a mechanism for desired motor pattern to proceed (selective facilitation) while inhibiting interference by competing motor patterns (surround inhibition). It has been hypothesized that there are increased areas of excitability within the basal ganglia (excessive facilitation) in Tourette syndrome with normal surround inhibition leading to exaggerated activity or spread to other body parts. Maturation of the circuitry may explain tendency for tics to diminish with puberty because dopamine in the basal ganglia is maximal at approximately 9 years of age.

The story is far from complete because there have been many overlapping and complementary hypotheses with conflicting supportive data that point to a variety of disturbances in dopaminergic and other neurotransmitter function. For example, neuropathologic studies in Tourette syndrome have shown a significant reduction in GABAergic and cholinergic interneurons in the caudate and putamen in addition to the globus pallidus externa with a marked increase in the globus pallidus interna. Extensive imaging investigations have been inconsistent and sometimes conflicting. Quantitative MRI has shown reduction in caudate volume, which correlated with tic severity in patients followed longitudinally. Other studies have demonstrated increased size of the hippocampus, amygdala, and thalamus in addition to the thinner sensory and motor cortex. Functional studies (fMRI) performed in patients trying to control tics demonstrated altered activity of various brain regions as well. Connectivity studies have revealed decreased projections between the caudate and the lateral frontal cortex, which support a cortical disinhibition model in addition to implying underlying aberrations in the striatum. Overall, the consensus that can be derived from these studies point to abnormalities of the basal ganglia and the motor and/or premotor regions. It makes sense, therefore, that pharmacotherapy should be aimed at these areas. This would explain the success of dopamine D2 receptor antagonists like the typical and atypical neuroleptics and dopamine-depleting agents such as tetrabenazine in control tics. However, the beneficial effects of drugs affecting other neural pathways, including serotoninergic, noradrenergic, histaminergic, glutaminergic, GABAergic, and cholinergic systems, are still to be explained.

COMORBIDITIES WITH FOCUS ON ATTENTION DEFICIT HYPERACTIVITY DISORDER AND OBSESSIVE-COMPULSIVE DISORDER

Ever since the time of the first description by Gilles de la Tourette, there has been awareness of other associated behavioral and emotional difficulties. A recent report from a multicenter genetic study involving over 1300 probands and 1100 unaffected family members showed that 86% of patients had other psychiatric diagnoses, with ADHD and OCD being the most common.[19] Of the cohort, 72% met criteria for OCD or ADHD; more than half (58%) had two or more psychiatric disorders. Other disorders, including mood, anxiety, and disruptive behavior, each occurred in approximately 30% of the participants. The age of greatest risk for the onset of most comorbid psychiatric disorders was between 4 and 10 years, with the exception of eating and substance use disorders, which began in adolescence. Similarly, in a large prospectively followed specialty clinic population, 53% also had OCD, 39% had ADHD, and 24% fulfilled criteria for both.[20] While the phenomenology of tic disorders is wide, the defining symptom of Tourette syndrome is the presence of both motor and phonic tics. This was supported by a community-based study that also showed that ADHD and OCD were significantly increased in the presence of tic disorders, as well as separation anxiety, overanxious disorder, simple phobia, social phobia, agoraphobia, mania, major depression, and oppositional defiant behavior.[21] In one of the largest international analyses of almost 7000 cases, the prevalence rate of ADHD in Tourette syndrome was 55%, within the range of many other reports.[22] If the proband was diagnosed with ADHD, a family history of ADHD was much more likely. Furthermore, ADHD was associated with earlier diagnosis of Tourette syndrome and a much higher rate of anger control problems, sleep problems, specific learning disability, OCD, oppositional defiant disorder, mood disorder, social skill deficits, sexually inappropriate behavior, and self-injurious behavior. Recognition of ADHD is crucial because there is cumulative evidence that its presence is not only contributory to adverse quality of life but actually is a greater determinant.[23,24]

At least one-third of patients with Tourette syndrome have obsessive-compulsive behaviors, and about 20% fulfill DSM-V criteria for OCD. Extensive studies that have addressed genetic, neurobiologic, and treatment responses have demonstrated differences in OCD coexisting with tics and OCD unrelated to tics. In one prospective study, it was reported that 41% of the Tourette syndrome cohort had experienced at least moderate OCD symptoms at one time.[25] These OCD symptoms were reported to have presented in late childhood or early adolescence, with their peak severity occurring approximately 2 years after the peak tic severity. When OCD presents in individuals with Tourette syndrome, there is a male preponderance, an earlier age of onset, a less robust response to medical treatment, and a greater likelihood that tics are present in first-degree relatives. The most common obsessive-compulsive symptoms involve symmetry, repetition rituals, counting compulsions, and need for sameness as opposed to OCD without tics, in which the patient has anxious thoughts with the need to do things right or avoid other thoughts or actions so that something bad does not happen. When they are comorbid, obsessive-compulsive behaviors are more likely to persist beyond adolescence than tics. Although OCD in the presence of Tourette syndrome is less likely to respond to selective serotonin reuptake inhibitor (SSRI) treatment and more likely to respond to neuroleptics, there is no apparent difference in response to cognitive behavioral therapy.

TREATMENT OF TOURETTE SYNDROME— GENERAL COMMENTS

There is overwhelming evidence that the spectrum of tic disorders (whether they fulfill all criteria for Tourette syndrome) has a neurobiologic basis rather than a purely psychologic origin. This allows for a rational basis for intervention that is potentially far more effective than some of the historical attempts from leeches to static electricity, spinal elongation, and herbal remedies. One might come to the erroneous conclusion that pharmacologic treatment is indicated for most affected children—although medications are appropriate for many moderately to seriously affected individuals, the majority will not require drug treatment if tics are mild and do not interfere with the child's ability to function at home or in school. However, all individuals with a tic disorder should be offered guidance to understand the basis of their condition and its potential impact on daily life; cognitive behavioral therapy is not only appropriate but also increasingly accessible to even children of elementary school age.[26] The child, his/her family, and others in the environment need to understand which symptoms can be considered involuntary and which are within voluntary control. It can be very difficult to separate compulsive mannerisms from impulsive behaviors from tics. For example, a child may impulsively make inappropriate comments but insist "I had to do it." It is important to educate the teacher and provide instruction to the entire class if a child's tics are severe enough to be noticed in school; this will lead to a greater understanding about Tourette syndrome and hopefully more acceptance of differences and less ridicule from peers. School issues in children with Tourette syndrome are often much more difficult when compounded by ADHD, learning disabilities, OCD, or behavioral disorders. Some affected children will benefit from special education to treat associated psychologic or educational problems. Many will also require more formal counseling or family therapy.

PHARMACOLOGIC TREATMENT OF TICS

As with all neuropsychiatric conditions, the decision to treat with a pharmacologic approach must be guided by clear indications that the symptoms are interfering with daily life. This is perhaps best summarized by European guidelines that give four reasons why one should consider moving beyond psychoeducation and proactively treating tics. These include subjective discomfort (e.g., pain or injury), sustained social problems (e.g., social isolation or bullying), social and emotional problems for the patient (e.g., reactive depressive symptoms), and functional interference (e.g., impairment of academic achievements).[27] If there are comorbidities, the choice of medication should be based on the target symptom, which is the source of the most significant impairment. This will vary from child to child—even in complex situations, it usually falls to one of the triad of tics, OCD, or ADHD. The challenging patient with more than one disabling symptom may eventually require more than one approach, but treatment should still begin by addressing the most severe problem without worsening other issues. Because the natural history of the disease includes wide variability over time (waxing and waning of symptoms), it is important that an adequate trial be given for each dosage of every medication.

The goal for treating tics should be reduction in tic severity (as well as less discomfort or social embarrassment) sufficient to allow normal functioning and not the complete elimination of all symptoms. The most effective agents to reduce tics include the typical and atypical neuroleptics, although there is evidence that adrenergics can be effective.[27] Dopamine D2 blockers, including haloperidol, were the first effective agents to reduce tic severity as early as the 1960s. Haloperidol and pimozide remained the only Food and Drug Administration (FDA)-approved neuroleptic drugs for the treatment of Tourette syndrome until recently when aripiprazole was added in 2014.[28] Comparative studies are few, but there is one randomized, double-blind controlled study that found pimozide to be superior to haloperidol in terms of efficacy and tolerability.[29] Since then, however, warnings have been raised about the safety of pimozide in terms of prolongation of QT interval. Despite lack of the FDA approval, clinical practice shifted to atypical neuroleptics, including risperidone and aripiprazole, although some find the typical neuroleptic fluphenazine to have the best balance of efficacy and safety.[30] All typical and atypical neuroleptic drugs are potent dopamine blockers, and they all help in approximately 75% of cases. However, undesirable side effects may include cognitive blunting, restlessness, weight gain, psychomotor retardation, and depressed mood.[31] There is also the long-term risk of tardive dyskinesia with these drugs; however, typical neuroleptics that target specifically dopamine (e.g., haloperidol and pimozide) are more likely to produce this adverse outcome than atypical neuroleptics such as risperidone and aripiprazole. Many clinicians will obtain EKG with all of these drugs, but it is specifically recommended that EKG be performed before treatment with pimozide, 3 months after initiating the drug and then yearly. Now that aripiprazole has been approved for children with Tourette syndrome, it has largely replaced other neuroleptics. Aripiprazole has been reported to have fewer side effects with respect to weight gain, QT interval alterations, extrapyramidal symptoms, and hyperprolactinemia when compared with other drugs in its class.

At this time, the most common initial pharmacologic treatment algorithm for most individuals with mild to moderate tics is the α-1 adrenergic antagonist guanfacine.[32] Doses of the immediate release preparation are usually 1–4 mg daily provided BID to avoid sedating side effects. The extended-release (ER) preparation marked blunts peak-trough variability even when given once daily. Studies have shown that optimal dosing often approaches 0.1 mg/kg/day and guanfacine ER is approved by the FDA up to 7 mg.[33] Despite widespread acceptance of guanfacine as a first-line agent to treat tics, a recent pilot, randomized double-blind placebo-controlled trial of guanfacine ER did not show meaningful effect in reducing tics.[34] Clonidine, originally developed as an antihypertensive agent, has been widely used for almost three decades.[35] Many clinicians find it useful, however, because it can be helpful in addressing other common coexisting issues, such as sleep resistance, anxiety disorders, and ADHD. Side effects typically include sedation and irritability with rare reports of orthostatic hypotension. Clonidine is most effective when administered at least TID. There is also an ER preparation that can be dosed BID and a patch preparation that only needs to be changed every 5–7 days. Doses are approximately 10 times lower than for guanfacine (0.1–0.6 mg daily), but clonidine is limited by the frequent incidence of sedating and hypotensive side effects.

Other drugs that have been reported to be useful in controlling tics include clonazepam, the nicotine patch, the nicotine receptor antagonist inversine, and dopamine agonists including pergolide. All of these approaches have had limited success and are generally no longer in common usage. In addition, there is evidence that antiepileptic drugs, including topiramate, can be effective. However, the most recent interest has been with dopamine-depleting agents, including tetrabenazine and deutetrabenazine.[36]

These VMAT2 inhibitors appear to be more effective and safer than neuroleptics, although there is no experience in children and there is still the risk of drowsiness, depression, restlessness, and parkinsonism.

In summary, an evidence-based Canadian guideline had a strong recommendation only for the use of guanfacine and clonidine in children. Weak recommendations were made for all other medical treatments, including neuroleptics, botulinum toxin, topiramate, and tetrabenazine, among others.[37]

Beyond daily medication, there is increasing experience over the past decade controlling intractable focal motor and vocal tics with local injection of botulinum toxin into the affected muscles.[38] This toxic denervation can ameliorate involuntary tics for months, and there is evidence that it can also eliminate the premonitory sensation that may be an integral part of the tic pathology. Enormous interest has been generated about the possibility of surgical treatment with deep brain stimulation, and the experience is rapidly growing. A recent consensus report has very carefully outlined the necessary steps to insure maximal safety in terms of identification of appropriate patients, treatment algorithms, and follow-ups.[39] Long-term results are too preliminary to consider this approach in the vast majority of pediatric patients who have a reasonable chance of outgrowing the disorder.

TREATMENT OF TICS AND ATTENTION DEFICIT HYPERACTIVITY DISORDER

It is impossible to discuss treatment of Tourette syndrome without directly considering coexisting behavioral symptoms. As mentioned earlier, general support with behavioral modification strategies and academic or other intervention in the classroom should be the first steps in controlling the psychologic effects and the associated behavioral problems with Tourette syndrome. It is always beneficial and often critically important to raise the child's self-esteem and improve motivation in addition to directly treating tics. However, a comprehensive discussion of the nonpharmacologic and drug management of behavioral problems is beyond the scope of this chapter.

When considering ADHD, stimulants, including the various immediate and ER preparations of methylphenidate and amphetamines, are the standard first-line treatment, and they often improve other associated symptoms from academic productivity to impulsive aggression, noncompliance, and also poor socialization.[40] The problem is that ADHD and Tourette syndrome commonly coexist with a prevalence rate of around 60%, and ADHD presents with a mean age of presentation before 5 years, while tics typically present several years later.[41] This leads to a dilemma in the determination of the role of stimulants in inducing tics. Because stimulants are the first-line agents for the treatment of ADHD, many children destined to develop tics at a later age are initially treated with methylphenidate or amphetamines. Conventional wisdom (and the Physicians' Desk Reference) states that stimulants are potentially unsafe in children with a personal history of tics or a family history of Tourette syndrome. However, most experts continue to recommend stimulants as a first-line treatment when all is taken into account, as long as families are provided sufficient education to

accept the possibility that medication can transiently induce or worsen tics, and sometimes resultant tics may be severe and chronic. A recent metaanalysis supports the safety of stimulants in this population.[42] It is necessary to emphasize the issue of relative risk and consider the safety and efficacy of alternative drug strategies, as well as the risk of not treating.

Even when ADHD symptoms are improved with stimulants, there can be worsening of tics, compulsions, or stereotypies. This can be apparently idiosyncratic at any dose but more often occurs in a dose-responsive fashion. Perhaps more subtle, but sometimes more important, is the misinterpretation of symptoms consistent with ADHD, which would better be explained by an alternative mechanism. Anxiety, OCD, or high-functioning autistic spectrum disorder can interfere with the ability to sustain attention or lead to hyperactivity. Children desperately trying to control tics, obsessing on a favorite topic, or in "shut down mode" from anxiety can be mislabeled with ADHD. Effective stimulants can even increase inner-directed focus and lead to withdrawal into their own world, especially in children with autism.[43]

Other medication approaches are available. Adrenergic nonstimulants, though less effective than stimulants in controlling the core symptoms of ADHD, have the advantage that they can also be effective in reducing tics.[44] A randomized controlled trial addressed the role of clonidine in children with Tourette syndrome and ADHD and compared it with methylphenidate alone or in combination.[45] Both clonidine and methylphenidate were individually effective in improving the primary outcome ADHD measure, and the combination produced the most robust effect. Interestingly, tic severity lessened in all active treatment groups, with the combination of clonidine and methylphenidate also being the most effective. However, side effects were common with clonidine administration. As mentioned earlier, although there is strong support for the value of guanfacine in the treatment of ADHD, a well-designed (albeit pilot) study of guanfacine ER did not show meaningful effect in reducing tics.[34]

Atomoxetine was released in early 2003 as a non-stimulant alternative for the treatment of ADHD in children and adults.[46] A randomized, placebo-controlled study of atomoxetine in children with comorbid tic disorder and ADHD demonstrated both efficacy and safety without exacerbating tics.[47] Although not statistically significant, there was a trend toward improved tic rating scales over the course of the study.

Tricyclic antidepressants can be used to treat ADHD, and they were once the drugs of second choice after stimulants until safety concerns limited their use except under special circumstances. All have potential cardiac toxicity (QT prolongation), and sudden death has been reported from desipramine. Sedation, weight gain, and anticholinergic effects are also common side effects.

There is little evidence that tricyclics are helpful in controlling tics, and there are even reports of tic exacerbation and the induction of other drug-induced movement disorders (dyskinesias).

TREATMENT OF TICS AND OBSESSIVE-COMPULSIVE DISORDER

Serotonin reuptake inhibitors and cognitive behavioral therapy are the most effective drugs to treat OCD in children and adults.[48] The greatest pediatric experience is with fluoxetine and sertraline, but similar benefits (and side effects) are seen with other drugs in the class, including fluvoxamine, paroxetine, citalopram, and escitalopram.[49] Not only can these drugs treat OCD, but they are also effective in controlling associated anxiety symptoms and social phobias. Clomipramine was the first agent shown to be effective in treating childhood OCD, and it may actually be the most effective. However, it also has all of the potential side effects of other tricyclics, including sedation, weight gain, tachycardia, dry mouth, and other anticholinergic toxicity. Venlafaxine, with combined serotonin and norepinephrine reuptake inhibition properties, is also effective in treating OCD symptoms. There has been much public discussion of the increased risks when SSRIs are prescribed to children and adolescents with depression, but little has been written about the risk of suicidal ideation in those with OCD. It is clear that SSRIs can produce overactivation, irritability, agitation, and even hypomania if introduced too quickly or administered at high doses; prudence would suggest careful risk-benefit analysis and a slow titration schedule. Although there are no long-term comparison trials of any of these drugs in children with comorbid OCD and Tourette syndrome, recent advances have been the subject of a careful review.[50]

DIFFERENTIAL DIAGNOSIS

Tourette syndrome is usually unmistakable when it presents in a typical fashion at the usual age in the context of a positive family history. Despite the tremendous increase in public awareness in the past two decades, Tourette syndrome is still frequently missed. Many affected individuals go undiagnosed or inappropriately treated for a wide variety of conditions from allergies,

asthma, and dermatitis to hyperactivity, nervousness, oppositional behavior, habits, and other conditions. Of course, all medical conditions, especially neuropsychiatric disorders, have a differential diagnosis. Most often, the obsessive-compulsive symptoms, anxiety disorders, or ADHD comes before the tics or is so overwhelmingly prominent that Tourette syndrome is not considered as a unifying diagnosis. Even when recognized, the repetitive nature of tics can sometimes be hard to tell apart and has led to the concept of "compulsive tics." Other underlying disorders must be considered especially when there are unusual features. Autistic spectrum disorder is sometimes a consideration because presenting behaviors of stereotyped hand flapping, bizarre posturing, elaborate compulsions, and the need to preserve sameness can be confused with tics. In addition, there is a definite increase in those who fulfill criteria for both autism and Tourette syndrome, reflecting the overlapping involvement of neural networks. Epilepsy can be a consideration, especially if automatisms, including eye movements and picking behaviors of complex partial seizures, are confused with tics. Careful history can usually distinguish tics from epilepsy because the former has no aura, preserved consciousness, and voluntary inhibition of movements; additionally, tics tend to disappear in sleep. It is deceptive to rely on EEG findings because nonspecific abnormalities can be seen in children with Tourette syndrome; epileptiform features are unusual but relatively common developmental findings such as rolandic spikes or brief generalized spike-wave discharges may occur in otherwise asymptomatic children. Neurodegenerative disorders presenting with abnormal movements may be difficult to distinguish in their early stages, but Wilson's disease and Huntington disorder have other characteristic clinical, laboratory, and imaging findings.

Among the most concerning differential diagnostic entities are PANDAS (pediatric autoimmune neuropsychiatric disorder associated with streptococcal infection) and PANS (pediatric neuropsychiatric syndrome). The hypothesis is that the dramatic onset of tics, obsessive-compulsive mannerisms, and other behavioral symptoms may be caused by an autoimmune disease related to (or similar to) Sydenham's chorea. PANDAS was first proposed by researchers at the National Institutes of Mental Health who described a group of children with OCD and tic disorders with acute, dramatic, and repeated exacerbations associated with group A β-hemolytic streptococcal infection.[51] In the past 20 years, there has been an explosion of mostly anecdotal reports as well as a few well-designed scientific studies to address the question. The concept of

PANS extended the hypothesis to viral and other infections and captured increasing public attention at the same time that autoimmune encephalitis (i.e., anti-NMDA receptor encephalitis) was recognized. Those who accept the hypothesis can look to guidelines for diagnostic assessment and treatment from the PANS Research Consortium.[52] What this has unfortunately resulted in is an abundance of primary care providers inappropriately testing for strep whenever a child presents with tics. With any suggestion of current or recent strep exposure, something common and considered normal within this age group, providers initiate treatment with prolonged courses of antibiotics and/or immunomodulation, including steroids, IVIG, plasmapheresis, and rituximab. This practice is representative of a lack of understanding of the literature and is both inappropriate and dangerous because there have been several nearly lethal outcomes with the above-referenced interventions.[53,54] It is widely accepted that the overwhelming evidence is against a streptococcal or other autoimmune mechanism as the etiology of Tourette syndrome or the explanation of an exacerbation in the vast majority of patients. It is important to maintain a clear vision and a risk-benefit analysis based on strong science even when there is a vocal lobby supporting aggressive treatment of putative infectious and autoimmune abnormalities.

CONCLUSIONS: COMMUNICATION AND COUNSELING

Tourette syndrome is a model disorder of the interaction of developmental, genetic, neurobiologic, and behavioral influences. Behavioral approaches are always appropriate, but they are often inadequate or inaccessible. There is no entirely safe psychopharmacologic agent, but one must also consider the risks of not getting treatment. Children with severe Tourette syndrome have difficulty learning due to the adverse impact of constant tics and other coexisting conditions, and they are often socially ostracized. It is clear that tic reduction and efforts to address serious comorbid conditions can dramatically improve quality of life. Medication treatment should never be the first approach and should always be performed in conjunction with behavioral and other supportive services. Adverse drug reactions should not discourage the clinician from considering other medication trials.

If one is looking for evidence-based guidelines, there is little information to help the clinician to prescribe medications for children with Tourette syndrome—whether for isolated, intractable psychiatric symptoms or with multiple disabling problems.[43] This is not to say that there is no experience. One of the first studies in children with Tourette syndrome and ADHD comparing methylphenidate, clonidine, and dual therapy with placebo showed both safety and efficacy, and even favored the combination treatment.[45] While there was much public concern several years ago about the safety of combining methylphenidate with tricyclic antidepressants, careful analysis demonstrated no synergistic toxicity. Combining SSRIs with other drugs, however, may require more caution. Atypical neuroleptics, for example, have serotonin reuptake inhibiting properties as well. This can lead to the "serotonin syndrome" with excessive sweating, tremor, myoclonus, diarrhea, and fever, in addition to agitation, confusion, and hypomania.

The natural history of Tourette syndrome in most cases includes stabilization or spontaneous remission during adolescence or young adulthood. Many patients are able to stop medication by this time. Although tics may improve with maturity, other symptoms associated with the disorder may continue and even become more problematic. It is not uncommon for depression, mood swings, and rage attacks to worsen during adolescence. Symptoms of OCD, ADHD, and learning disabilities do not typically improve even when tics go into remission. There is much optimism in the field based on the combination of research advances in the underlying pathophysiology, effective treatment, and new understanding of the genetic basis of Tourette syndrome coupled with the demystification of and growing recognition of the disorder as a developmental neurobiologic condition with behavioral and emotional dimensions.[55]

REFERENCES

1. Lajonchere C, Nortz M, Finger S. Gilles de la Tourette and the discovery of Tourette syndrome. *Arch Neurol.* 1996;53:567–574.
2. Frundt O, Woods D, Ganos C. Behavioral therapy for Tourette syndrome and chronic tic disorders. *Neurol Clin Pract.* 2017;7:148–156.
3. Jancovic J. Medical progress: Tourette's syndrome. *N Engl J Med.* 2001;345:1184–1192.
4. Kurlan R. Tourette's syndrome. *N Engl J Med.* 2010;363:2332–2338.
5. Robertson MM. The Gilles de la Tourette syndrome: the current status. *Arch Dis Child Edu Pract.* 2012;97:166–175.
6. McNaught KSP, Mink JW. Advances in understanding and treatment of Tourette syndrome. *Nat Rev.* 2011;7:667–676.
7. Leckman JF, Zhang H, Viatale A, et al. Course of tic severity in Tourette syndrome in the first two decades. *Pediatrics.* 1998;102:14–19.

8. Groth C, Debes NM, Rask CU, et al. Course of Tourette syndrome and comorbidities in a large prospective clinical study. *J Am Acad Child Adolesc Psychiatry.* 2017;56:304–312.

9. Freeman RD, Zinner SH, Muehler-Vahl KR, et al. Coprophenomena in Tourette syndrome. *Dev Med Child Neurol.* 2009;51:218–227.

10. Kwak C, Dat Vuong K, Jankovic J. Premonitory sensory phenomenon in Tourette's syndrome. *Mov Disord.* 2003;18:1530–1533.

11. Lehman LL, Gilbert DL, Leaach JL, et al. Vertebral artery dissection leading to stroke caused by violent neck tics. *Neurology.* 2011;77:1706–1708.

12. Kurlan R, McDermott MP, Deeley C, et al. Prevalence of tics in schoolchildren and association with placement in special education. *Neurology.* 2001;57:1383–1388.

13. Scahill L, Sukhodolsky DG, Williams SK, et al. Public health significance of tic disorders in children and adolescents. *Adv Neurol.* 2005;96:240–248.

14. Centers for Disease Control and Prevention (CDC). Prevalence of diagnosed Tourette syndrome in persons aged 617 years – United States, 2007. *Morb Mortal Wkly Rep.* 2009;58:581–585.

15. Robertson MM, Eapen V, Cavanna AE. The international prevalence, epidemiology and clinical phenomenology of Tourette syndrome: a cross-cultural perspective. *J Psychosom Res.* 2009;67:475–483.

16. Deng H, Gao K, Janovic J. The genetics of Tourette syndrome. *Nat Rev Neurol.* 2012;26:1–11.

17. Willsey AJ, Fernandez TV, Yu D, et al. De novo coding variants are strongly associated with Tourette disorder. *Neuron.* 2017;94:486–499.

18. Leckman JF, Bloch MH, Smith ME, et al. Neurobiological substrates of Tourette's disorder. *J Child Adolesc Psychiatry.* 2010;20:237–247.

19. Hirschtritt ME, Lee PC, Pauls DL, et al. Lifetime prevalence, age of risk, and genetic relationships of comorbid psychiatric disorders in Tourette syndrome. *JAMA Psychiatry.* 2015;72:325–333.

20. Lebowitz ER, Motlagh MG, Katsovich L, et al. Tourette syndrome in youth with and without obsessive compulsive disorder and attention deficit hyperactivity disorder. *Eur J Child Adolesc Psychiatry.* 2011;21:451–457.

21. Kurlan R, Como PG, Miller B, et al. The behavioral spectrum of tic disorders: a community-based study. *Neurology.* 2002;59:414–420.

22. Freeman RD. Tic disorders and ADHD: answers from a world-wide clinical dataset on Tourette syndrome. *Eur Child Adolesc Psychiatry.* 2007;16(suppl 1):15–23.

23. Schuerholz LJ, Baumgardner TL, Singer HS, et al. Neuropsychological status of children with Tourette's syndrome with and without attention deficit hyperactivity disorder. *Neurology.* 1996;46:958–965.

24. Sukhodolsky DG, Landeros-Weisenberger A, Sahill L, et al. Neuropsychological functioning of children with Tourette syndrome with and without attention deficit/hyperactivity disorder. *J Am Acad Child Adolesc Psychiatry.* 2010;49:1155–1164.

25. Bloch MH, Peterson BS, Scahill L, et al. Adulthood outcome of tic and obsessive-compulsive symptom severity in children with Tourette syndrome. *Arch Pediatr Adolesc Med.* 2006;160:65–69.

26. Piacentini J, Woods DW, Scahill L, et al. Behavior therapy for children with Tourette disorder: a randomized controlled trial. *J Am Med Assoc.* 2010;303:1929–1937.

27. Roessner V, Plessen KJ, Rothenberger A, et al. European clinical guidelines for Tourette syndrome and other tic disorders. Part II: pharmacological treatment. *Eur J Child Adolesc Psychiatry.* 2011;20:173–196.

28. Liu Y, Hong NI, Wang C, et al. Effectiveness and tolerability of Aripiprazole in children and adolescents with Tourette's disorder: a meta-analysis. *J Child Adolesc Psychopharmacol.* 2016;26:436–441.

29. Gilbert DL, Batterson JR, Sethuraman G, Sallee FR. Tic reduction with risperidone versus pimozide in a randomized, double-blind crossover trial. *J Child Adolesc Psychopharmacol.* 2004;43:206–214.

30. Wijemanne S, Wu LJC, Jankovic J. Long-term efficacy and safety of fluphenazine in patients with Tourette syndrome. *Mov Disord.* 2014;29:126–130.

31. Pringsheim T, Pearce M. Complications of antipsychotic therapy in children with Tourette syndrome. *Pediatr Neurol.* 2010;43:17–20.

32. Scahill L, Chappell PB, Kim VS, et al. A placebo-controlled study of guanfacine in the treatment of children with tic disorders and attention-deficit/hyperactivity disorder. *Am J Psychiatry.* 2001;158:1067–1074.

33. Biederman J, Melmed RD, Patel A, et al. A randomized, double-blind, placebo-controlled study of guanfacine extended release in children and adolescents with attention-deficit/hyperactivity disorder. *Pediatrics.* 2008;121:e73–84.

34. Murphy TK, Fernandez TV, Coffey BJ, Rahman O, et al. Extended-release guanfacine does not show a large effect on tic severity in children with chronic tic disorders. *J Child Adolesc Psychopharmacol.* 2017;20:1–9.

35. Leckman JF, Hardin MR, Riddle MA, et al. Clonidine treatment of Gilles de la Tourette's syndrome. *Arch Gen Psychiatry.* 1991;48:324–328.

36. Pringsheim T, Doja A, Gorman D, et al. Canadian guidelines for the evidence-based treatment of tic disorders: pharmacotherapy. *Can J Psychiatry.* 2012;57:133–143.

37. Marras C, Andrews D, Sime E, Lang AE. Botulinum toxin for simple motor tics: a randomized, double-blind, controlled trial. *Neurology.* 2001;56:605–610.

38. Jankovic J, Jimenez-Shahed J, Budman C, et al. Deutetrabenazine in tics associated with Tourette syndrome. *Tremor Other Hyperkinet Mov.* 2016;6. https://doi.org/10.7916/D8M32W3H.

39. Schrock LE, Mink JW, Woods DW, et al. Tourette syndrome deep brain stimulation: a review and updated recommendations. *Mov Disord.* 2015;30:448–471.

40. Wolraich M, Brown L, Brown RT, et al. ADHD: clinical practice guideline for the diagnosis, Evaluation and treatment of Attention-Deficit/Hyperactivity Disorder in children and adolescents. *Pediatrics.* 2011;128:1007–1022.

41. Martino D, Ganos C, Pringsheim TM. Tourette syndrome and chronic tic disorders: the clinical spectrum beyond tics. *Int Rev Neurobiol.* 2017;134:161–190.
42. Cohen SC, Mulqueen JM, Ferracioli-Oda E, et al. Meta-analysis: risk of tics associated with psychostimulant use in randomized, placebo-controlled trials. *J Child Adolesc Psychiatry.* 2015;54:728–736.
43. Gilbert DL, Jankovic J. Pharmacological treatment of Tourette syndrome. *J Obsessive Compuls Relat Disord.* 2014;3:407–414.
44. Banaschewski T, Roessner V, Dittmann RW, et al. Non-stimulant medications in the treatment of ADHD. *Eur Child Adolesc Psychiatry.* 2004;13(suppl 1):102–116.
45. Tourette syndrome study Group. Treatment of ADHD in children with tics: a randomized, controlled trial. *Neurology.* 2002;58:527–536.
46. Allen AJ, Kurlan RM, Gilbert DL, et al. Atomoxetine treatment in children and adolescents with ADHD and comorbid tic disorders. *Neurology.* 2005;65:1941–1949.
47. Michelson D, Faries D, Wernicke J, et al. Atomoxetine in the treatment of children and adolescents with ADHD: a randomized, placebo-controlled, dose-response study. *Pediatrics.* 2001;108:e83–92.
48. Franklin ME, Sapyta J, Freeman JB, et al. Cognitive behavior therapy augmentation of pharmacotherapy in pediatric obsessive-compulsive disorder: the Pediatric OCD Treatment Study II (POTS II) randomized controlled trial. *JAMA.* 2011;306:1224–1232.
49. Krebs G, Heyman I. Obsessive-compulsive disorder in children and adolescents. *Arch Dis Child.* 2015;100:495–499.
50. Lombroso PJ, Scahill L. Tourette syndrome and obsessive-compulsive disorder. *Brain Dev.* 2008;30:231–237.
51. Swedo SE, Leonard HL, Garvey M, et al. Pediatric autoimmune neuropsychiatric disorders associated with streptococcal infections: clinical description of the first 50 cases. *Am J Psychiatry.* 2008;155:264–271.
52. Swedo S, Leckman J, Rose N. From research subgroup to clinical syndrome: modifying the PANDAS criteria to describe PANS (pediatric acute-onset neuropsychiatric syndrome). *Pediatr Ther.* 2012;2:1–8.
53. Kang J, Frankovich J, Cooperstock M, Cunningham MW, et al. Clinical evaluation of youth with pediatric acute-onset neuropsychiatric syndrome (PANS): recommendations from the 2013 PANS Consensus Conference. *J Child Adolesc Psychopharmacol.* 2015;25:3–13.
54. Frankovich J, Swedo S, Murphy T, et al. Clinical management of pediatric acute-onset neuropsychiatric syndrome: Part II – use of immunomodulatory therapies. *J Child Adolesc Psychopharmacol.* 2017;27:1–16.
55. Gunduz A, Okun MS. A review and update on Tourette syndrome: where is the field headed? *Curr Neurol Neurosci Rep.* 2016;16:37–50.

FURTHER READING

1. Weisman H, Qureshi IA, Leckman JF, et al. Systematic review: pharmacological treatment of tic disorders – efficacy of antipsychotic and alpha-2 adrenergic agonist agents. *Neurosci Biobehav Rev.* 2013;37:1162–1171.
2. Kurlan R, Johnson D, Kaplan EL. Streptococcal infection and exacerbations of childhood tics and obsessive-compulsive symptoms: a prospective blinded cohort study. *Pediatrics.* 2008;121:1188–1197.

Management of ADHD in Youth With Comorbid Epilepsy

GAURAV MISHRA, MD • JAY SALPEKAR, MD

KEY SUMMARY POINTS

- It is important to be vigilant clinically to recognize the presence of epilepsy in patients with attention deficit hyperactivity disorder (ADHD), and vice versa.
- The longer the duration of seizures or subclinical epileptiform discharges, higher the likelihood of finding ADHD or its symptoms.
- In cases with subclinical seizures and ADHD, identification of the underlying epilepsy and type will guide treatment. In some cases, appropriate use of antiepileptic drugs may significantly reduce ADHD symptoms, thus eliminating the need for being on multiple medications.
- The quality of sleep along with seizure control is greatly predictive of cognitive and behavioral outcomes.[1] Thus, correcting sleep is a big part of improving the quality of life and prognosis.
- In the majority of cases, cautious stimulant usage is safe and appropriate for ADHD comorbid with epilepsy.

INTRODUCTION

Epilepsy is a common illness in children and adolescents. Although epilepsy is often considered a neurologic condition, psychiatric comorbidities are associated with epilepsy well beyond the prevalence in the general pediatric population. Of all psychiatric comorbid conditions, management dilemmas are perhaps most prominent in the association of attention deficit hyperactivity disorder (ADHD) and pediatric epilepsy. Children with epilepsy as many as 40% or more will also have ADHD. However, clinicians are often stymied in terms of treating these comorbidities because of long-standing fears of altering the seizure threshold with stimulants or other available medication treatments. Unfortunately, the evidence base guiding the use of stimulants in the context of epilepsy is underdeveloped, and, in many ways, insufficient to dispel long-standing conventional wisdom, discouraging the use of stimulants in persons with epilepsy. As a result, many clinicians undertreat ADHD in this population, leading to additional morbidity. This chapter will review pertinent details of this comorbidity and offer reasoned approaches to treating ADHD in the context of epilepsy. In doing so, clinicians may be better able to provide comprehensive care in this population and improve quality of life.

Attention Deficit Hyperactivity Disorder

ADHD is the most common pediatric psychiatric illness. It affects about 5%–6% of the pediatric population.[2] Children with ADHD are first recognized because of multiple social impairments such as frequent conflicts with peers, poor frustration tolerance, and physically being unable to remain seated in a classroom setting. Academic impairments such as poor learning and low grades are common. These symptoms tend to be the most apparent in school-age children and appear twice as often in boys. However, the gender differences are less in older children and the prevalence may be equal in both genders by adulthood.[2–4]

According to the *Diagnostic and Statistical Manual of Mental Disorders, Fifth Edition*, ADHD is diagnosed when the youth presents with symptoms of inattention and with/without hyperactivity and impulsivity, in two or more settings, causing significant problems in social, school, or work functions.[3] The illness presents in multiple different permutations and combinations, but the interrater reliability of the diagnostic criteria for ADHD far surpasses the level obtained in diagnosing most other psychiatric illnesses.[5] Specific diagnostic criteria are outlined in Box 5.1.

The diagnosis of ADHD requires the onset of at least six inattention symptoms and six hyperactive-impulsive

BOX 5.1
DSM-5 Criteria for Attention Deficit Hyperactivity Disorder (ADHD)

People with ADHD show a persistent pattern of inattention and/or hyperactivity-impulsivity that interferes with functioning or development:

1. Inattention: six or more symptoms of inattention for children up to age 16 years, or five or more symptoms for adolescents 17 years and older and adults; symptoms of inattention have been present for at least 6 months, and they are inappropriate for developmental level:

   - Often fails to give close attention to details or makes careless mistakes in schoolwork, at work, or with other activities.
   - Often has trouble holding attention on tasks or play activities.
   - Often does not seem to listen when spoken to directly.
   - Often does not follow through on instructions and fails to finish schoolwork, chores, or duties in the workplace (e.g., loses focus, side-tracked).
   - Often has trouble organizing tasks and activities.
   - Often avoids, dislikes, or is reluctant to do tasks that require mental effort over a long period (such as schoolwork or homework).
   - Often loses things necessary for tasks and activities (e.g., school materials, pencils, books, tools, wallets, keys, paperwork, eyeglasses, mobile telephones).
   - Is often easily distracted.
   - Is often forgetful in daily activities.

2. Hyperactivity and impulsivity: six or more symptoms of hyperactivity-impulsivity for children up to age 16 years, or five or more symptoms for adolescents 17 years and older; symptoms of hyperactivity-impulsivity have been present for at least 6 months to an extent that is disruptive and inappropriate for the person's developmental level:

   - Often fidgets with or taps hands or feet, or squirms in seat.
   - Often leaves seat in situations when remaining seated is expected.

   - Often runs about or climbs in situations where it is not appropriate (adolescents or adults may be limited to feeling restless).
   - Often unable to play or take part in leisure activities quietly.
   - Is often "on the go" acting as if "driven by a motor."
   - Often talks excessively.
   - Often blurts out an answer before a question has been completed.
   - Often has trouble waiting for his/her turn.
   - Often interrupts or intrudes on others (e.g., butts into conversations or games).

In addition, the following conditions must be met:

   - Several inattentive or hyperactive-impulsive symptoms were present before age 12 years.
   - Several symptoms are present in two or more setting (e.g., at home, school or work; with friends or relatives; in other activities).
   - There is clear evidence that the symptoms interfere with or reduce the quality of social, school, or work functioning.
   - The symptoms do not happen only during schizophrenia or another psychotic disorder. The symptoms are not better explained by another mental disorder (e.g., mood disorder, anxiety disorder, dissociative disorder, or a personality disorder).

Based on the types of symptoms, three kinds (presentations) of ADHD can occur:

Combined presentation: if enough symptoms of both criteria inattention and hyperactivity-impulsivity were present for the past 6 months.

Predominantly inattentive presentation: if enough symptoms of inattention, but not hyperactivity-impulsivity, were present for the past 6 months.

Predominantly hyperactive-impulsive presentation: if enough symptoms of hyperactivity-impulsivity, but not inattention, were present for the past 6 months.

From American Psychiatric Association, DSM-5 Task Force. *Diagnostic and Statistical Manual of Mental Disorders: DSM-5*. 5th ed. Washington, D.C.: American Psychiatric Association; 2013. vol. xliv, 947 p., with permission.

symptoms by the age of 12 years.[3] Inattention impairments include an inability to attend to detail, making careless mistakes in schoolwork, having trouble sustaining attention, not listening when spoken to directly, not following through on instructions, being disorganized, losing important things, getting easily distracted, and being forgetful.[3] The hyperactive-impulsive impairments include fidgeting/tapping hands or feet, squirming or

restless physical movement, running around class, routinely getting out of their seat, climbing furniture, and appearing to be always "on the go." Children with ADHD may also talk excessively, have difficulty waiting for their turn, and interrupt or intrude on others' conversations or activities.[3] The core impairments in ADHD often lead to additional problems with executive functions such as working memory, self-regulation, internalization of speech, and processing of information.[6,7] ADHD leads to impairments in areas other than only academics and behavior. High impulsivity, hyperactivity, and inattention also result in children needing repeated reminders to stay on task and to behave both at home and school. These children also frequently find it hard to establish friendships with their peer group because of inability to engage in the back and forth of conversation that children who can focus are able to do. Self-esteem is also affected because of these children struggling for social acceptance and academic success as compared with peers who can focus well and follow directions better, thus integrating into the mainstream of their peer groups.

Epilepsy

Epilepsy is the most common pediatric neurological illness present in about 1% of youth between the ages of 0 and 17 years.[8] The International League Against Epilepsy, 2014, defined epilepsy as at least two unprovoked seizures occurring more than 24 h apart, *or* one unprovoked seizure and a probability of further seizures. Epilepsy is considered resolved for children who are older than the age criteria for their specific epilepsy subtype *or* for those who have remained seizure-free for 10 years and with no anticonvulsant medicines for the last 5 years[9] (see Box 5.2).

Nomenclature for seizures has changed through the years. At this time, seizures are described as either focal or generalized, involving disrupted consciousness or not. Some seizures may start from one part of the brain (focal) and spread, becoming secondarily generalized. Common seizure disorders include childhood absence epilepsy (CAE), a primary generalized seizure disorder, or temporal lobe epilepsy, a focal seizure disorder commonly involving structures such as the amygdala or hippocampus. Features of relevant seizure types are described in Table 5.2.[9]

The presence of epilepsy predisposes children to a much higher likelihood of being diagnosed with psychiatric illnesses such as depression, anxiety, ADHD, conduct disorder, developmental delay, or autistic spectrum disorder.[10] Some reports indicate that nearly 80% of children with epilepsy have neurobehavioral comorbidities.[11] About 40% of children with epilepsy have an intellectual disability, 33% have ADHD, and 21% are on the autism spectrum.[6] The two major distinctions of ADHD in children with epilepsy and those presenting in the general population are the preponderance of the inattentive subtype, compared with the combined type that is more common in the general population. Also distinctive is a nearly equal prevalence of ADHD in boys and girls with epilepsy versus the predominance among males in school-aged children without epilepsy.[6,12,13] The presentation of ADHD in these patients with epilepsy is more severe in

---

> **BOX 5.2**
> **International League Against Epilepsy (ILAE) 2014 Definition**
>
> Epilepsy is a disease of the brain defined by any of the following conditions:
> 1. At least two unprovoked (or reflex) seizures occurring >24 h apart.
> 2. One unprovoked (or reflex) seizure and a probability of further seizures similar to the general recurrence risk (at least 60%) after two unprovoked seizures, occurring over the next 10 years.
> 3. Diagnosis of an epilepsy syndrome.
>
>   Epilepsy is resolved for individuals who had an age-dependent epilepsy syndrome but are now past the applicable age or those who have remained seizure-free for the last 10 years, with no seizure medicines for the last 5 years.

From Fisher RS, et al. ILAE official report: a practical clinical definition of epilepsy. *Epilepsia*. 2014;55(4):475–482, with permission.

---

the presence of other psychosocial risk factors.[14] Children with complicated epilepsy and those with higher seizure frequency have a higher likelihood to have a diagnosis of ADHD. Hyperactivity is seen more commonly in children with intractable epilepsy.[15,16]

ADHD and epilepsy have a special relationship encompassing their etiology, symptomatology, diagnosis, and treatment. Their relationship cannot be explained just by the fact that children with epilepsy are more likely to have an evaluation for ADHD.[6] Austin et al. demonstrated that the longer a child had seizures, the higher likelihood there was of them presenting with ADHD symptoms.[17] Higher rates of ADHD were noted in children with longer periods of unrecognized seizures versus children with new onset seizures, both, however, being much higher than the average population.[17] The common finding of subclinical seizures and abnormal electroencephalogram (EEG) spikes in patients with ADHD points to a possible common etiology. These commonalities and points of differentiation are further discussed in this chapter.[5,9]

COMORBIDITY OF ATTENTION DEFICIT HYPERACTIVITY DISORDER AND EPILEPSY[9]

ADHD and epilepsy have been found to be overrepresented, each in the presence of the other. In other words, patients with epilepsy are more likely to be diagnosed with ADHD, and interestingly, the converse is also true. ADHD is found in about 30%–40% of patients with epilepsy compared with 5%–6% in the general population.[12] Ott et al. showed an incidence of nearly 60%–70% of ADHD in patients with medically refractory epilepsy.[18] The inattentive subtype of ADHD is more common than hyperactive-impulsive subtype. The gender ratio of 2:1 for males:females in patients with ADHD appears to be less prominent in the context of epilepsy.[12] It has also been observed that patients with ADHD between 5% and 60% have abnormal or even frank epileptiform EEG discharges. One report suggests that nearly 14% of children with ADHD eventually develop seizure disorders.[19]

Socanski et al. showed that nearly 35% of patients with ADHD had abnormal EEG findings. In another study with 517 children, about 7.5% of patients had epileptiform discharges. They also found 2.3% of the children with ADHD to have epilepsy. This is more than double the average rate in the population.[20–22] Table 5.1 demonstrates findings in studies evaluating the comorbidity of ADHD and epilepsy.

PATHOLOGY

There also appears to be a direct pathologic relationship between epilepsy and ADHD. Children with epilepsy are much more likely to have ADHD, and children with ADHD are much more likely to have abnormal epileptiform discharges on an EEG and eventually develop a seizure disorder than those without ADHD. These rates are also higher than those seen in siblings of these patients.[17] Marston et al. determined that the longer a child has had epilepsy, the larger the likelihood of being diagnosed with ADHD—15.8% for those with a remote versus 8.1% of those with a recent diagnosis of epilepsy. This was further compared with 3.1% seen in normal siblings. This would point to seizures and subclinical epileptiform activity having a role in the development of attention problems.[26] Dunn et al. also found kids with new onset seizure to have had increased attention and behavior issues 6 months before their first recorded seizure.[12] Thus, the longer the duration of seizures or subclinical epileptiform discharges, the higher the likelihood of finding ADHD or its symptoms.

The pathophysiology of the association between ADHD and epilepsy is difficult to elucidate with confidence; however, Kaufman et al.[27] presented the three possible comorbidity hypothesis to explain the over-representation between the two conditions.

1. The first hypothesis is that there are independent circumstantial factors. The fact is that ADHD is a common psychiatric illness in childhood, and epilepsy is also a common neurological illness; thus they are bound to cooccur at a higher level.

2. The second hypothesis is that ADHD and epilepsy may have common genetic factors, biochemical factors, or key genetic-environmental interactions. This common etiology would then explain why the two conditions are so often found in the same patient.

3. Finally, a direct effect of epilepsy may relate to attention function. Chronic seizures and subepileptiform discharges, peri-ictal and post-ictal phases, all present with effects on focus and processing speeds. Antiepileptic medications also can have a negative effect on focus and processing speeds.[27] In that way, it may be that epilepsy itself, maybe even beyond discrete seizures, has direct effects on focus that will rise to the level of diagnostic significance in affected children.

Other Pathogenic Mechanisms

The attention function has been found to be associated with the dorsolateral prefrontal cortex and orbital prefrontal cortex. The symptoms of ADHD, which possibly arise from dysfunction of the dorsolateral prefrontal cortex, include organization, planning, attention, and working memory. Dysfunction of the orbital cortex appears to affect the social responses and impulse control segments of the ADHD symptom cluster.[27] Castellanos et al. showed in their brain volume studies that, when development was tracked, children with ADHD showed smaller total cerebral and cerebellar volumes than controls. They showed that any structural or developmental impacts of ADHD on the brain caused by genetic or environmental factors do not change in response to stimulant treatment.[28]

Disinhibition is a key characteristic of ADHD, and one suggested mechanism of ADHD medication efficacy is that they increase the inhibitory influence of frontal cortex on subcortical structures,[29] particularly caudate nucleus. The caudate nucleus is implicated in motor disinhibition syndromes such as Huntington's chorea and may similarly be awry in other conditions involving disinhibition or impulsivity. Some academicians consider that the caudate nucleus dysfunction is particularly involved in ADHD as thought output from the prefrontal cortices is not efficiently inhibited.

Effect of subclinical epileptiform activity

Epilepsy presents with unprovoked seizures, which are uncontrolled electrical impulses spreading through the brain. The extent of this spread determines if they are partial or generalized.[9,27] Many of the times, the seizure activity is limited to subclinical epileptiform discharges. However, these are also known to affect attention and brief cognitive deficits.[30] Children with ADHD are also found to have a much higher incidence

TABLE 5.1
Comorbidity of Attention Deficit Hyperactivity Disorder (ADHD) and Epilepsy

References	Study Type	Study Details	Results	Conclusions
Zhang et al.[23]	Retrospectively selected.	161 patients aged 6.2–18 years, who were diagnosed with frontal lobe epilepsy.	59% (95/161) of patients were subsequently diagnosed with ADHD.	Interestingly, the presence of sustained abnormalities on the electroencephalogram (EEG) was associated with a statistically significantly higher incidence of ADHD than a normal EEG (89.4% compared with 25% in this patient population). Patients in this study were treated with carbamazepine, valproic acid, or both, and 63% of patients became well controlled on these medications.
Socanski et al.[21]	Retrospective chart review. Children with ADHD who were evaluated in their clinic between 2000 and 2005.	Factors compared: age, sex, disorders of psychological development, cognitive level, pharmacologic treatment for ADHD, initial response to treatment, and ADHD subtype with and without epilepsy. In addition, compared data with a Norwegian study in a large general pediatric population.	Of the 607 children with ADHD (age 6–14 years; 82.4% males), 14 (2.3%) had a history of epilepsy and 13 of these had active epilepsy. This is a higher occurrence than expected in the general pediatric population (0.5%). Most patients had mild epilepsy and they were more likely to be seizure-free (79%) compared with the patients with epilepsy in general pediatric population.	• The ADHD patients with and without epilepsy did not differ regarding age, gender, disorders of psychologic development, IQ level <85, or ADHD subtype. • The patients had been diagnosed with epilepsy 1.8 years before the ADHD assessment. • All patients with epilepsy were treated with methylphenidate (MPH), and initial response to MPH was achieved in 85.7%.
Davis et al.[24]	Population-based case-control study of the 1976–82 Rochester birth cohort.	The objective here was to compare the incidence and characteristics of epilepsy with the population. Cohorts of children with (n=358) and without ADHD (n=728) based on medical record review to age 20 years.	• Cases were 2.7 times more likely than controls to have epilepsy (95% confidence interval [CI]=0.94–7.76; $P=.066$), had earlier seizure onset (median age, 5.5 vs. 15 years; $P=.020$), and exhibited a trend toward more frequent seizures (more than monthly, 63% vs. 17%). • Among children who met the research criteria for ADHD, those with epilepsy tended to be less likely to have received a clinical diagnosis of ADHD (63% vs. 89%; $P=.052$) or to be treated with stimulants (50% vs. 85%; $P=.025$).	• The findings suggest a higher incidence of epilepsy among children with ADHD than those without. • Epilepsy in children with ADHD appears to be more severe than in those without. • There appears to be a reluctance to diagnose and initiate treatment for ADHD in children with epilepsy.
Hersdorffer et al.[25]	Population-based case-control study.	Newly diagnosed unprovoked seizures among Icelandic children aged 3–16 years. 109 cases and 218 controls. Children with seizures were matched to the next two same-sex births from the population registry.	Forty-six cases were identified with a single incident unprovoked seizure and 63 with incident epilepsy. Most cases were male. A history of ADHD was 2.5-fold more common among children with newly diagnosed seizures than among control subjects (95% CI, 1.1–5.5).	The association was restricted to ADHD predominantly inattentive type (odds ratio [OR], 3.7; 95% CI, 1.1–12.8), not ADHD predominantly hyperactive-impulsive type (OR, 1.8; 95% CI, 0.6–5.7) or ADHD combined type (OR, 2.5; 95% CI, 0.3–18.3).

of subclinical epileptic activity.[27] These transient cognitive deficits are seen in 50% of epileptic patients with subepileptiform discharges. Transient cognitive deficits are also more common in generalized 3 Hz spike and wave discharges that are typical discharges involved with absence seizures.[30,31] Children with absence epilepsy may have cognitive dysfunction and inattention that could result from the cumulative impact of repeated absence seizures.[32] Holtmann et al. also found an increased incidence of rolandic spikes at 5.6% in children with ADHD compared with 2.4% seen in the regular population.[33]

CLINICAL PRESENTATION

The significant overlap of the common finding of inattention in both, patients with ADHD and epilepsy, makes it imperative to establish whether the ADHD symptoms were present before the onset of seizures. The key clinical features of ADHD are distractibility, inattention, and disorganization. These, however, are also common features in subclinical seizures, peri-ictal and post-ictal periods, thus leading to possible confusion in accurate diagnosis.[5] Even if a patient has a confirmed diagnosis of epilepsy, the side effects of many antiepileptic drugs (AEDs) have negative effects on cognition, disinhibition, irritability, and poor concentration Table 5.5.

Despite many of the symptoms of ADHD and epilepsy being common, there are some differences in how they present.[5] ADHD symptoms of inattention and distractibility are generally seen throughout the day and at multiple settings; however, in patients with epilepsy, these are generally seen in the peri-ictal phase. Hyperactivity and impulsivity are very commonly seen in ADHD and even more so in unstructured environments. Impulsivity is not a common feature of epilepsy. Disorganization is more commonly seen in ADHD than in epilepsy. Social relations tend to be affected in ADHD because of the inability to appropriately engage in the back-and-forth interactions that normal conversations are comprised of. However, in epilepsy the social difficulties tend to arise more from anxiety about seizures, isolation, and stigma[5].

The diagnosis and treatment of ADHD comorbid with epilepsy would need, to begin with, a detailed clinical interview. The proposed steps of evaluation include the following (see Box 5.3):

- A detailed evaluation of presenting symptoms of ADHD. The history of seizures or diagnosis of epilepsy. Clarifying the temporal relationship between onset of seizures and ADHD symptoms.

- Obtaining history of ADHD symptoms, being present in at least two or more locations, e.g., home and school. This can be supported by the Vanderbilt or Swanson, Nolan and Pelham (SNAP) IV Questionnaire SNAP-IV scale.[34]
- ADHD symptoms being present at times other than only peri-ictal or post-ictal periods.
- If the history or time course of symptoms is unclear, consider further evaluation with an EEG to rule out any subclinical seizures, which may explain the symptoms.[35]
- A neuropsychologic examination may also point to a diagnosis of ADHD for further clarity about academic deficiencies.
- Detailed evaluation of sleep quality/fragmentation can also give a clear idea of symptom etiology. A video polysomnography study may aid detection of subclinical seizures in cases indicated.
- Assess for additional comorbid illnesses, such as anxiety and learning disorders.
- If the patient has a diagnosis of epilepsy and is on AEDs, evaluate to see if these drugs are causing any significant effects on cognition/ability to stay focused. Check drugs levels and other metabolic abnormalities causing these symptoms.

BOX 5.3
The Diagnosis and Treatment of Attention Deficit Hyperactivity Disorder (ADHD) Comorbid With Epilepsy

- A detailed psychiatric and neurologic evaluation. Clarifying the temporal relationship between onset of seizures and ADHD symptoms.
- Obtaining history of ADHD symptoms being present in at least two or more locations.[34]
- ADHD symptoms being present at times other than only peri-ictal or post-ictal periods.
- If the history is unclear, consider evaluation with EEG to rule out any subclinical seizures.[35]
- Neuropsychologic assessment to evaluate for ADHD versus learning disabilities.
- Detailed evaluation of sleep quality/fragmentation— video polysomnography study.
- Assess for additional comorbid illnesses, such as anxiety and learning disorders.
- Evaluate if antiepileptic drugs are causing any significant effects on cognition/ability to stay focused. Check for drugs levels and other metabolic abnormalities.

Frequent epileptiform activity on an EEG would make an independent diagnosis of ADHD less likely, especially if the epilepsy is untreated. Some common epilepsy types that may also have some symptoms that mimic ADHD include the following:

1. **CAE** presents commonly with inattention, poor focus, daydreaming, staring, difficulty in visual sustained attention, problems with verbal and nonverbal attention, and memory. Despite a good response to antiepileptic medications, these patients often take a long time to get diagnosed and at times could be treated with stimulants for ADHD before finally receiving a diagnosis for absence seizures.[36] Caplan et al. found about 61% of CAE patients having some form of psychiatric comorbidity.[37] About 26% had ADHD and 11% had ADHD combined with anxiety/affective disorders.[38]

2. **Frontal lobe epilepsy (FLE)** is another common epilepsy syndrome associated with ADHD. About 70% of patients with FLE have ADHD.[23] Clinically, FLE and ADHD have many common symptoms such as impulsivity, irritability, and disinhibition.[1,39] The frontal lobes are involved in motor function, problem-solving, initiation, judgment, impulse control, and social and sexual behavior. Hermann et al. found that children with FLE with ADHD presenting together have a much poorer executive functioning compared with controls or FLE without ADHD.[40]

The first hypothesis includes children having impaired frontal cortical function, thus having a higher incidence of ADHD and epilepsy. A second hypothesis suggests that multiple epileptiform discharges impair normal brain development, thus also preventing normal learning.[23]

3. **Rolandic epilepsy/benign childhood epilepsy with centrotemporal spikes** is associated with 21%–30% of patients having ADHD.[36] These patients show a greater susceptibility to distractors occurring in their visual field and less efficient attentional control.

In a study of 145 children by Kanazawa et al., about 48.3% of patients had abnormal EEG findings and 22.1% had epileptiform discharges.[41] They also found that the about half of the focal discharges were central and frontal and occipital was the next most frequently encountered.[41]

4. **Sleep-related epilepsies**: Poor sleep has been associated with lesser ability to focus, lower retention, irritability, and learning problems in children, especially in the context of ADHD. Clinically sleep fragmentation is also associated with attentional deficits and hyperactivity.[42] Electrical status epilepticus during slow-wave sleep presents with prolonged focal epileptic activity and this interferes with cognitive functions and learning. Nocturnal seizures are known to increase time to rapid eye movement sleep and lead to drowsiness, thus reducing sleep efficiency[42,43] (see Table 5.2).

TREATMENT

The first line of treatment of ADHD without epilepsy is stimulant medication—methylphenidate (MPH) and amphetamine preparations. There is a concern, however, that stimulants may cause a worsening of preexisting seizure disorders, or even precipitate seizures in a person who is susceptible or has subclinical epileptiform discharges, by lowering the seizure threshold.[27]

In our clinical experience, patients with epilepsy, controlled well on one antiepileptic medication, were in general able to be started on MPH without any new seizure onset or complication. Evidence does exist that shows that patients who have less than one seizure per month appear to have no greater risk of seizure exacerbation than the general population when taking stimulants.[50] This information should offer clinicians confidence in treating children and adolescents with ADHD in the context of epilepsy. For patients with less stable epilepsy, stimulants may still be reasonable options, though should be used more cautiously. The risk factors for a chronic stimulant prescription use causing seizures include complicated ADHD and epileptiform discharges in EEG. This risk is especially high in patients with centrotemporal spikes.[35] Gonzalez and Heydrich noted that the factor determining a positive/negative response on stimulants was in fact the presence of a comorbid developmental delay rather than the presence or absence of seizures in the past 6 months[13] (see Table 5.3).

1. **MPH**: In the presence of a diagnosis of epilepsy, MPH has emerged as the first-line medication for ADHD. It is recommended to be used in a therapeutic dose range of 20–60 mg/day or 0.3–1 mg/kg/day.[51] MPH prevents the reuptake of noradrenaline and dopamine into neurons, thus stimulating cortical and subcortical regions that affect attention.[52] FDA warning still exists for MPH potentially lowering seizure threshold, advising against its use in patients with uncontrolled seizure disorders. The commonly available preparations of this medication include MPH—brands Concerta, Ritalin, Metadate, Daytrana, and Methylin—and dexmethylphenidate—brand Focalin.[53] These are all available in oral immediate- or extended-release and some

TABLE 5.2
Seizure Disorders With Comorbid Attention Deficit Hyperactivity Disorder (ADHD)[44]

Seizure Disorder	Neurological Features	ADHD Symptoms
Absence seizures/Petit mal seizures[45]	Absence seizures cause lapses in awareness and staring. They are generalized onset seizures. They begin and end abruptly, lasting only a few seconds. Mistaken for daydreaming and may not be detected for months. Common in children.	Inattention, poor focus, daydreaming, staring behaviors, difficulty in visual-sustained attention, verbal and nonverbal attention, and memory, despite a good response to antiepileptic medications.[37]
Landau-Kleffner syndrome[46]	Begins between 3 and 7 years of age. Progressive loss of speech. Seizures occur during sleep. This syndrome includes a loss of IQ, language impairment, and acquired epileptic aphasia.	Behavioral issues, hyperactivity, and a decreased attention span (80%). Impaired short-term memory, rage, aggression, and anxiety.
Generalized tonic-clonic seizures[47]	Present between 5 and 40 years of age. Happen most often within 1–2 h of waking up from sleep. Common triggers for seizures include sleep deprivation, fatigue, alcohol, fever, menstrual cycle, and flashing lights. Treatment with seizure medications is usually needed long term.	Deficits of attention.
Childhood absence epilepsy[36,45]	Seizures are usually staring spells during which the child is not aware or responsive. Each seizure lasts about 10 s–20 s and ends abruptly. Two-thirds of children respond to treatment. The seizures usually disappear by mid-adolescence.	Cognitive deficits, linguistic difficulties, and the onset of ADHD antedated the diagnosis of epilepsy in 82% of patients.
Benign childhood epilepsy with centrotemporal spikes[48]	Involves twitching, numbness, or tingling of the child's face or tongue. Seizures last for <2 min and usually occur at night. Child remains fully conscious. These comprise 15% of all epilepsies in children. Seizures usually stop on their own by age 15 years.	Susceptible to distractors occurring in their visual field; poor sustained attention; and more aggressive behaviors.
Electrical status epilepticus during slow-wave sleep[49]	Rare epilepsy syndrome, starts in mid-childhood. Children affected usually already have a diagnosis of epilepsy. The first sign of any problem is usually that the rate of a child's learning appears to slow down significantly.	Attentional deficits, hyperactivity, and learning disorders.
Nocturnal frontal lobe epilepsy	Frontal lobe epilepsy produces brief seizures possibly accompanied with startling and screaming. These seizures may occur in clusters. Treatment includes medication and sometimes surgery.	Inattention, hyperactivity, and impulsivity.
Temporal lobe epilepsy[36]	Localization-related epilepsy.	Higher risk for memory and mood difficulties.

From Ryvlin P, Rheims S, Risse G. Nocturnal frontal lobe epilepsy. *Epilepsia*. 2006;47(suppl 2):83–86, with permission.

TABLE 5.3
Treatment Algorithm

#	Medication Classes	Group and Preparations	Target Symptoms	Potential Side Effects
1	Stimulants	Methylphenidate and dexmethylphenidate • Immediate release • Extended release • Patch	Inattention Hyperactivity Impulsivity	Appetite suppression Mood changes Insomnia Cardiac arrhythmias
		Amphetamine • Mixed amphetamine and dextroamphetamine salts, lisdexamfetamine. • Immediate release • Extended release	Inattention Hyperactivity Impulsivity	Appetite suppression Mood changes Insomnia Cardiac arrhythmias
2	Norepinephrine noradrenaline reuptake inhibitor	Atomoxetine	Inattention Anxiety	Insomnia Irritability
3	α 2a Agonists	Guanfacine • Immediate release • Extended release	Hyperactivity Impulsivity Insomnia	Dizziness Rebound hypertension, and rebound headaches, if taken inconsistently Cardiac arrhythmias
		Clonidine • Immediate release • Extended release	Hyperactivity Impulsivity Insomnia	Dizziness Rebound hypertension, and rebound headaches, if taken inconsistently Cardiac arrhythmias
4	Antidepressant	Bupropion • Extended release	Inattention Anxiety	Lowered seizure threshold—more commonly seen with immediate-release versions Insomnia Irritability
5	Tricyclic antidepressant[65]	Desipramine Imipramine Nortriptyline	Nonstimulant medication with most evidence for treatment of ADHD	Possible effect on seizure threshold at high doses
6	Selected mood stabilizers	Valproic acid	Impulsivity	Inattention and hyperactivity Raises serum levels of methylphenidate
		Lamotrigine	Attention Behavior	Rash—Stevens-Johnson syndrome Suicidal ideations
		Carbamazepine	Improves attention, alertness, and mood Behavior	Irritability Sedation Toxic epidermal necrolysis Stevens-Johnson syndrome
7	Second-generation antipsychotics	Risperidone	Aggression Impulsivity Irritability	Weight gain, metabolic syndrome, tremors, tardive dyskinesia, hyperprolactinemia
		Aripiprazole	Aggression Impulsivity Irritability	Weight gain, metabolic syndrome, tremors, tardive dyskinesia, akathisia

ADHD, attention deficit hyperactivity disorder.

TABLE 5.4
Studies Involving Methylphenidate and Its Efficacy

Group	Study Type	Study Size	Intervention	Results
Feldman et al.[57]	Double-blind, placebo-controlled crossover study.	Children (N=10; age 6–10 years) with well-controlled epilepsy and ADHD. Patients received a single antiepileptic drug throughout the study.	MPH 0.3 mg/kg per dose given at 8 a.m. and 12 p.m. on school days for 4 weeks.	ADHD symptoms improved. No patient experienced a seizure during the study.
Gross-Tsur et al.[58]	Double-blind, placebo-controlled crossover study.	Children (N=30; age 6–16 years) with seizure disorders and ADHD. Patients received antiepileptic drug for the first 2 months of study.	MPH 0.3 mg/kg was added as a single dose in the morning for the next 2 months.	ADHD symptoms improved. Seizure-free patients did not have any seizures during MPH treatment. 3 of the 5 children with active seizures experienced an increased seizure frequency.
Hemmer et al.[59]	Retrospective study.	Reviewed medical records of nonepileptic children with ADHD.	EEG performed before stimulant treatment (most received MPH 0.3–1.0 mg/kg/day).	Seizures occurred in 2% of the stimulant-treated group (N=205). 3 of the 30 patients with epileptiform EEGs experienced a seizure; 1 of the 175 patients with a normal EEG experienced a seizure.
Gucuyener et al.[60]	12-month cohort study.	Children with ADHD and either epilepsy (N=57) or abnormal EEG but no seizure activity (N=62).	Patients received MPH 0.3–1.0 mg/kg/day; epileptic patients also received antiepilepsy drugs.	ADHD symptoms improved in both groups. No seizures were experienced by patients with abnormal EEGs; seizure frequency unchanged in patients with epilepsy.

ADHD, attention deficit hyperactivity disorder; *EEG*, electroencephalogram; *MPH*, methylphenidate.

liquid (Quillivant) and transdermal (Daytrana) preparations.

Some studies have pointed to an association of MPH precipitating epilepsy in patients with preexisting subclinical epileptiform discharges and causing more seizures in patients with poorly controlled epilepsy to start with.[54] However, Santos et al. demonstrated that use of MPH up to 1 mg/kg/day was safe even in youth with active seizure disorders.[50] In many patients, even if this benefit is just for symptom reduction, it can be useful for families.[55]

In a chart review of a small sample of 36 patients presented by Gonzalez and Heydrich, patients with MPH responded better than patients placed on amphetamine preparation.[13]

Ravi et al. in a review comparing different studies to evaluate effects of MPH on consolidation found that 92% of patients had no increase in seizures from MPH treatment and 71% showed a positive response[13,27,56] (see Table 5.4).

2. **Amphetamines**: These are indicated for monotherapy of ADHD along with MPH preparations. Dextroamphetamine and mixed amphetamine salts are the two most commonly used preparations, used in both immediate- and extended-release forms. Their mechanism of action is similar to that of MPH—binding to norepinephrine and dopamine transporter and preventing reuptake of dopamine and norepinephrine from the synapse.[61] Despite the above similarities, Gonzalez-Heydrich found

that the amphetamine preparations were effective in only 24% of patients with epilepsy and comorbid ADHD versus 63% in MPH preparations.[13]

3. **Atomoxetine**: It is commonly a second-line option for treating ADHD and tried if MPH and amphetamine preparations cannot be used because of side effects or worsened seizure frequency. Its mechanism is a noradrenergic reuptake inhibitor. Michelson et al. found an effect size of 0.7 at about 6 weeks of starting treatment.[62] Atomoxetine has an effect size of 0.7 compared with 0.95 in stimulants and it's seen to reduce about 40% of ADHD core symptoms.[62,63] Commonly, patients with ADHD may also present with some anxiety, and this medication is seen to have a positive effect on both.[6] Torres et al. did not find any increased risk of seizures with atomoxetine.[64] The indications boil down to situations of severe epilepsy, patients with multiple medications, high comorbidity, and multiple failures to stimulants.[64] The treatment response rate with atomoxetine, however remains significantly lower than stimulants.

4. **α2a Agonists—Guanfacine and Clonidine**: These medications have emerged as important monotherapy and adjunct medications for children with ADHD. They work on the α2 adrenoceptors in the prefrontal cortex and basal ganglia. They seem to be less effective than stimulants, especially for the focus and inattention symptoms; however, they may work well as monotherapy and as adjuncts for impulsivity and hyperactivity.[6]

5. **Bupropion extended release**: Bupropion is also used in the treatment of ADHD when the above options have been exhausted. Immediate-release forms, themselves, have been known to lower seizure threshold and cause seizures in about 0.4% of the patients.[65] This side effect is, however, generally seen at high doses of the immediate-release formulation, in patients with eating disorders and in those with a history of seizures.[65] These side effects are generally not found in the extended-release preparations of bupropion because of steady blood levels seen. The immediate-release preparation causes a blood level spike, thus more likely to precipitate seizures.

6. **Mood stabilizers/antiepileptic drugs**: These agents are a common thread between the treatment of epilepsy and mood disorders, impulsivity, and aggression in psychiatry. There are, however, two scenarios for consideration of AEDs for ADHD in the context of epilepsy. First would be clinical presentation with uncontrolled epilepsy, presenting with inattention

and confusion apart from seizures. In some situations, the inattention symptoms are not clearly discernible, and AEDs help with diagnostic clarification also. Adjustment of AED doses or use of appropriate antiseizure medication can significantly improve the ADHD symptoms.

The second situation to consider AEDs is when ADHD symptoms are not amenable to treatment by traditional stimulant or α2a receptor agonist preparations; the next option could be the use of mood stabilizers. Valproic acid can be used to control symptoms of impulsivity in ADHD.[66] Carbamazepine and lamotrigine are known to improve attention and alertness and help with behavioral difficulties.[67] This beneficial effect of lamotrigine was found to be associated with its ability to reduce epileptic discharges.[68] In some cases of straightforward ADHD, mood stabilizers/AEDs could be considered first-line treatments, especially if additional medications outside of the anticonvulsant are not desired by patients or families (see Table 5.5).

7. **Second-generation antipsychotics**: Usage of this class of medicine is uncommon in ADHD. Mechanistically, reduction of dopamine function does not seem to enhance attention. However, this class of medicine has been used in combination to treat severe uncontrolled ADHD, especially when presenting with aggression.

Case Report

The patient AN, is an 11-year-old Caucasian girl who presents to the outpatient child and adolescent psychiatry clinic after having been referred by neurology for difficulties in school. She describes having problems with focus in class, as well as some problems with losing items necessary to complete schoolwork. She is distractible at school and often loses track of planned activities at home. She has difficulties following three-step instructions and sometimes seems to not pay attention when she is spoken to. She has some friends but has a reputation of being "spacy" and as a result has been excluded from peer activities. She has a history of rolandic epilepsy (BECTS) and was reported by the referring neurologist to have seizures every 6–8 weeks, usually occurring at night. She has been stable taking a therapeutic dosage of oxcarbazepine, although the dose has not changed in about 6 months. She has no other relevant medical or psychiatric history.

At this point, a high index of suspicion is present for ADHD—the predominantly inattentive subtype. The epilepsy is mostly stable, at least to the degree where ADHD symptoms seem to occur independent of

TABLE 5.5
Attention and Behavioral Effects of Antiepileptic Drugs

Antiepileptic Drug	Potential Psychiatric Effects
Benzodiazepines	Confusion, disinhibition, cognitive impairment, irritability. Can also improve anxiety.
Carbamazepine[31]	Improves attention, alertness, and mood. Also helps in behavioral difficulties. May cause irritability, sedation.
Lacosamide	Memory impairment, behavioral dysregulation.
Oxcarbazepine	Impaired concentration, somnolence. Possible improvement in impulse control.
Lamotrigine[31]	Improvement in attention and behavior. Possible antidepressant effect and may cause activation.
Phenobarbital[31]	Hyperactivity, poor attention, aggression. Cognitive impairment worsens with higher doses.
Phenytoin[16]	Confusion, cognitive impairment affecting memory, motor, and mental speed. Inattention and hyperactivity.
Gabapentin/pregabalin	Cognitive impairment, behavioral difficulties, poor attention.
Rufinamide	Agitation.
Topiramate[31]	Word-finding difficulty, poor attention, confusion.
Vigabatrin	Agitation, somnolence.
Zonisamide	Irritability, aggression, sedation.
Levetiracetam	Irritability, mood fluctuation.
Valproic acid[16]	Decreases impulsivity. Inattention and hyperactivity. May raise serum levels of methylphenidate.[69]

From Dadson S. Psychiatry & epilepsy: a century of evolving understanding. In: Bautista RED, ed. *Epilepsy: A Century of Discovery*. Nova Science Publisher; 2012:23.

seizure episodes. In that sense, independent treatment of ADHD may reasonably proceed.

AN was diagnosed with provisional ADHD, and rating scales were sent to school to get independent verification of symptoms. Additionally, the neurologist was contacted, and it was determined that a blood test had not been performed for over 6 months. A blood test for oxcarbazepine as well as complete blood count and comprehensive metabolic profile were also ordered, and the patient was instructed to return to the office in 1–2 weeks. Upon return, it was determined that the oxcarbazepine level was therapeutic and that teacher ratings for ADHD symptoms were confirmatory. Extended-release MPH was cautiously begun at the lowest possible dose and titrated up over the next few weeks. AN was described to have an excellent response and continued follow-up with the child psychiatrist every 2 months.

Key points of this history include establishing seizure frequency, assessing the therapeutic level of the anticonvulsant drug, and seeking corroborating information to verify the diagnosis. If the anticonvulsant blood level was low, it may have been preferable to first increase the anticonvulsant dosage before considering treatment with stimulant medication. Additionally, if the symptoms could not be verified by teacher ratings, then referral to neuropsychology for comprehensive assessment may have been preferable, as there could be learning disabilities or problems with executive function that existed beyond ADHD. Finally, seizure frequency and monitoring need to be the job of the child psychiatrist and the neurologist. If seizures have occurred recently, then assessment of the utility of stimulant medication is more nuanced.

DISCLOSURE STATEMENT

Dr Mishra has no relevant financial disclosures. Dr Salpekar receives research funding from Lundbeck for an investigator-initiated clinical trial.

REFERENCES

1. Parisi P, et al. Attention deficit hyperactivity disorder in children with epilepsy. *Brain Dev.* 2010;32(1):10–16.
2. CDC. *Attention-Deficit/Hyperactivity Disorder (ADHD)*; 2017. [Data & Statistics: Children with ADHD] https://www.cdc.gov/ncbddd/adhd/data.html-ref1.
3. American Psychiatric Association, DSM-5 Task Force. Diagnostic and Statistical Manual of Mental Disorders: DSM-5. 5th ed. vol. xliv. Washington, D.C.: American Psychiatric Association; 2013. 947 pp.
4. Dunn DW, Kronenberger WG. Childhood epilepsy, attention problems, and ADHD: review and practical considerations. *Semin Pediatr Neurol.* 2005;12(4):222–228.
5. Salpekar JA, Mishra G. Key issues in addressing the co-morbidity of attention deficit hyperactivity disorder and pediatric epilepsy. *Epilepsy Behav.* 2014;37:310–315.
6. Williams AE, Giust JM, Kronenberger WG, Dunn DW. Epilepsy and attention-deficit hyperactivity disorder: links, risks, and challenges. *Neuropsychiatr Dis Treat.* 2016;12: 287–296.
7. Willcutt EG, et al. Validity of the executive function theory of attention-deficit/hyperactivity disorder: a meta-analytic review. *Biol Psychiatry.* 2005;57(11):1336–1346.
8. Epilepsy fast facts | epilepsy | CDC. *Epilepsy.* 2017. Available from: https://www.cdc.gov/epilepsy/basics/fast-facts.htm.
9. Fisher RS, et al. ILAE official report: a practical clinical definition of epilepsy. *Epilepsia.* 2014;55(4):475–482.
10. Russ SA, Larson K, Halfon N. A national profile of childhood epilepsy and seizure disorder. *Pediatrics.* 2012;129(2):256–264.
11. Reilly C, Atkinson P, Das KB, et al. Neurobehavioral co-morbidities in children with active epilepsy: a population-based study. *Pediatrics.* 2014;133(6):e1586–e1593.
12. Dunn DW, Austin JK, Harezlak J, Ambrosius WT, et al. ADHD and epilepsy in childhood. *Dev Med Child Neurol.* 2003;45(1):50–54.
13. Gonzalez-Heydrich J, Hsin O, Gumlak S, et al. Comparing stimulant effects in youth with ADHD symptoms and epilepsy. *Epilepsy Behav.* 2014;36:102–107.
14. Ekinci O, Okuyaz C, Gunes S, et al. Understanding sleep problems in children with epilepsy: associations with quality of life, Attention-Deficit Hyperactivity Disorder and maternal emotional symptoms. *Seizure.* 2016;40: 108–113.
15. McCusker CG, et al. Adjustment in children with intractable epilepsy: importance of seizure duration and family factors. *Dev Med Child Neurol.* 2002;44(10):681–687.
16. Kwan P, Brodie MJ. Neuropsychological effects of epilepsy and antiepileptic drugs. *Lancet.* 2001;357(9251):216–222.
17. Austin JK, Harezlak J, Dunn DW, Huster GA, Rose DA, Ambrosius WT. Behavior problems in children before first recognized seizures. *Pediatrics.* 2001;107(1):115–122.
18. Ott D, et al. Measures of psychopathology in children with complex partial seizures and primary generalized epilepsy with absence. *J Am Acad Child Adolesc Psychiatry.* 2001;40(8):907–914.
19. Richer LP, Shevell MI, Rosenblatt BR. Epileptiform abnormalities in children with attention-deficit-hyperactivity disorder. *Pediatr Neurol.* 2002;26(2):125–129.
20. Socanski D, Herigstad A, Thomsen PH, Dag A, Larsen TK. Epileptiform abnormalities in children diagnosed with attention deficit/hyperactivity disorder. *Epilepsy Behav.* 2010;19(3):483–486.
21. Socanski D, Aurlien D, Herigstad A, Thomsen PH, Larsen TK. Epilepsy in a large cohort of children diagnosed with attention deficit/hyperactivity disorders (ADHD). *Seizure.* 2013;22(8):651–655.
22. Socanski D, Aurlien D, Herigstad A, Thomsen PH, Larsen TK. Attention deficit/hyperactivity disorder and interictal epileptiform discharges: it is safe to use methylphenidate? *Seizure.* 2015;25:80–83.
23. Zhang DQ, Li FH, Zhu XB, Sun RP. Clinical observations on attention-deficit hyperactivity disorder (ADHD) in children with frontal lobe epilepsy. *J Child Neurol.* 2014;29(1):54–57.
24. Davis SM, Katusic SK, Barbaresi WJ, et al. Epilepsy in children with attention-deficit/hyperactivity disorder. *Pediatr Neurol.* 2010;42(5):325–330.
25. Hesdorffer DC, Ludvigsson P, Olafsson E, Gudmundsson G, Kjartansson O, Hauser WA. ADHD as a risk factor for incident unprovoked seizures and epilepsy in children. *Arch Gen Psychiatry.* 2004;61(7):731–736.
26. Marston D, et al. Effects of transitory cognitive impairment on psychosocial functioning of children with epilepsy: a therapeutic trial. *Dev Med Child Neurol.* 1993;35(7):574–581.
27. Kaufmann R, Goldberg-Stern H, Shuper A. Attention-deficit disorders and epilepsy in childhood: incidence, causative relations and treatment possibilities. *J Child Neurol.* 2009;24(6):727–733.
28. Castellanos FX, et al. Developmental trajectories of brain volume abnormalities in children and adolescents with attention-deficit/hyperactivity disorder. *JAMA.* 2002;288(14):1740–1748.
29. Zametkin AJ, Rapoport JL. Psychopharmacology: the third generation of progress. In: Meltzer HY, ed. New York: Raven Press; 1987.
30. Schwab RS. A case of status epilepticus in petit mal. *Electroencephalogr Clin Neurophysiol.* 1953;5(3):441–442.
31. Schubert R. Attention deficit disorder and epilepsy. *Pediatr Neurol.* 2005;32(1):1–10.
32. Besag F, Caplan R, Sillanpää M, Aldenkamp A, Dunn DW. Psychiatric and behavioural disorders in children with epilepsy (ILAE task force report): epilepsy and ADHD. *Epileptic Disord.* 2016. https://doi.org/10.1684/epd.2016.0811.
33. Holtmann M, Becker K, Kentner-Figura B, Schmidt MH. Increased frequency of rolandic spikes in ADHD children. *Epilepsia.* 2003;44(9):1241–1244.
34. Wolraich ML, Bard DE, Neas B, Doffing M, Beck L. The psychometric properties of the Vanderbilt attention-deficit hyperactivity disorder diagnostic teacher rating scale in a community population. *J Dev Behav Pediatr.* 2013;34(2):83–93.

35. Brown MG, Becker DA, Pollard JR, Anderson CT. The diagnosis and treatment of attention deficit hyperactivity disorder in patients with epilepsy. *Curr Neurol Neurosci Rep.* 2013;13(6):351.

36. Nolan MA, et al. Memory function in childhood epilepsy syndromes. *J Paediatr Child Health.* 2004;40(1–2):20–27.

37. Barnes GN, Paolicchi JM. Neuropsychiatric comorbidities in childhood absence epilepsy. *Nat Clin Pract Neurol.* 2008;4(12):650–651.

38. Caplan R, Siddharth P, Stahl L, et al. Childhood absence epilepsy: behavioral, cognitive, and linguistic comorbidities. *Epilepsia.* 2008;49(11):1838–1846.

39. Delgado-Escueta AV, Swartz BE, Walsh GO, Chauvel P, Bancaud J, Broglin D. Frontal lobe seizures and epilepsies in neurobehavioral disorders. *Adv Neurol.* 1991;55:317–340.

40. Hermann B, Jones J, Dabbs K. The frequency, complications and aetiology of ADHD in new onset paediatric epilepsy. *Brain.* 2007;130(Pt 12):3135–3148.

41. Kanazawa O. Reappraisal of abnormal EEG findings in children with ADHD: on the relationship between ADHD and epileptiform discharges. *Epilepsy Behav.* 2014;41:251–256.

42. Stores G. Electroencephalographic parameters in assessing the cognitive function of children with epilepsy. *Epilepsia.* 1990;31(suppl 4):S45–S49.

43. Foldvary N. Sleep and epilepsy. *Curr Treat Options Neurol.* 2002;4(2):129–135.

44. Ryvlin P, Rheims S, Risse G. Nocturnal frontal lobe epilepsy. *Epilepsia.* 2006;47(suppl 2):83–86.

45. Kiriakopoulos E, Shafer PO. *Absence Seizures;* 2017. http://www.epilepsy.com/learn/types-seizures/absence-seizures.

46. Holmes GL. *Landau-Kleffner Syndrome;* 2013. http://www.epilepsy.com/learn/types-epilepsy-syndromes/landau-kleffner-syndrome.

47. Hernandez AW. *Generalized Tonic-Clonic Seizures;* 2016. http://www.epilepsy.com/learn/types-epilepsy-syndromes/epilepsy-generalized-tonic-clonic-seizures-alone.

48. Volkl-Kernstock S, Bauch-Prater S, Ponocny-Seliger E, Feucht M. Speech and school performance in children with benign partial epilepsy with centro-temporal spikes (BCECTS). *Seizure.* 2009;18(5):320–326.

49. Appleton DR. *Electrical Status Epilepticus During Slow-Wave Sleep (ESESS);* 2017. https://www.epilepsy.org.uk/info/syndromes/electrical-status-epilepticus-during-slow-wave-sleep-esess.

50. Santos K, Palmini A, Radziuk AL, et al. The impact of methylphenidate on seizure frequency and severity in children with attention-deficit-hyperactivity disorder and difficult-to-treat epilepsies. *Dev Med Child Neurol.* 2013;55(7):654–660.

51. Greenhill LL, Pliszka S, Dulcan MK, et al. Practice parameter for the use of stimulant medications in the treatment of children, adolescents, and adults. *J Am Acad Child Adolesc Psychiatry.* 2002;41(2 suppl):26S–49S.

52. Volkow ND, Fowler JS, Wang G, Ding Y, Gatley SJ. Mechanism of action of methylphenidate: insights from PET imaging studies. *J Atten Disord.* 2002;6(suppl 1):S31–S43.

53. PDR, T. *Physician's Desk Reference.* 7th ed; 2007. Montvale, NJ.

54. Torres AR, Whitney J, Gonzalez-Heydrich J. Attention-deficit/hyperactivity disorder in pediatric patients with epilepsy: review of pharmacological treatment. *Epilepsy Behav.* 2008;12(2):217–233.

55. Shalev R. Good news: methylphenidate for ADHD in epilepsy. *Dev Med Child Neurol.* 2013;55(7):590–591.

56. Ravi M, Ickowicz A. Epilepsy, attention-deficit/hyperactivity disorder and methylphenidate: critical examination of guiding evidence. *J Can Acad Child Adolesc Psychiatry.* 2016;25(1):50–58.

57. Feldman H, Crumrine P, Handen BL, Alvin R, Teodori J. Methylphenidate in children with seizures and attention-deficit disorder. *Am J Dis Child.* 1989;143(9):1081–1086.

58. Gross-Tsur V, Manor O, van der Meere J, Joseph A, Shalev RS. Epilepsy and attention deficit hyperactivity disorder: is methylphenidate safe and effective? *J Pediatr.* 1997;130(4):670–674.

59. Hemmer SA, Pasternak JF, Zecker SG, Trommer BL. Stimulant therapy and seizure risk in children with ADHD. *Pediatr Neurol.* 2001;24(2):99–102.

60. Gucuyener K, Erdemoglu AK, Senol S, Serdaroglu A, Soysal S, Kockar AI. Use of methylphenidate for attention-deficit hyperactivity disorder in patients with epilepsy or electroencephalographic abnormalities. *J Child Neurol.* 2003;18(2):109–112.

61. Kuczenski R, Segal DS. Effects of methylphenidate on extracellular dopamine, serotonin, and norepinephrine: comparison with amphetamine. *J Neurochem.* 1997;68(5):2032–2037.

62. Michelson D, Allen AJ, Busner J, et al. Once-daily atomoxetine treatment for children and adolescents with attention deficit hyperactivity disorder: a randomized, placebo-controlled study. *Am J Psychiatry.* 2002;159(11):1896–1901.

63. Faraone SV, Biederman J, Spencer TJ, Aleardi M. Comparing the efficacy of medications for ADHD using meta-analysis. *MedGenMed.* 2006;8(4):4.

64. Torres A, Whitney J, Rao S, Tilley C, Lobel R, Gonzalez-Heydrich J. Tolerability of atomoxetine for treatment of pediatric attention-deficit/hyperactivity disorder in the context of epilepsy. *Epilepsy Behav.* 2011;20(1):95–102.

65. Budur K, Mathews M, Adetunji B, Mathews M, Mahmud J. Non-stimulant treatment for attention deficit hyperactivity disorder. *Psychiatry (Edgmont).* 2005;2(7):44–48.

66. Golden AS, Haut SR, Moshe SL. Nonepileptic uses of antiepileptic drugs in children and adolescents. *Pediatr Neurol.* 2006;34(6):421–432.

67. Dadson S. Psychiatry & epilepsy: a century of evolving understanding. In: Bautista RED, ed. *Epilepsy. A Century of Disocvery.* Nova Science Publisher; 2012:23.

68. Pressler RM, Robinson RO, Wilson GA, Binnie CD. Treatment of interictal epileptiform discharges can improve behavior in children with behavioral problems and epilepsy. *J Pediatr.* 2005;146(1):112–117.

69. Gara L, Roberts W. Adverse response to methylphenidate in combination with valproic acid. *J Child Adolesc Psychopharmacol.* 2000;10(1):39–43.

CHAPTER 6

Evolution From Feeding Disorders to Avoidant/Restrictive Food Intake Disorder

IRENE CHATOOR, MD • REBECCA BEGTRUP, DO, MPH

INTRODUCTION

Eating disorders in young children and infants are generally referred to as "feeding disorders," to emphasize the relationship between caregiver and child that may be strained or dysregulated in these conditions. This term includes a variety of conditions ranging from food refusal and disinterest to food aversions, overeating, undereating, fear of eating, pica (or the eating of nonfood substances), and rumination. Approximately 20%–30% of infants and young children have been perceived to have feeding problems that encompass a broad range, from mild (so-called picky eating) to severe as may be seen in autism.[1] One difficulty in pinpointing the incidence and prevalence of these disorders lies in their naming and categorization. The definitions and diagnostic classifications of feeding disorders have varied greatly among clinicians. However, identifying feeding disorders in infants and young children is critical because the disorders adversely affect the entire family, not just the individual. In addition, if left untreated, these disorders can persist into adolescence and adulthood.

DEFINITIONS OF FEEDING DISORDERS

There has been much controversy over the appropriate categorization of Feeding Disorders of Infancy and Early Childhood. DSM-IV-TR[2] criteria were too restrictive, leading to many young children going undiagnosed and untreated. For these reasons, alternative classifications have been used to increase the specificity of the DSM-IV-TR diagnosis, most notably the "Feeding Behavior Disorder" section in DC: 0-3R (2005),[3] which defined six different feeding disorders based on the classifications by Chatoor.[4] The *DSM-5*[5] then grouped these feeding disorder subtypes under one heading, "Avoidant/Restrictive Food Intake Disorder" (ARFID). Of note, the ARFID diagnostic criteria can be applied to individuals of all ages, which is key as this psychopathology can persist from childhood and early infancy into adolescence and even adulthood, as previously mentioned.

The *DSM-5* describes three main types of ARFID: those with an apparent lack of interest in food and eating, those with sensory aversions to specific food characteristics, and those with a conditioned negative association and fear of eating due to or in anticipation of an aversive experience. These DSM-5 varieties are also described in DC: 0-3R (2005). The DSM-5 ARFID subtype, "apparent lack of interest in food or eating" is described in DC: 0-3R as "Infantile Anorexia"; the DSM-5's "avoidance based on the sensory characteristics of food" is described in DC: 0-3R as "Sensory Food Aversions"; the DSM-5's "concern about aversive consequences of eating" is described in DC: 0-3R as "Feeding Disorder Associated with Insults to the Gastrointestinal Tract" and was termed "Posttraumatic Feeding Disorder" by Chatoor in 2002.

The DSM-5 classification also allows for the diagnosis of the three remaining DC: 0-3R Feeding Disorder subtypes, including those of state regulation, those of caregiver-infant reciprocity, and those associated with concurrent medical condition. The *DSM-5* differentiates ARFID from more common feeding difficulties by requiring at least one of the following: (1) significant weight loss (or failure to achieve expected weight gain or faltering growth in children), (2) significant nutritional deficiency, (3) dependence on enteral feeding or oral nutritional supplements, and (4) marked interference with psychosocial functioning.

HISTORY AND COMPARATIVE NOSOLOGY

Previously, there was much confusion over the criteria for the diagnosis of feeding disorders in infants and young children. There were no recognized standards resulting in naming and criteria variability among clinicians, researchers, and authors. Some of the terminology utilized in the past included: "picky," "choosy," "selective," or "problem" eaters, food "refusal," "selectivity," or "aversion," and dysphagia.[1] With the inclusion of "Feeding Disorders of Infancy or Early Childhood" in *DSM-IV* in 1994, the classification of feeding disorders began to clarify.

To further complicate issues, the terms "feeding disorder" and "failure to thrive" (FTT) have been used interchangeably for several years. FTT refers to weight gain that is inadequate based on standardized growth charts. It generally is broken down into organic and nonorganic causes. Organic causes are due to a diagnosable medical condition, such as heart disease, milk allergy, reflux, cerebral palsy, Down syndrome, and metabolic disorders. Nonorganic causes of FTT have historically been blamed on maternal deprivation or neglect. While these causes certainly can cause FTT, there are several other nonorganic causes of FTT that have since been recognized. The last category of FTT (which was added later) is due to a combination of organic and nonorganic contributing factors. The use of the term FTT as an overarching diagnosis for all patients with feeding disorders is misleading, as not all patients with feeding disorders have FTT and vice versa. In addition, the term "failure to thrive" does not describe the underlying feeding disturbance, but rather indicates the symptomatology only. Despite the agreement among many clinicians, researchers, and authors that FTT should be used to describe symptoms only, rather than used as a diagnostic term, "failure to thrive" persists as a diagnosis in both the psychologic and pediatric literature.

Given the limitations of the DSM-IV diagnostic criteria for Feeding Disorders of Infancy or Early Childhood, DC: 0-3R diagnostic criteria served as a template for the updated DSM-5 classification, ARFID. This classification system was initially published by Chatoor in 2002 and then modified in 2003 by the Task Force for Research Diagnostic Criteria for Infants and Preschool Children.[6] The six Feeding Disorder subtypes were then published in the 2005 DC: 0-3R. In addition, an American Psychiatric Association supported work group further revised the criteria that were then published in "Age and Gender Considerations in Psychiatric Diagnosis" in 2007.[7]

The six subtypes include (1) feeding disorder of state regulation, (2) feeding disorder of caregiver-infant reciprocity, (3) **infantile anorexia**, (4) **sensory food aversions**, (5) feeding disorder associated with a concurrent medical condition, and (6) **feeding disorder associated with insults to the gastrointestinal**

tract. Numbers 1 through 4 have onset at specific times in a child's development (arranged chronologically), whereas the last two may have onset at any time. Those in bold will be discussed in further detail in this chapter. For the sake of clarity, these subtypes will be described using both the DSM-5[5] and DC: 0-3R[3] classifications.

SPECIFIC FEEDING DISORDERS SUBTYPES OF AVOIDANT/RESTRICTIVE FOOD INTAKE DISORDER (DSM-5)

I. ARFID Subtype: "Apparent Lack of Interest in Eating or Food" (DSM-5)

Infantile Anorexia (DC: 0-3R)

DC: 0-3R criteria: Requires all six of the following:

1. The infant/young child refuses to eat adequate amounts of food for at least 1 month.
2. Onset of the food refusal occurs before 3 years of age.
3. The infant/young child does not communicate hunger cues or lacks interest in food but shows strong interest in exploration, interaction with caregiver, or both.
4. The child demonstrates significant growth deficiency.
5. Food refusal does not follow a traumatic event.
6. Food refusal is not due to an underlying medical condition.

Clinical features

Infantile anorexia (IA) is characterized by poor appetite, lack of interest in eating, and poor growth in an otherwise active and engaged child. Chatoor first described this clinical picture in the 1980s after treating malnourished patients, following their medical hospitalization, who had been diagnosed with FTT nonorganic type with the assumption of maternal neglect, despite having fully engaged mothers who were desperate to get their children to eat and gain weight. IA was later described as a subtype of Feeding Behavior Disorder in DC: 0-3R (2005). Onset of IA is usually within the first 3 years of life, most commonly between ages 9 and 18 months. This is the time when infants are becoming more physically independent, learning to talk and walk, and beginning the transition to spoon and self-feeding. These children tend to be quite active and engageable. They are often interested in everything but eating, which may appear to bore them. They are resistant to stopping their activities to be placed in their high chairs and often refuse to even open their mouths to be fed, many times throwing their food and utensils. Parents of these infants and young children become worried by the poor food intake and growth. They try a variety of things in an attempt to coax the children into eating, including distraction, bribes, feeding on the go (i.e., offering bites of food while the child is playing, running by, or otherwise engaged in noneating activities), and sometimes even resorting to force feeding. These parents become fixated on getting food into their children, feeling that every calorie counts. This raises the tension between the child and parent, which increases the distress for all parties and often results in making meal times almost unbearable for the entire family.

Risk factors

Chatoor and Lucarelli et al. independently identified risk factors for the development of IA. These include both risk factors related to the infant or young child (i.e., the identified patient) and those related to the primary caregiver (generally the patient's mother). Difficult temperament in the infant may result in irregular sleeping and feeding patterns, high physiologic arousal and poor regulation, and intense stress responses, such as severe temper tantrums.[8,9] The risk factors related to the mother's psychopathology include an insecure or disorganized attachment style, maternal eating disorder, and maternal depression and/or anxiety.[10,11] In addition, both overly controlling and overly permissive parenting styles are also risk factors for the development of IA. The transactional model of feeding disorders demonstrates the negatively reinforcing interactions between the child who is refusing food and the caregiver who becomes distressed by this food refusal and therefore attempts to become more controlling of the child's food intake, which further results in the child's refusal to eat, thereby further increasing the caregiver's anxiety and distress, etc.

Differential diagnosis

IA must be differentiated from other feeding disorders that result in food refusal. The ARFID subtype "concern about aversive consequences" generally has a more sudden onset and follows a traumatic event to the gastrointestinal tract or oropharynx. Such traumas may result from choking, gagging or severe vomiting, or placement of endotracheal or nasogastric tubes. Depending on the type of traumatic experience, these children may refuse all foods, only solids, or only liquids/the bottle. The ARFID subtype "avoidance based on the sensory characteristics of food" results in children refusing specific foods, but eating well when offered foods they prefer.

Etiology and course

Toddlers with IA tend to have higher levels of physiologic arousal, including more difficulty downregulating their arousal.[8,9] They enjoy talking and stay very

engaged in play. They struggle with ending their play when it is time to eat and often have little to no awareness of their hunger cues. Various studies have demonstrated a strong correlation between difficult child temperament, irregular sleeping and feeding patterns, negative/willful behaviors, and mother-child conflict during feeding time.[12] This conflict is also significantly correlated with mother's insecure attachment to her own parents, drive for thinness, bulimia, anxiety, and depression. The conflict between the mother and child during eating was inversely correlated to the child's weight; the higher the conflict, the lower the child's weight.[10-12] However, these correlations should be used with caution in explaining the etiology of these feeding disorders. The lack of interest in eating and lack of appetite in these children tend to lead to increased anxiety and feelings of helplessness in their parents. The parents attempt to engage the children in eating by bribing, distracting, etc. When this does not result in increased food intake by the child, it results in increased anxiety in the parents, which allows the child to gain more control over this tension-filled power struggle. This leads to the parents feeling even more helpless, which allows the child to execute even more control over the feeding situation and results in the parents feeling even less effective, as they are unable to set appropriate limits during mealtimes. This is a trap of maladaptive engagement patterns.

Research[13] demonstrated that toddlers with IA had normal cognitive development, on average. The Mental Developmental Index (MDI) score for the control group of healthy eaters was 11 points higher than that of the group with IA though. On further examination, it was revealed that the mother-child interactions related to feeding and play, not the child's weight, were the main contributing factor involved in the differences of MDI scores. The toddlers with lower scores on cognitive performance demonstrated more conflict in the mother-child relationship, particularly with regard to control, and also showed more significant intrusiveness by the mothers during their play interactions.

Lucarelli and colleagues conducted a natural course longitudinal study of children with IA,[14] from 2 to 11 years of age. These children had received minimal interventions at the time of diagnosis and no further treatment. At 11 years of age, approximately 70% of these children demonstrated various degrees of malnutrition, ranging from mild to severe, and higher scores, compared with the control group, on screens for anxiety, moodiness, aggressiveness, and somatic complaints. Correlations were also noted between continuing maternal eating and psychopathology, particularly depression and anxiety, and internalizing problems in the children. This study points to the seriousness of this feeding disorder and the importance of early diagnosis and intervention in this patient population.

In a treatment follow-up study of 20 children who were between ages 6 months and 2 years at the time of diagnosis with IA,[15] 17 of the participants (85%) made significant progress in their recovery. There was resolution of the parent-child conflict over eating. In addition, the children had learned to recognize their hunger cues, improved their food intake, and improved their growth. Even so, these children continued to lose their appetites when excited or overstimulated. However, once emotionally reregulated, their appetites returned and they generally made up for the missed meals. The three who did not do as well as others had continued struggles with their parents with regard to eating. In all three cases, the environments during mealtimes, either at home or at the children's day care centers, were too stimulating or disorganized to allow these children to relax enough to experience their appropriate hunger cues. This overstimulation decreased their appetites and reinforced the disinterest in eating, leading to a continuation of food refusal.

Another follow-up study of children treated for IA,[16] in which parents helped their children learn internal regulation of eating, demonstrated a decrease in mother-toddler conflict, a decrease in the struggle for control during feeding, an improvement in the children's growth, and a decrease in maternal isolation and depression. Because feeding one's children is such a significant part of the family culture in most societies, any difficulty in this arena can reflect negatively on the parents, particularly the mother, whom society has deemed the primary caregiver. Many societies equate food with love. A well-fed child is considered a well cared for and loved child, whereas a child who is underweight is considered neglected by his/her parents. While this may be the case at times, and certainly was believed to be the underlying cause of nonorganic FTT for many years, it is simply not true that the parents (including the mothers) of children with IA are neglectful of their children. In fact, many times these mothers are desperate to get their children to eat, as was the case for the patients in whom Dr. Chatoor first identified the illness. However, these societal pressures frequently result in depression and isolation of the children's mothers. It can be difficult to explain that one's child simply does not want to eat, particularly when other mothers appear to have an easier time nourishing their children. In fact, many mothers of children with IA note that in trying to discuss their child's feeding difficulties with other mothers

who have not experienced such difficulties, the other mothers tend to dismiss their concerns, stating that the child must simply not be hungry at this time or that the child will grow out of it. Just as IA affects the mental health and well-being of the entire family due to the conflict it creates around eating, something that must be done multiple times a day, so too can the treatment benefit the entire family, relieving the pressure, isolation, anxiety, and depressed mood from the child's caregivers.

Chatoor's 5- to 10-year follow-up study of children with IA[16] demonstrated no correlation between the children's IQ scores at the time of follow-up and their percentage of ideal body weight at the time of diagnosis, suggesting that the malnutrition, which led to low weight at the time of diagnosis, did not adversely affect their cognitive abilities later on. When looking at eating behaviors stratified by good or poor growth at the time of follow-up (good growth >−2.5 z on height and weight; poor growth ≤−2.5 z on height and weight), it is notable that nearly all participants in the control group of healthy eaters (93%) and most of those in the IA better growth group (75%) completed most of their lunches at school, whereas only 40% of those in the IA poor growth group completed most of their lunches at school. A similar pattern emerged for family dinners. Whereas most of the families of the control children, and those who were doing well, had regular family dinners, only 50% of the children in the poor weight group reported to have regular family dinners. In addition, although both height and weight were correlated at the time of follow-up with whether the child ate lunch at school and whether the family ate dinners together, the family dinners had a significantly greater impact on both height and weight than did the child's completion of lunch at school. There were also statistically significant differences between the two groups with IA diagnoses, good growth and poor growth, regarding food-related behaviors. The enjoyment of food was lower in the poor growth group, and slowness in eating, emotional undereating, and food fussiness were all more pronounced in the poor growth group. Early satiety was also greater in the poor growth group. This group of children also demonstrated a propensity toward talking instead of eating during meal times, forgetting to eat, playing instead of eating, resistance to sit at the table, and a tendency to leave the table when they did not want to eat. Of note, the children with IA did not show any increased signs of anorexia nervosa or bulimia nervosa.

Clinically, it appears that the earlier a child with IA presents for treatment, the shorter the recovery course.

Children who do not present for evaluation and treatment of IA until they are older tend to be small for their age, both in weight and height. Their head circumferences and intellectual abilities generally appear normal for their ages though. In Chatoor's follow-up study of children treated for IA as toddlers,[16] two-thirds outgrew the feeding disorder, whereas one-third did not. There was no correlation between their weights (at the time of diagnosis or at the time of follow-up) and their intellectual functioning. In fact, one-third of these children functioned in the superior range.

IA often runs in families, so it is important to ask parents of children with suspected IA about their own eating behaviors, as well as those of their immediate family members. The questions should include investigation into both current and childhood eating behaviors. Adults with IA demonstrate similar signs and symptoms as those that present in the infants and young children; however, the adults are more likely to be aware of the need to eat to maintain their health. For example, these adults are just as likely as the children with IA to lose their hunger cues when physiologically aroused, such as when they are feeling overly stressed or anxious. They also forget to eat when they are distracted by more interesting matters and may be very chatty at mealtimes. However, owing to their improved awareness of societal expectations, these individuals will often push themselves to make time for meals, particularly when eating in a social setting, such as a meal with friends or colleagues.

Treatment

The treatment for IA is based on the transactional model mentioned previously. Understanding how the child's difficult temperament interacts with the caregiver's insecurities in parenting techniques and anxieties, which results in conflict over control and autonomy, is key to the treatment of this feeding disorder. The goal of the treatment is to assist the parent in changing his/her behaviors, which then results in changes in the child's behaviors and facilitates the development of internal regulation of eating according to hunger and fullness cues in the child.

The treatment begins with discussion of the child's temperament with his/her parents. It is important to help parents understand that their child experiences an increased level of arousal, which supports the child's intense curiosity and emotionality, but which interferes with his/her hunger cues, making the child less aware of hunger. These children often have learned that refusing to eat is a powerful way to gain their parents' attention, which frequently results

in the parents working to entertain and distract the strong-willing infant. As the parent works to coerce the child into eating, the child becomes more physiologically aroused and is less able to recognize his/her hunger. Unfortunately, these efforts on the part of the parents only serve to reinforce these negative patterns of interaction and struggles for control between the parent and child. These children have not only an increased level of arousal, but they also have difficulty down-regulating, which is necessary for them to relax, to eat, and to go to sleep. This explains why they often not only have difficulty eating but also struggle with going to sleep and calming themselves when upset. As one father aptly put, "The turn off button is not working." However, on a positive note, these children are often great learners and exceptionally bright. The challenge is to help them learn to self-regulate so that they can feel their hunger cues and can go to sleep in the evening.

The next step is to explore the parents' reticence in limit setting. Perhaps the parents have lost prior pregnancies, struggled with infertility, or experienced harsh discipline during their own childhoods, which causes them to be more lenient in their own parenting style. Whatever the dynamic, this issue must be explored first, before the parents can be helped to work on setting appropriate limits with their own children.

Once this groundwork has been laid, the work can begin to change the behaviors in the parents and child and to facilitate the development of internal regulation of hunger and fullness in the child. The following **feeding guidelines**[17] are explained:

1. Feed your child at regular times, spacing meals and snack approximately 3–4 h apart. Your child should have no food or drinks outside these set meal/snack times, aside from water if thirsty. This allows your child to experience physiologic hunger at mealtimes and prevents him/her from filling up in-between meals due to snacking.

2. Eat all meals and snacks in the kitchen or dining room, rather than in front of the TV or while the child is playing. This minimizes distractions and allows your child to focus on his/her hunger and fullness cues.

3. Offer your child small portions and allow him/her to have more until he/she is full and does not want to eat anymore. This will help engage your child in the feeding process and prevent him/her from becoming bored or overwhelmed by large amounts of food. It will also allow your child to learn to eat until sated.

4. Occasionally offer your child "special foods" along with the meal. These items may include desserts, candies, or "junk" foods. Allow your child to eat these items first, if desired. This will help to remove the special value of these foods. Some parents find it helpful to have 2 or 3 designated "dessert days" every week. This will prevent the child from asking for a dessert at each meal.

5. Do not praise of criticize your child based on the amount that he/she eats. Eating is not meant to be a performance. Rather, your child should learn to regulate his/her intake based on hunger and fullness cues. Instead of praising the amount of food consumed, you can praise your child's feeding skills. That is, rather than saying, "Wow! You ate so much!," try saying, "Wow! You got the spoon to your mouth all by yourself!"

6. Do not use food as a reward, special gift, expression of your affection, or a way to calm your child. Do not restrict food intake or withhold food as a threat or punishment for your child. This will keep your child from learning to eat due to emotional reasons.

7. Teach your child to sit at the table until "Mommy's and Daddy's tummies are full," rather than leaving when he/she is "done." If one is disinterested in eating, one can be "done" with a meal even before it begins. However, keeping the child at the table until the parents' are sated allows the child to recognize his/her own hunger and to reengage in the meal.

8. The meal should last only 20–30 min, regardless of how much or little the child has eaten. The child will learn to make up for the lacking intake at the next meal.

9. Discourage your child from playing with the food or talking excessively at the meal. Instead, set a special time for playing and talking with your child after the meal is completed.

10. If your child gets up from his/her chair, throws food or utensils, or is otherwise misbehaving, give one warning. If the behavior does not resolve, administer a "time-out." The "time-out" procedure should not be viewed as a punishment. It has two main goals: to help the child stop the behaviors that interfere with eating and to help the child learn self-calming when upset or not getting his/her way.

In addition to providing the parents with the feeding guidelines, it is also important to help them with limit setting and teach them a time-out procedure that emphasizes helping the child to accept limits and learn self-calming when they cannot have their way. Teaching parents the feeding guidelines and the "time-out" procedure is best done in two sessions lasting approximately 2 h each. These intense therapeutic sessions assist in promoting trust between the parents and therapist. This trust can go a long way in allowing the parents to make behavioral changes that they were otherwise disinclined to make. These shifts in interactional patterns between parents and young children often require only a few sessions (more if the children are older when they start treatment). However, some maladaptive parent-child interaction patterns are more deeply engrained than others and therefore may require longer treatment. In addition, some patients may present with severe malnourishment, requiring more intensive therapeutic intervention or even hospitalization. Given the dyadic nature of IA with conflicts over control and autonomy, dysregulated eating in both caregivers and children, the difficult temperament of the children, and the frequent anxiety in the caregivers, it is paramount that the treatment focus both on the child and the caregivers. Referring to the feeding guidelines and regular family meals, the parents are given the message that "what is good for the child is also good for the parents."

II. ARFID Subtype: Avoidance Based on the Sensory Characteristics of Food (DSM-5)

Sensory Food Aversions (DC: 0-3R)

DC: 0-3R criteria: Requires all four of the following:

1. The child consistently refuses to eat specific foods with specific tastes, textures, and/or smells.
2. Onset of the food refusal occurs during the introduction of a novel type of food.
3. The child eats without difficulty when offered preferred foods.
4. The food refusal causes specific nutritional deficiencies or delay of oral motor development.

Clinical features

Sensory food aversions (SFAs) are common. Some children refuse to eat a few select foods, whereas others will refuse most foods, only accepting a few select foods. The onset of this feeding disorder occurs when a new food or foods are introduced. For example, an infant with SFA may nurse and take breast milk in a bottle fine but may balk when offered formula. Or they may do well with both formula and breast milk, but reject solid foods of certain textures, tastes, or temperatures. Some children will become so selective that they will only eat one or two brands of a particular type of food. They will reject the same type of food made by another company, even if it is disguised in the container from their preferred brand. Many toddlers and young children can be "picky" when it comes to their dietary preferences, so the diagnosis of SFA should only be made if the food selectivity is so severe that it leads to nutritional deficiencies, oral motor or speech delays, and/or social anxiety surrounding eating, which causes interference in psychosocial functioning in older children. The oral motor and speech delays can occur because these children are not engaging their oral muscles in chewing, as they otherwise would when eating a more varied diet.

Children with SFA eat well when it is their preferred food but refuse to eat if offered food that is aversive to them with regard to the taste, smell, texture, or temperature of the food. When fed foods that the infant does not tolerate, the reactions can vary from grimacing to spitting out the food, wiping the tongue/mouth, gagging, and/or vomiting. After the initial aversive experience, the infants usually refuse to continue eating that particular food. In addition, they may generalize the experience and then refuse to eat any food item of similar color, smell, or appearance. The most common time for presentation of SFA is when the infant begins to eat solids with differing textures or at age 2 years, when they begin to try table foods. The aversive reaction can be so intense that the child will cut out entire categories of food from his/her diet, such as all vegetables, all fruits, or all meats. In particularly extreme cases, the child may refuse to eat a preferred food if it has even touched another food item, even a preferred food, but particularly one of his/her feared foods. Diets lacking fruits and vegetables may be deficient in certain vitamins. Milk and meat refusal can lead to deficiencies in zinc, protein, iron, and calcium. As noted above, the removal of these chewier foods from the diet may also result in oral motor delays, which can cause articulation difficulties.

Many of these children also struggle with hypersensitivities to sensory experiences outside of mealtimes. Children with SFA may not tolerate messes on their hands or clothing; may avoid walking barefooted on grass, sand, or other uneven surfaces; may avoid certain fabrics, clothing tags, or seams in socks and shoes; and may not tolerate strong smells or loud sounds well.

Risk factors

Risk factors in the development of SFA fall into two categories, those inherent to the child and those inherent to the environment. The risk factors inherent to the child include general neophobia (fear of change and the unknown), general sensory integration problems (such as sensitivities to touch, sounds, and bright lights), and a propensity toward anxiety. The risk factors inherent to the environment include food choices that are restricted by parents who

themselves struggle with SFA, coercive methods utilized by parents in an attempt to convince their child to eat (e.g., "You'll sit at this table until you eat your vegetables!"), and excessive praise by parents when the child eats a new food. This last factor may seem counterintuitive at first but can be understood when considering that turning the child's eating into a performance for the parents inevitably gives the control over mealtime to the child who can then choose to eat or not based on the effect he/she desires to evoke in the parents.

There are varying models of genetic transmission regarding SFA. Morton et al.[18] described multilocus and multiallelic models in 1981. A two locus model was proposed by Olson et al.[19] In 2003, Kim et al.[20] described a bitter receptor gene, $Tas2r$, on chromosome 7q with a nontasting haplotype recessive to the tasting haplotype. Studies have shown that individuals who avoid eating vegetables are more sensitive to the bitter taste and have been described as supertasters. Supertasters actually have been found to have more taste buds on their tongues than nontasters. This causes them to experience food tastes, textures, etc., more strongly, which can result in an aversive reaction and subsequent refusal of said food.

Differential diagnosis

As noted earlier, many times toddlers are "picky" eaters or enjoy the relative sense of control they can wield when realizing that refusing to eat will cause their parents distress and may result in extra attention or entertainment by the parent desperate to convince the toddler to eat. In this circumstance, the food avoidance is inconsistent. The child may eat broccoli well at one meal, then refuse it altogether at the next, for example. It is the child's mood and the wish for control that drives this sort of food refusal. However, in children with SFA, they consistently refuse the same foods or categories of foods, regardless of their emotional state. Children in both categories may become distressed when offered a food they do not want to eat, but the toddlers with SFA do this consistently every time that particular food is offered. A child with SFA can also refuse to eat based on mood, but generally this child will eat well when offered preferred foods and will only become distressed and refuse to eat when offered nonpreferred foods. However, a child refusing based solely on emotional state will refuse the food regardless of whether it is preferred or not.

SFA must also be distinguished from ARFID subtype: concern about the aversive consequences of eating (DSM-5) (a.k.a. "posttraumatic feeding disorder" [PTFD]). Children with this latter category of feeding disorder (to be described in more detail shortly) refuse to eat all solids or drink anything from a bottle, depending on the mode in which the feeding-related trauma occurred. Children with SFA may develop secondary PTFDs if their aversive reaction to a given food is so strong that it results in gagging or vomiting and/or the parents force the child to consume one of his/her aversive foods. They may become fearful of eating altogether. Unlike children with IA, those with SFA have normal hunger and satiety cues.

Etiology and course

Research done with preschoolers, older children, and adults has related taste sensitivities to the bitter substance, propylthiouracil, to strong food preferences, as well as the number of taste buds on one's tongue. Those with more taste buds, the "supertasters," demonstrated stronger taste preferences than the "nontasters."[21-23] Cooke et al.[24] studied food neophobia in a large twin study with participants ages 8–11 years. This study showed that 78% was heritable and 22% was due to nonshared environmental factors. Kim et al.'s study[20] demonstrated that certain polymorphisms on the taste receptor gene family, Tas2r, differentiate supertasters from nontasters. There is evidence of heritability, as some parents share food sensitivities with their biologic children.

As noted above, the eating environment can also influence development of SFA. If the parents are restrictive in their food intake, due to food sensitivities, dietary constraints, their own eating disorders, etc., they may offer only a limited variety of foods to their children, thus making it less likely for the children to be comfortable in trying new foods when offered. Attempts at coaxing or forcing children to eat can also result in restrictive food intake, as they become oppositional and subsequently more anxious about trying new foods. Children need appropriate supports when attempting to overcome these fears of trying new foods. A longitudinal study by Nicholas et al.[25] demonstrated a link between selective eating and anxiety, obsessive-compulsive symptoms, social difficulties, and school problems.

Skinner et al.[26] completed a longitudinal study of children ages 2–8 years. This study found that the numbers of foods the child liked at age 4 years predicted the number of foods liked by a child at age 8 years. Children were more likely to accept new foods between ages 2 and 4 years compared with school ages. School-aged children with SFA may experience social anxiety around eating and therefore avoid social engagements involving food, such as birthday parties and sleepovers.

During adolescent and young adult years, these individuals may learn to overcome their SFA to be able to engage in food-related social events. Clinically, it appears that girls are motivated by social engagement to overcome their fear of new foods at younger ages than their male counterparts. Girls may feel these social pressures as young as 7 or 8 years, whereas their male peers with SFA do not feel subject to the social pressures until early adolescence.

Possible comorbidities of SFA include sensory integration disorder and autism spectrum disorder, both of which involve hypersensitivity to sensory inputs. In addition, anxiety disorders may cooccur with SFA. Much of the basis of SFA lies in the fear of trying new foods and the fear of the sensory experience the new foods create.

Treatment

The treatment of SFA requires a desensitization of the taste buds through repeated exposure. However, the challenge for the therapist remains how to motivate children of different ages and with different temperaments to allow and seek the exposure to new and feared foods.

Birch et al.[27] conducted research that demonstrated that infants would accept new foods and related foods following repeated exposures. With toddlers, the number of exposures required before ready acceptance of a new food may be 10 or more. Toddlers can be notoriously stubborn regarding trying new foods. Birch's study found that threats to complete food items or to take away privileges did not work well. However, toddlers are quite responsive to modeling behaviors by their caregivers. When parents eat new foods, but do not offer it to the toddlers, the children are more likely to become interested and want to try that food.

The same feeding guidelines utilized for IA are again applied in the treatment of SFA. In addition, the work focuses on repeated exposure to feared foods. No one enjoys all foods. Therefore, it is less important to have the child eat every food offered, and more important to focus on expanding their dietary variety, keeping in mind the need to compensate for nutritional deficiencies caused by the feeding disorder. If a particular food causes the infant or child to gag or vomit, parents should not offer that food again because the child may develop an intense fear of that food and generalize to other foods of the same color or appearance. Instead, the parents should move on to other foods. If the infant merely grimaces or spits the food out, that food can be offered again in the future, but in smaller amounts and followed by a sip or bite of a preferred drink/food item. The amount of the disliked food is gradually increased over time.

Modeling by parents is a key aspect to the treatment of SFA in toddlers. Rather than offering the toddler a new food, the parents should eat the new food themselves and wait for the child to ask for a bite. The parent can then give the child a small sample of it while explaining that this is special food just for mommies and daddies. By lending a sense of specialness to the food, it makes the food item more attractive to the child. Parents can also interest the toddlers by giving special names to the new foods, such as "magic noodles" or "princess apple," and by preparing the food items in fun or exciting ways, such as pancakes with smiley faces made of fruit. The parents should remain neutral regarding whether or not the child likes the new food. This will allow the child to remain neutral with regard to trying new foods as well. The fear of trying new foods can significantly limit a child's diet.

By age 3 years, the modeling of trying new foods by parents becomes less effective. However, when starting preschool, children are sometimes willing to try a new food in that setting that they would not have tried otherwise in the home setting. As preschoolers have a rich sense of fantasy and make-believe, focused play therapy can also be useful. The therapy consists of playing "feeding the baby dolls." The practitioner models for patient and parents in the clinic setting, then the parents continue the work at home. Everyone is given a baby doll, including the child. Each baby doll receives a toy plate, plastic ware, and cup. Plastic foods are used. The practitioner talks about how his/her baby doll is hungry, but afraid of trying a new food. The child and parents also talk about what their baby dolls are feeling. The practitioner then notes that her baby doll wants to be brave and try the new food anyway. Using the play food, the practitioner feeds her baby doll until the baby doll's tummy is full. The child and parents do the same. This type of play therapy can be reenacted in the home environment focusing on how brave the baby dolls are to try new foods. While during mealtimes the parents are to avoid making direct comments about the child's eating, the child may subconsciously desire to be brave like his/her baby doll and try new foods, as well.

School-aged children can be engaged more directly in their treatment, as they may have better understanding of the importance of expanding their diets. They are helped by learning that they are supertasters and that they have more taste buds on their tongue than other children, that these taste buds give them a stronger experience of the taste and texture of some foods, but

that they can desensitize their taste buds by repeated exposure. With these children, a hierarchy of 10 feared foods is developed, ordering them from least to most scary based on the child's assessment. A behavioral plan is then developed, which includes earning one point of courage for every bite of a given feared food the child consumes. The least scary food on the list is the first food worked with. The child can earn small prizes for reaching 10, 30, and 50 points of courage. The prizes may increase in specialness as the child progresses through the bites. The prizes should be agreed upon by parents together with the child to ensure that they will motivate the child. The prizes do not need to be costly. Examples may include allowing the child to pick what movie the family will watch or having a special one-on-one play "date" with one of the parents, perhaps going to a particular museum or park, etc., to play. The prizes are used as a way to reward the child for being "brave." Once a child has eaten 50 bites of a feared food, he/she can usually incorporate it into his/her regular diet. The child can then move on to the next feared food on the list.

III. ARFID Subtype: Concern About the Aversive Consequences of Eating (DSM-5)

Feeding Disorder Associated with Insults to the Gastrointestinal Tract (DC: 0-3R)

Posttraumatic Feeding Disorder (Chatoor, 2007)

DC: 0-3R criteria: Requires all four of the following:

1. Food refusal follows a major aversive event or repeated noxious insults to the oropharynx or gastrointestinal tract that trigger intense distress in the infant or young child.
2. The infant or young child's consistent refusal to eat takes one of the following forms:
   a. The infant or young child refuses to drink from the bottle but may accept foods offered by spoon.
   b. The infant or child refuses solid food but may accept liquids.
   c. The child refuses all oral feedings.
3. Reminders of the traumatic event(s) cause distress, as manifested by one or more of the following:
   a. The infant shows anticipatory distress when positioned for feeding.
   b. The infant of young child resists intensely when a caregiver approaches with a bottle or food.
   c. The infant or young child shows intense resistance to swallowing food placed in his/her mouth.
4. The food refusal poses an acute or long-term threat to the child's nutrition.

Clinical features

PTFD may present with refusal of solids, refusal of the bottle, or refusal of all food intake, depending on the type of traumatic insult. The onset of PTFD is sudden, following a traumatic insult to the oropharynx and/or GI tract. Examples of traumatic events may include choking, severe gagging, vomiting, gastroesophageal reflux (GER), insertion of a nasogastric feeding tube, endotracheal intubation, or other instrumentation of the oropharynx. Forced feeding can also be a traumatic experience that results in PTFD. PTFD affects an estimated 4% of infants with GER who do not have a history of esophageal surgery, but up to 40% of those who do have esophageal surgery.[28] Parents are not always aware of the inciting event because they may not consider it to be traumatic because many other children may experience similar events without developing a PTFD. Children who develop PTFD may be more prone to anxiety and have lower pain thresholds than those who do not. Older children who develop PTFD following an episode of choking or gagging have explained their subsequent food refusal by describing a fear that food would become stuck in their throats causing them to choke to death.[29] Infants and young children demonstrate this fear by becoming distressed and crying in anticipation of being fed or when seeing their high chairs, bottles, or spoons. Some infants will allow the food in their mouths but will refuse to swallow, instead cheeking the food or spitting it out.[30] In the severest of instances, the infant or child will refuse to eat altogether. This places the children at acute risk of dehydration, as their fear overrides their drive for hunger or thirst.

The intense food refusal causes significant anxiety in the child's parent. The fear of dehydration and malnourishment drives these parents to attempt to coax or force their children to eat. They may attempt to offer a wide variety of foods, offering them at all times of the day and night. These attempts are largely unsuccessful and may further intensify the child's fear and food refusal. Infants with PTFD who refuse the bottle may be able to take the bottle while asleep, as the suck reflex while asleep persists until approximately 10 months of age. However, if they wake and see the bottle, they will often become distressed and push the bottle away. Overall, the significance of the food refusal poses a serious threat to the child's health and requires acute intervention.

Risk factors

Risk factors include an underlying separation anxiety disorder. In addition, episodes of choking, gagging, and vomiting may trigger a PTFD. Medical instrumentation of the oropharynx and insertion of nasogastric tubes may also trigger PTFD. Unfortunately, some infants and children with this feeding disorder may end up requiring a feeding tube due to the severity of their food refusal and subsequent malnutrition.

Differential diagnosis

PTFD must be differentiated from IA and SFA. With IA, the child has inconsistent food refusal, which is dependent on the child's mood. These children are not afraid to eat but rather do not have the hunger drive compelling them to eat. In addition, they have no particular limits on the types of foods they will eat. With SFA, the food avoidance is more predictable and is based on an aversion to a particular taste, texture, temperature, smell, or look of the food, rather than the more overarching food refusal seen with PTFD. Children with SFA may sometimes develop PTFD as well, following an extreme aversive reaction, such as severe gagging or vomiting, or when forced to eat the aversive foods that then trigger gagging and vomiting.

Etiology and course

Infants with PTFD appear to refuse to eat or drink from the bottle because of fear. They have associated eating food and/or drinking from the bottle with pain and therefore avoid it. It is unclear why the same experience (i.e., choking, gagging, nasogastric tube placement) may cause a PTFD in some infants and children, but not in others. Although there are no longitudinal studies on the natural course of PTFD, clinical experience informs us that with treatment most children eventually outgrow it. However, in extreme cases, it may be necessary to place a nasogastric or even a gastrostomy tube to provide adequate hydration and nutrition while the child works to overcome the PTFD. Some children remain dependent on tube feedings for years.

A study by Lucarelli et al.[31] demonstrated that children with PTFD scored in the clinically significant range for aggressive behaviors. These include angry moods, temper tantrums, stubbornness, excessive screaming, low frustration tolerance, and attention-seeking behaviors. This emotional dysregulation, when coupled with a traumatic feeding event, likely perpetuates the feeding disorder. The mothers of these children also scored significantly higher on anxiety screens, some even receiving a diagnosis of an anxiety disorder. There appears to be a reciprocal relationship between the anxiety of the mothers and the emotional dysregulation of the infants/children with PTFD. The mother's anxiety may more directly contribute to the development of PTFD by preventing said mother from adequately addressing her child's distress at the time of the inciting event, resulting in the child experiencing the event as traumatic and lacking skills to downregulate his/her emotional distress.

Possible comorbidities of PTFD include anxiety disorders, GER, eosinophilic gastroenteritis, and SFAs.

Treatment

A multidisciplinary team approach is best in dealing with these complex cases. The team should consist of a pediatrician and/or gastroenterologist, nutritionist, occupational or speech therapist, and a psychiatrist and/or psychologist. When the children refuse all food intake, they are at risk for dehydration, as well as malnourishment. It is critical that their medical needs are addressed first, before the psychiatric intervention is implemented. Owing to the acuity of the medical situation, IV fluids or nasogastric tube feedings may be required. The child may also require medication to treat GER, for example. Once the child's hydration and nutritional requirements have been addressed, the work to undo the PTFD can begin.

For infants who are avoiding bottle feeds, a regular sleep schedule must be established so that sleep feeds can be administered. As previously noted, most infants maintain the suck reflex in their sleep through 10 months of age. Parents can take advantage of this to nourish their child while he/she sleeps, thereby avoiding the child's distress over seeing the bottle. If the child wakes, he/she will likely initially begin to cry and refuse to continue. However, over time, the infant may allow the feeding to continue even upon awakening during a feed. At the start of the intervention, while awake, the parents should avoid attempts at feeding or even showing the bottle to the infant, as this will only reinforce the child's fear. Over time, an empty bottle may be given to the child to play with during waking hours. Eventually, the child's association between bottle feeds and pain will have dissipated, and wakeful feeds can be reintroduced.

If nasogastric or gastrostomy tube feedings are required to sustain the child's health, they are best administered at night, while the child sleeps. During the day, meals should occur every 3–4 h with no feedings in-between. Again, the feeding guidelines[17] can be utilized, although an exception is made for these children with regard to distractions at the meal. Although normally no TV or other distractions would be allowed at mealtime, for children with PTFD, the fear of eating may be so severe that such distractions are necessary during the initial phase of treatment to assist the child in overcoming their eating-related fears. If the

child still drinks from the bottle, the regular feedings should occur first, followed by bottle feeds, also in the high chair. There should be no bottle feedings at other times to reinforce hunger cues at the set mealtimes. These hunger cues may assist the child in overcoming his/her fear of eating. It is helpful to encourage self-feeding skills in these infants as the mastery over these skills may assist in lessening the anticipatory fear of eating. Once the child begins eating solids, the texture must be advanced slowly to avoid episodes of gagging that may reinforce the fear of eating and set-back the child's progress. Although external reinforcers, such as a favorite toy or TV show, are useful at the start of this therapeutic intervention, once the child has begun to overcome the fear of eating, these reinforcers should be phased out so that the child can begin to learn to respond to internal cues of hunger and fullness.

The process of reintroducing food for older children begins with asking the child to make a list of foods that he/she wants to start eating again. A behavioral plan is developed in which the child starts with the least scary food on his/her list and is rewarded with a "courage point" for each bite of food he/she completes. As the "courage points" accumulate, prizes can be awarded to reinforce the progress the child makes. The foods should be gradually introduced, advancing slowly from thickened liquids to purees, then soft foods, and finally chewy foods, such as nuts, granola and, finally, meats. The underlying anxiety can also be treated with a liquid SSRI.

Inpatient hospitalization for treatment of a PTFD may be necessary if the child is unable to overcome his/her fear of eating and therefore remains dependent on bottle or nasogastric/gastrostomy tube feeds. There are two main parts of the inpatient hospital intervention: manipulation of the child's appetite and contingency management. For children with tube feeds, water or Pedialyte are utilized to manipulate caloric intake while ensuring adequate hydration. The goal is to allow the child to become hungry. Behavioral interventions include use of both positive and negative reinforcements for food acceptance of refusal. These interventions must be tailored to the particular child. Thus, a skilled and cohesive team is required when treating these more extreme cases of PTFD. Again, the overarching goal is to assist the child in overcoming his/her fear of eating and to facilitate a return to internal hunger/fullness regulation by the child. Psychologic interventions and counseling are also important for the parents to support them in dealing with their child's difficult and often stressful feeding disorder, as well as to teach them how to best support their child in the recovery process.

COMORBIDITIES OF FEEDING DISORDERS

A validation study of five feeding disorders classified by Chatoor,[32] and later published in DC: 0-3R (2005),[3] demonstrated that although the majority of children had a single feeding disorder diagnosis, out of 444 young children who participated in the study, 135 had two feeding disorders and 10 children carried three diagnosis. The most frequent comorbidities were between IA and SFA. This is important to keep in mind, because to successfully treat these children each feeding disorder has to be addressed. A child who presents with a poor appetite and lack of interest in eating and food, and who also experiences sensory aversions to certain foods and becomes very selective, poses a big challenge for the parents. This child will go without eating anything if presented with an aversive food and often refuses a preferred food if upset about being asked to eat a feared food. It is very important for parents to understand both feeding disorders and how they can compound the problem of getting the child to eat. The parents need to adhere to the feeding guidelines and structure regular mealtimes so that the child experiences hunger at mealtimes. In addition, the parents need to offer only foods that the child accepts without protest. Coaxing these children to try new foods can be so upsetting for them that they may stop eating altogether.

Another comorbidity of two feeding disorders can be seen in children with SFA who may have experienced severe gagging or vomiting when exposed to a new aversive food and who become so traumatized by the experience that they not only refuse to eat the identified aversive food, but they generalize to other foods of similar color, smell, texture, or appearance. These children may develop severe anticipatory anxiety when approached with food and may be unable to eat an adequate diet, resulting in a PTFD that compounds the original SFA feeding disorder.

COMORBIDITIES OF FEEDING, SLEEP, AND ANXIETY DISORDERS

Major developmental tasks for young children are the regulation of feeding, sleep, and emotions. They are clearly connected, and children who have difficulty with self-calming have difficulty settling down at the table and find it hard to transition to sleep. These children become controlling and dependent on their parents to modulate their emotional state, and they often are given to temper tantrums when they cannot get their way. Children with IA are particularly vulnerable in this way because of their heightened physiologic arousal and their difficulty downregulating their arousal. This

heightened physiologic arousal drives their curiosity and facilitates their learning, but it also becomes a vulnerability if these children do not learn self-calming when they are young. As they grow older, they struggle with having difficulty going to sleep, laying awake for an hour or more, feeling tired in the morning, and often experiencing anxiety and fears that overshadow their lives.

In addition, children with SFA often present with severe anticipatory anxiety when challenged by new or feared foods, which has been described in the literature as neophobia. In some children the anxiety spreads to other areas of their lives as well. Some older children often experience anxiety when meals are part of social events, such as birthday parties or sleepovers.[33]

Children who present with a PTFD often struggle with some underlying anxiety that becomes activated by the traumatic event, e.g., choking, severe gagging, or vomiting. They become highly anxious and may have difficulty not only with eating but with sleeping as well. The anxiety in these children can become so debilitating that they have difficulty functioning in their daily lives.

TREATMENT OF COMORBID ANXIETY AND SLEEP DISORDERS

Regular meal and bed times are very important for these children. Parents need to be helped to establish a set bedtime routine to facilitate relaxation and to help the child to fall asleep. However, some children continue to struggle and medication may be indicated. Because most of these children experience a heightened level of arousal, the SSRI medications often activate these children even more, and Imipramine, a tricyclic, seems more helpful in regulating their sleep and helping with their anxiety during the day.

Children with IA, who have a poor appetite, are highly anxious, and have difficulty going to sleep, are often helped with the combination of a tricyclic and olanzapine. Olanzapine has been used with adolescents with anorexia nervosa, and it clearly helps these children to become more aware of their hunger.[34] It increases their appetite and helps with weight gain in addition to decreasing their anxiety. However, both medications need to be monitored closely for possible side effects.

CONCLUSION

Considering the importance of regulating feeding, sleep, and emotions in the first 3 years of life, early diagnosis and treatment of feeding disorders is critical to preventing ongoing problems with eating and the frequent comorbidities of sleep disturbance and anxiety disorders in these children. Picky eating and feeding difficulties are not uncommon in young children, but many times feeding disorders go untreated due to lack of knowledge or understanding of these illnesses. Worse yet, many times parents are blamed for their children's low appetite or selectivity, creating more shame and isolation in those parents, which leads to more anxiety and perpetuates the dysfunctional cycle of negative parent-child interactions. The severity of PTFDs, at least, tends to bring children into treatment more rapidly because their refusal to eat can result in serious and rapid dehydration and/or overall malnutrition, whereas children with IA or SFA may take longer to present for treatment. Children with IA may present with low weight and/or stature. Those with SFA may appear healthy with regard to their growth curves but may have significant nutritional deficits. While children with PTFD tend to outgrow their illnesses, IA and SFA are more likely to persist into adulthood if left untreated. In addition, the longer the feeding disorder has been going on, the more ingrained the negative feeding behaviors become and the longer it takes to therapeutically reverse them. Therefore, it is important that children with feeding disorders are identified and begin treatment as early as possible so that both the children and their parents can come to better understand the issues contributing to the feeding difficulties and so that they can be successful in overcoming these barriers to their bright and healthy futures.

REFERENCES

1. Kerzner B, Milano K, MacLean WC, Berall G, Stuart S, Chatoor I. A practical approach to classifying and managing feeding difficulties. *Pediatrics*. 2015;135(2):344–353.
2. First MB, Tasman A. *DSM-IV-TR Mental Disorders: Diagnosis, Etiology and Treatment*. J. Wiley; 2004.
3. Chatoor I. Diagnostic classification of feeding disorders. In: *Diagnostic Classification of Mental Health and Developmental Disorders of Infancy and Early Childhood. Revised Edition (DC: 0–3R)*. Washington, DC: Zero to Three Press; 2005.
4. Chatoor I. Feeding disorders in infants and toddlers: diagnosis and treatment. *Child Adolesc Psychiatr Clin N Am*. 2002;11(2):163–183.
5. American Psychiatric Association. *Diagnostic and Statistical Manual of Mental Disorders, 5th Edition: DSM-5*. 5th ed. Washington, D.C.: American Psychiatric Publishing; 2013.
6. Scheeringa M. Research diagnostic criteria for infants and preschool children: the process and empirical support. *J Am Acad Child Adolesc Psychiatry*. 2003;42(12):1504–1512.
7. Chatoor I, Ammaniti M. A classification of feeding disorders in infancy and early childhood. In: Narrow WE, First MB, Sirovatka PJ, Regier DA, eds. *Age and Gender Considerations in Psychiatric Diagnosis: A Research Agenda for DSM-5*. Arlington, VA: American Psychiatric Association; 2007.
8. Chatoor I, Ganiban J, Hirsch R, Borman-Spurrell E, Mrazek DA. Maternal characteristics and toddler temperament in infantile anorexia. *J Am Acad Child Adolesc Psychiatry*. 2000;39(6):743–751.
9. Chatoor I, Ganiban J, Surles J, Doussard-Roosevelt J. Physiological regulation and infantile anorexia: a pilot study. *J Am Acad Child Adolesc Psychiatry*. 2004;43(8):1019–1025.
10. Ammaniti M, Lucarelli L, Cimino S, D'olimpio F, Chatoor I. Maternal psychopathology and child risk factors in infantile anorexia. *Int J Eat Disord*. 2010;43(3):233–240.
11. Chatoor I, Ganiban J, Colin V, Plummer N, Harmon RJ. Attachment and feeding problems: a reexamination of nonorganic failure to thrive and attachment insecurity. *J Am Acad Child Adolesc Psychiatry*. 1998;37(11):1217–1224.
12. Chatoor I, Hirsch R, Ganiban J, Persinger M, Hamburger E. Diagnosing infantile anorexia: the observation of mother-infant interactions. *J Am Acad Child Adolesc Psychiatry*. 1998;37(9):959–967.
13. Chatoor I, Surles J, Ganiban J, Beker L, Paez LM, Kerzner B. Failure to thrive and cognitive development in toddlers with infantile anorexia. *Pediatrics*. 2004;113(5):e440–e447.
14. Ammaniti M, Lucarelli L, Cimino S, D'olimpio F, Chatoor I. Feeding disorders of infancy: a longitudinal study to middle childhood. *Int J Eat Disord*. 2012;45(2):272–280.
15. Chatoor I, Hirsch R, Persinger M. Facilitating internal regulation of eating: a treatment model for infantile anorexia. *Infants Young Child*. 1997;9(4):12–22.
16. Chatoor I, Sill A, Barber N, Kerzner B. Infantile Anorexia treated during early childhood: 5-10 years later. In: *Scientific Programs and Abstracts*. Edinburgh, Scotland. 2011:111.
17. *Understanding Early Childhood Feeding and Eating Problems*. Dr. Chatoor. http://drchatoor.com/.
18. Morton CC, Cantor RM, Corey LA, Nance WE. A genetic analysis of taste threshold for phenylthiocarbamide. *AMG Acta Genet Med Gemellologiae Twin Res*. 1981;30(1):51–57.
19. Olson JM, Boehnke M, Neiswanger K, Roche AF, Siervogel RM, MacCluer JW. Alternative genetic models for the inheritance of the phenylthiocarbamide taste deficiency. *Genet Epidemiol*. 1989;6(3):423–434.
20. Kim U, Jorgenson E, Coon H, Leppert M, Risch N, Drayna D. Positional cloning of the human quantitative trait locus underlying taste sensitivity to phenylthiocarbamide. *Science*. 2003;299(5610):1221–1225.
21. Reed DR, Nanthakumar E, North M, Bell C, Bartoshuk LM, Price RA. Localization of a gene for bitter-taste perception to human chromosome 5p15. *Am J Hum Genet*. 1999;64(5):1478.
22. Essick GK, Chopra A, Guest S, McGlone F. Lingual tactile acuity, taste perception, and the density and diameter of fungiform papillae in female subjects. *Physiol Behav*. 2003;80(2):289–302.

23. Miller IJ, Reedy FE. Variations in human taste bud density and taste intensity perception. *Physiol Behav.* 1990;47(6): 1213–1219.

24. Cooke LJ, Haworth CM, Wardle J. Genetic and environmental influences on children's food neophobia. *Am J Clin Nutr.* 2007;86(2):428–433.

25. Nicholls D, Christie D, Randall L, Lask B. Selective eating: symptom, disorder or normal variant. *Clin Child Psychol Psychiatry.* 2001;6(2):257–270.

26. Skinner JD, Carruth BR, Bounds W, Ziegler PJ. Children's food preferences: a longitudinal analysis. *J Am Diet Assoc.* 2002;102(11):1638–1647.

27. Birch LL. Development of food preferences. *Annu Rev Nutr.* 1999;19(1):41–62.

28. Dellert SF, Hyams JS, Treem WR, Geertsma MA. Feeding resistance and gastroesophageal reflux in infancy. *J Pediatr Gastroenterol Nutr.* 1993;17(1):66–71.

29. Chatoor I, Conley C, Dickson L. Food refusal after an incident of choking: a posttraumatic eating disorder. *J Am Acad Child Adolesc Psychiatry.* 1988;27(1):105–110.

30. Chatoor I, Ganiban J, Harrison J, Hirsch R. Observation of feeding in the diagnosis of posttraumatic feeding disorder of infancy. *J Am Acad Child Adolesc Psychiatry.* 2001;40(5):595–602.

31. Lucarelli L, Cimino S, Zavaroni D, Ammaniti M. Infantile post-traumatic feeding disorder and infantile anorexia: a clinical evaluation on maternal and child risk psychopathological factors. *Infant Ment Health J.* 2011;32:7. Wiley-Blackwell 111 River St, Hoboken 07030-5774, NJ USA.

32. Chatoor I, Hirsch R, Wonderlich S, Crosby R. Validation of a diagnostic classification of feeding disorders in infants and young children. In: *Developing an Evidence Based Classification of Eating Disorders: Scientific Findings for DSM-5.* Arlington, VA: American Psychiatric Association; 2011:185–202.

33. Timimi S, Douglas J, Tsiftsopoulou K. Selective eaters: a retrospective case note study. *Child Care Health Development.* 1997;23(3):265–278.

34. Norris ML, Spettigue W, Buchholz A, et al. Olanzapine use for the adjunctive treatment of adolescents with anorexia nervosa. *J Child Adolesc Psychopharmacol.* 2011;21(3):213–220.

CHAPTER 7

Eating Disorders

LAUREL WEAVER, MD, PHD • ALIX TIMKO, PHD

In this chapter, we will focus on the four primary pediatric eating disorders: anorexia nervosa (AN), bulimia nervosa (BN), binge eating disorder (BED), and avoidant-restrictive food intake disorder (ARFID). Eating disorders are severe psychiatric illnesses that begin in adolescence and have the potential to become chronic if not treated swiftly. Although there are similarities across these four disorders, there are also differences in presentation, treatment, and the depth of our understanding of their pathophysiology. What is not in doubt is that these illnesses are severe, debilitating, life-threatening, and have medical and psychosocial sequelae that are significantly underappreciated by many in the behavioral health and medical fields.

DIAGNOSTIC CRITERIA AND EPIDEMIOLOGY

Before the *Diagnostic and Statistical Manual of Mental Disorders, Fifth Edition* (*DSM-5*), the only diagnosable eating disorders were AN, BN, and a residual category referred to as "eating disorder not otherwise specified" or EDNOS. The frequency and heterogeneity of EDNOS were high. To help reduce the number of individuals diagnosed with EDNOS, the diagnostic criteria for AN and BN were changed; BED and ARFID were added. Replacing EDNOS is the other specified feeding or eating disorder. Eating disorders that fall into this category are clinically severe but do not meet diagnostic criteria for one of the other eating disorders (e.g., atypical AN or BN, subclinical BED, night eating syndrome, and purging disorder). Generally speaking, the alterations in diagnostic criteria were successful in reducing the number of cases of AN and BN that were classified as EDNOS in the *DSM-IV*. Adding BED and ARFID further reduced the incidence of patients who would have been diagnosed with EDNOS.[1]

Anorexia

AN is characterized by a significantly low body weight, a fear of becoming fat/gaining weight or engaging in behaviors to avoid weight gain, and a disturbance in the way in which one experiences their body. The latter aspect of the diagnostic criteria can reflect body dissatisfaction, the role of body shape in self-evaluation, or a denial of how serious their low weight is. Patients can be diagnosed with restrictive-type anorexia or anorexia with binge/purge behaviors. In the latter, patients can either binge or purge, or they do both. They must have been engaging in this binge/purge behavior for at least 3 months. In the *DSM-5*, the amenorrhea criterion was removed and there is no longer a weight criterion. Instead, the amount of underweight is determined via age, gender, and developmental trajectory. There is also a greater focus on behavioral aspects of anorexia (such as engaging in behaviors to avoid weight gain) as opposed to cognitive symptoms. In our experience, younger patients frequently do not endorse the traditional cognitive symptoms; thus, the addition of behavioral aspects of AN is very helpful for diagnosis in a pediatric population.

From an epidemiologic standpoint, much of the clinic and population data have focused on adults or not differentiated adults from adolescents in the sample. When only research on the epidemiology of AN in adolescent samples is examined, then 0.10%–1.7% of adolescents are diagnosed with AN.[2-6] Of note, available studies typically use DSM-IV criteria, which may not be as diagnostically sensitive in youth. Although low prevalence rates are often used to support the idea that AN (and eating disorders, in general) is a rare illness, this is likely not the case. In a community sample of German youth, the 12-month prevalence rate for AN was 0.40%; however, a significant percentage of males and females reported cognitions and behaviors typical of anorexia. The most common symptoms reported were being underweight and/or refusal to gain weight (in 27% of females and 24% of males).[5] When cases determined by DSM-IV criteria are reexamined using DSM-5 criteria, there is a 50% increase in the lifetime prevalence rate for anorexia in adolescents.[6] In one clinical sample, the rate of adolescents presenting for treatment with AN increased from 29.3% with DSM-IV criteria to 40% with DSM-5 criteria.[7]

Although typically considered a primarily female disorder, an analysis of data in the National Comorbidity Survey Replication Adolescent Supplement indicated that the ratio of females to males with DSM-IV anorexia was 1:1. However, subthreshold AN was more common in females than males.[3] Generally speaking, more females than males are diagnosed with anorexia although the rates vary from study to study; however, the most commonly cited ratio is 10:1.[8] The onset of anorexia may have a slightly different course in males than females; more research is needed to understand the similarities and differences between males and females. Anorexia occurs in all ethnicities[9]; however, Caucasian females tend to be overrepresented in many samples.

Overall, the median age of onset for AN is 12.3 years of age.[3] Impairment is high, with 97.1% of adolescents with AN reporting high impairment; of those 24.2% indicated severe impairment. In AN, social impairment was significant: 88.9% of adolescents reported social impairment, 19.6% indicated that social impairment was related to the eating disorder.[3] Over half of adolescents with AN (55%) have a comorbid disorder. Anxiety is most common, with high rates of comorbid social anxiety, obsessive-compulsive disorder (OCD), and specific phobia.[10] Depression also cooccurs. Both depression and anxiety can be a side effect of starvation or, if already present, can be worsened by starvation.[11] AN is also significantly associated with oppositional defiant disorder.[3] Almost one-third of adolescents with AN reported suicidal ideation. Of those who expressed suicidal thoughts, 2.3% indicated having a plan and 8.2% reported a suicide attempt. Anorexia has the highest mortality rate of all psychiatric illnesses and is the third most common chronic illness in adolescents. Almost two-thirds of adolescents with AN seek out treatment; however, only 25% of those receive specialty treatment.[3]

Bulimia

BN is characterized by weekly episodes of binge eating and a subsequent compensatory behavior for 3 months. Objectively, binge eating is considered consuming a large amount of food within a 2-h period while experiencing a lack of control over what or how much one is consuming. This binge is followed by a compensatory behavior (e.g., vomiting, use of diuretics or laxatives, excessive exercise, fasting). Individuals with bulimia typically overvalue shape and weight. Key to a diagnosis of bulimia is that it cannot occur during a period of anorexia. If someone is underweight, meets all criteria for AN, and engages in binging/purging, this is binge/purge-type AN, *not* bulimia.

The epidemiology of bulimia is subject to the same adult bias as studies of the epidemiology of anorexia. Swanson and colleagues[3] found a prevalence rate of 0.9%; however, rates range from 0.10% to 1.1% in other studies.[4,5,12] Bulimia does appear to be more common in females, specifically females who identify as Hispanic. Like anorexia, bulimia begins in adolescence. Although some research indicates that bulimia has a later age of onset than anorexia,[13] other reports indicated that the median age of onset is 12.4 years of age.[3] The majority of individuals with bulimia engage in two or more types of compensatory behaviors.[14] Males are more likely to engage in excessive exercise. In adults, there is some evidence that males will exercise not to compensate for calories consumed during a binge but rather to reduce fat and increase muscle definition.[15] Bulimia does appear to be more common in females; however, the rates in boys are not regularly reported. The female to male ratio for bulimia has ranged from 3:1 to as high as 25:1.[16]

Impairment is high in bulimia, with 78% of adolescents in the National Comorbidity Study Replication reporting impairment, 10.7% of these adolescents reported severe impairment. Youth with BN also reported that their eating disorder negatively affected their social and family relationships.[3] Comorbidity rates are approximately 83% in bulimia. Depression is the most common comorbid condition.[10] Impulsive and self-harm behaviors are often observed.[17] Over half affected individuals express suicidal ideation; of those 25.9% have a plan and over a third (35.1%) of adolescents with bulimia have attempted suicide.[3] These rates are the highest among adolescents with eating disorders and higher than in adolescents with other psychiatric diagnoses.[18] Only 60% of adolescents and their families seek out treatment, and 21.5% seek out specialty treatment.[3]

Binge Eating Disorder

BED was formally recognized with the adoption of the *DSM-5* in 2013. To meet criteria, individuals must have recurrent episodes of binge eating (as defined in bulimia) but do not engage in compensatory behaviors. As this is a new diagnosis, there is not a great deal of information about the epidemiology of BED. It does appear to be more common in females,[3,19] and there is limited evidence that it may be observed more in ethnic minorities.[3] Lifetime prevalence is 1.4%. The median age of onset is 12.6 years of age[20]; however, some research notes an age of onset that corresponds to emerging adulthood.[21] Of the adolescents who are diagnosed with BED, almost two-thirds

(62.6%) report impairment. One-third (34.4%) report suicidal ideation; of those 5.1% have a plan and 15.1% report having attempted suicide.[3] Comorbidities are high, with 83% of adolescents presenting with a cooccurring psychiatric disorder; depression and anxiety are common. Binge eating predicts weight gain and obesity; the loss of control associated with a binge is more strongly associated with eating disorder cognitions than the amount of food consumed.[19] A high percentage of children and adolescents seek out treatment for BED (60%); however, this may be due to the association of BED with overweight and obesity. Of those seeking treatment, 11% receive specialty treatment.[3]

Avoidant-Restrictive Food Intake Disorder

ARFID is characterized by avoidance or restriction of food, leading to significant weight loss or failure to thrive, nutritional deficiency, dependence on enteral feeding or oral nutritional supplements, or marked interference with psychosocial functioning. Diagnostic criteria categorize several subtypes of ARFID, which include food restriction based on sensory-based avoidance, lack of interest, or anxiety-based avoidance. Body image disturbance is typically not observed in ARFID. Given the newness of the diagnostic category, there are no epidemiologic studies of ARFID. However, rates of ARFID in pediatric eating disorder programs range from 5% to 22.5%.[22] Although ARFID has popularly been thought to be "less severe" than AN, patients with ARFID have a harder time with weight regain, more reliance on enteral nutrition, longer hospital stays, the same remission and readmission rates as AN,[23] and a longer duration of illness.[24]

Differentiating avoidant-restrictive food intake disorder from anorexia

It can be difficult to distinguish between the diagnosis of ARFID and AN, particularly in young children. On face value, children can meet criteria for both ARFID and AN simultaneously. If weight/shape concerns are thought to underlie the illness, AN is diagnosed. However, children and adolescents with anorexia may not express body weight or image concerns, and DSM-5 criteria reflect this fact. As a lack of body disturbance also occurs in ARFID, it is often assumed that when there is a differential to make between anorexia and ARFID and there is no body disturbance—the correct differential is ARFID. In our clinical experience this is not necessarily the case; there is often an impulse in clinicians to name the "less serious" illness, such as ARFID as the primary diagnosis. Given that outcomes of ARFID may not be

more positive than those of AN,[23] this impulse may be misguided. It can also interfere with determining the best treatment plan.

It cannot be stressed enough that in a clinical scenario where a child presents with malnutrition, engages in behaviors that interfere with weight gain, and has a lack of insight into the seriousness of the situation, anorexia must be considered as a potential diagnosis. Our clinical rule of thumb is to consider AN when a youngster presents with malnutrition and to reserve final diagnosis until treatment begins/full recovery from malnutrition is made. Treatment for the eating disorder can also function as a probe to help with diagnosis. Children or adolescents with AN will frequently struggle with weight gain, and during this process more typical eating disorder cognitions may become apparent. For other children or adolescents, it may not be until time passes, or weight gain is required, which cognitions that are more clearly related to AN may be expressed, if at all.

DIFFERENTIAL DIAGNOSIS OF EATING DISORDERS AND DIAGNOSTIC DILEMMAS

The differential diagnosis of eating disorders includes both psychiatric and medical differentials. Age of the child can make the differential diagnosis more difficult. Many nonspecialist healthcare providers inaccurately assume that children younger than 12 years cannot be diagnosed with an eating disorder. This is not the case. Most of the research on children with eating disorders focuses on those with restrictive eating disorders. Children below the age of 12 years with an eating disorder can be frequently misdiagnosed as having an anxiety disorder, primary feeding problem, or a gastrointestinal (GI) problem. In fact, those children who do not express eating disorder cognitions are more likely to have somatic symptoms and anxiety,[25] which could delay the diagnosis of an eating problem. In a clinical sample of young children (5–12 years) with restrictive eating disorders, 62.1% were diagnosed with AN.[25] Almost half were medically unstable and required hospitalization, and rates of restrictive eating disorders in boys were high. Extrapolated from this study, rates of restrictive eating disorders in young children and adolescents exceed those of medical conditions that are considered to be an epidemic.[25]

Another variable that can make a differential diagnosis difficult is the determination as to whether or not a child or adolescent is underweight. Using a fixed body mass index criterion is not appropriate for children and adolescents because they are in a period of growth and development. Instead, when calculating a child or adolescent's expected body weight, one needs to take into consideration the child's historical growth curves and anticipated growth and weight gain. Furthermore, adolescents with atypical anorexia may be in the normal weight range (due to a history of being overweight and losing weight) but may be below the weight that is appropriate for them and allows for medical and psychiatric stability.

There can sometimes be confusion between the diagnoses of AN and BN. The confusion is understandable given the phenomenon of diagnostic crossover. Individuals with eating disorders may move from one diagnosis and back again over the course of the illness. Anywhere from 20% to 50% of individuals with AN will eventually cross over to BN,[26-29] whereas only 10%–30% of individuals diagnosed with BN will later meet criteria for AN.[20,30] Individuals with AN will also switch back and forth between different subsets of AN throughout the course of their diagnosis, with studies citing that this occurs for about 50%–65% of individuals with AN.[26,31] However, if criteria for malnutrition are present, and there is the presence of purging behaviors, the correct diagnosis is binge/purge-type AN.

Another key differential is between eating disorders and anxiety disorders. As noted earlier, young children with eating disorders are often initially misdiagnosed as having an anxiety disorder. The distinction can be difficult to make because anxiety disorders are frequently comorbid with eating disorders, particularly AN. When children develop an eating disorder, they become distressed upon presentation of food, which may be mistaken for an anxiety disorder. Furthermore, both anxiety and depression can be the result of or worsen with malnutrition.[11] As an example, a child with generalized anxiety disorder, when malnourished, may more frequently verbalize worries and somatic complaints. If the focus of the impairing distress is on eating, an eating disorder would be diagnosed; the clinician would then decide whether ARFID or AN is the best diagnosis. If the child describes other symptoms of a primary anxiety disorder such as social anxiety disorder or OCD, this disorder would be diagnosed as comorbid, particularly if it preceded the malnutrition or persisted in the renourished state.

Obsessive-Compulsive Disorder Differential

Obsessive-compulsive behaviors are commonly observed in anorexia, so much so that it has also been suggested that AN may belong to a spectrum of compulsive behaviors.[32] A large population–based study

indicates that males with OCD have a 37-fold risk of comorbid AN, whereas females with OCD have a 16-fold risk of comorbid AN.[33] OCD and AN also appear to increase the risk for each other[34]; longitudinally, individuals who are diagnosed with OCD have a 4-fold higher risk of developing AN later and individuals with AN have a 10-fold increase in risk for developing OCD later.[33] Adults with AN often report that OCD predated the onset of the eating disorder.[35] Premorbid OCD predicts poorer outcome in AN, particularly in cases where AN began early in childhood or adolescence.[35-37] Despite the frequent cooccurrence of these disorders, diagnosing one in the context of the other can be difficult. There is increasing evidence that the cooccurrence of these disorders impedes treatment.[38,39] The presence of obsessions and compulsions is a significant moderator of treatment outcome in adolescents with AN; those who have high levels of obsessionality require longer treatment course and have poorer outcome.[40,41] Standard treatment for pediatric OCD is not effective when children or adolescents are underweight,[42] highlighting the need for rapid weight restoration and the development of new treatments that can target both OCD symptoms and eating disorder symptoms.

Social Anxiety

Social anxiety is a common disorder in adolescents.[43] Eating disorders are socially isolating and are associated with impairment in social domains.[3] Anorexia is hypothesized to be characterized by some difficulties in the area of social cognition (e.g., reading social signals, understanding emotion),[44,45] which may also overlap with social anxiety. Adults with eating disorders frequently report a history of social anxiety: 55% of adults with anorexia reported a lifetime diagnosis of social anxiety; the social anxiety predated the onset of anorexia in 75% of those patients. In bulimia, 59% of adults reported a diagnosis of social anxiety, which predated the onset of the eating disorder on 88% of those women.[46] Social anxiety is the most common anxiety disorder to still be present at long-term follow-up.[47] Adolescents with anorexia or bulimia will report anxiety around eating in front of others, can have difficulty reintegrating into friend groups after missing school due to treatment, and may be overly sensitive to negative feedback or have a more inhibited temperament.

Clinical Implications

When malnutrition is present in an apparently anxious child and if the child or adolescent engages in behaviors that interfere with weight gain, and/or if there is a lack of insight into the seriousness of the situation, AN is the de facto primary diagnosis. Although anxiety may be present, it is important to clearly define anorexia as the primary diagnosis. Malnutrition often causes or exacerbates preexisting anxiety and depression. However, the phenomenology between anxiety disorders and eating disorders is different, and the treatments are different. A good rule of thumb is to focus on weight restoration in any adolescents who has lost weight or failed to gain sufficient weight. It is important to note that during the weight restoration period, anxiety may increase. After weight restoration is completed, the child or adolescent can be reassessed for the presence or exacerbation of anxiety symptoms that are independent of those experienced during eating. At this point in time, clinical decisions can be made to determine whether or not psychosocial or pharmacologic treatment for the anxiety should be added to the treatment plan.

Medical Differential

When assessing a child or adolescent who is malnourished, medical illnesses causing malnutrition must be ruled out. Malnutrition frequently causes symptoms of depression, anxiety, and rigidity around food, even when the primary cause of the malnutrition is medical.[48] Medical illnesses must therefore be carefully considered and ruled out in the malnourished child or adolescent, including (but not limited to) primary GI illnesses such as Crohn's disease or Celiac disease, endocrine causes such as thyroid disease or Addison's disease, and oncologic or inflammatory causes.[49] However, primary GI illnesses can coexist with eating disorders, and leanness is thought to be a risk factor for the development of eating disorders.[50] It is important not to attribute all weight loss automatically to medical etiologies or comorbid conditions.

Eating disorders and resultant malnutrition affect all major organ systems. Laboratory workup should include measurements of kidney and liver function, electrolytes (particularly in patients who are purging), thyroid function, hematologic/cell line measurements, hormonal/endocrine assessment, and assessment of the cardiovascular system.[51] Amenorrhea in females and pubertal disruption in males are common and may underlie the development of osteopenia and osteoporosis. Major causes of death are from sudden death from cardiac causes, implicated in one-third of cases,[52] and suicide, implicated in 20%–30% of cases.[53] Major long-lasting sequelae after weight restoration include osteoporosis[54] and possibly reversible structural brain abnormalities.[55,56]

During regular care of adolescents with anorexia, physical exam should be performed and orthostatic vital signs should be evaluated. Bradycardia, hypotension, orthostasis, and hypothermia are common.[51] Electrocardiogram readings can show QTc prolongation and other arrhythmias.[57] Physical manifestations common in restrictive eating disorders may include lanugo, acrocyanosis, and yellow-orange palms from hypercarotenemia.[58] In disorders involving purging, Russell's sign upon dermatologic exam (a callus on the hand or knuckle where there is reflexive biting of the hand during induced vomiting), discoloration and erosion of enamel on teeth, and swollen parotid glands can result from persistent vomiting.[59] Clinical suspicion for an eating disorder must be high when a youngster's abnormal vital signs are determined to be due to malnutrition or any of the aforementioned physical exam abnormalities are present.

TREATMENT OF EATING DISORDERS

Given the severity eating disorders, there have been surprisingly few randomized clinical trials examining treatments. Nonetheless, we do have enough information about treatment to know that family-based approaches have the most empirical support.[60,61] Treatment is primarily behavioral in nature but can include psychopharmacology. Treatment for all eating disorders should be multidisciplinary. Typically, a therapist and physician who specialize in eating disorders are needed. If the treating therapist is not a psychiatrist, then one may need to be added to the team to assess for or monitor medication. If needed, dieticians can be part of the team; however, family-based protocols (see below) typically do not include them.

A useful concept when formulating a treatment plan for children and adolescents with eating disorders is that of the "three-legged stool" from evidence-based medicine.[62] This metaphor highlights that effective treatment incorporates clinical expertise, research data, and patient preference. Given the paucity of treatment trials in children and adolescents with eating disorders, clinical expertise and patient preference may become important when formulating a treatment plan. When reviewing research below on the treatment of pediatric eating disorders, we will only review treatments that have sufficient evidence to be considered efficacious or probably efficacious. Those with less evidence are considered to be possibly efficacious or experimental in nature.

Although psychosocial/behavioral treatments are the most effective, in our clinical experience parents often want to explore the possibility of medication in treatment. Medication treatment of eating disorders in children and adolescents is not a sole modality of treatment but rather must be viewed as part of a multimodal treatment plan. It is important that patients and parents understand this point because a focus solely on medication will likely not yield positive results without ancillary psychosocial treatments. Indeed, in our experience in a majority of cases there is no need for medication. Despite the dearth of extant evidence for their efficacy, psychotropic medications are commonly prescribed clinically in pediatric patients with eating disorders, at rates as high as 60%.[63,64] In this chapter, we will review medications commonly prescribed for AN, BN, BED, and ARFID.

Most of what is known about pharmacologic treatment in eating disorders in children and adolescents comes from short-term trials in adults with eating disorders.[64,65] What will be successful in the medication treatment of eating disorders in children and adolescents must be inferred from what has been successful in adult trials. The difficulty with doing so is that adults have likely been ill for a significant period of time; thus their illness represents one that has had a more chronic course. It is possible that eating disorders in adults may be qualitatively different (e.g., with a different neurobiology) from the illness that has a new onset in a child or adolescent. Information from adult trials tells us more about what may or may not be helpful for severe and enduring or chronic eating disorders; there may be a role for some pharmacologic agents in the treatment of eating disorders in children and adolescents that is not evident in adults. When discussing the practice of evidence-based medication management for psychiatric illness in children and adolescents, it is important to note that it is often "off-label," that is, without approval from the US Federal Drug Administration. The treatment of eating disorders is no exception.

TREATMENT OF ANOREXIA NERVOSA
Behavioral Treatments

Anorexia is the only eating disorder for which we have an empirically supported treatment in adolescence (note, there is no empirically supported treatment for adults with anorexia). Family treatment is recommended, with foundational clinical care techniques developed at the Philadelphia Child Guidance Center in the 1970s[66] and refined by the Maudsley Hospital in London. A manualized treatment approach based on this earlier work, family-based treatment (FBT), has received the most research support.[67] FBT is agnostic in terms of the etiology of the disorder and views parents as a key member of the treatment team. FBT is explicit in that it does not blame the parents for the development of anorexia.[57] Viewing parents as a resource and key to recovery instead of an obstacle or complicit with the eating disorder is frequently viewed as a key shift in the treatment of anorexia.[59] Other key characteristics of FBT include viewing the adolescent as separate from the eating disorder, assuming that parents have all the skills they need to get their child healthy and assuming that the adolescent is encumbered only by the eating disorder.[68]

The purpose of FBT is to restore weight and return the adolescent to their appropriate developmental track. FBT is an outpatient treatment; adolescents must be medically stable to participate. If adolescents become medically unstable during treatment, a brief hospital stay can be used to stabilize any medical concerns. FBT is typically delivered in 20 sessions over 12 months and has three distinct phases.[57] Phase 1 typically lasts for 10 sessions and focuses on weight restoration. In this phase, parents take full responsibility for renourishing their child. That is, parents make all decisions about meals, portion and plate all meals and snacks, observe the youth eating the meal, and ensure that all necessary calories are consumed. This phase can also include continued observation to ensure that any physical activity is appropriately reduced or eliminated and prevent any purging from occurring. Siblings play supportive role and are protected from the job assigned to the parents.

FBT has two key interventions that occur during Phase I: orchestrating an intense scene and the family meal. In the former, the severity of the illness is highlighted and parents face the gravity of the situation they are currently in. The purpose is to stimulate the family to help the parents organize to support their child through renourishment. In the family meal, the parents are tasked with bringing meal to session that they feel will nourish their child. The family eats the meal while the therapist observes and asks questions. Weight gain of approximately 4 lbs during the first 4 weeks of Phase 1 is predictive of a better outcome (i.e., full weight restoration).[69] In Phase 2, parents turn responsibility over food and eating back to their child in a developmentally and culturally appropriate way. Finally, in Phase 3 any issues of development are discussed.

FBT is effective for many families; remission rates range from 21.8% to 42% at the end of treatment and from 29% to 49% by 12-month follow-up.[70]

Although many families benefit from FBT, not all do. Early research indicated that families who tend to cope with illness with a more critical communication style (known as expressed emotion) do not do as well in treatment. A separated form of FBT where the therapist sees the adolescent individually followed by the parent may be more appropriate for families with high expressed emotion.[71–73] FBT is also less likely to be successful when there is severe parental psychopathology and/or serious discord between parents. It has been hypothesized that symptom accommodation in anorexia could maintain the illness and interfere with treatment; however, there has not been any empirical work on this.[74] FBT does not focus on the etiology of the illness nor does it focus on maintenance factors. Treatment is hypothesized to be effective via increases in parental self-efficacy and potentially via parent-facilitated exposure.[68]

There are now a number of variants of FBT, and it has been successfully disseminated to nonresearch settings.[75] A shorter trial of FBT (10 sessions over 6 months) is effective for adolescents with low levels of compulsivity.[41] If families are not doing well by week 4 in treatment, an adaptive form of FBT has shown to be effective.[76] In this treatment, adaptation, after session 4 if the adolescent has not gained sufficient weight, three additional sessions are inserted into the protocol. In the first session, the seriousness of failure to gain 4 lbs in the first 4 weeks is stressed. The session is intended to create a crisis atmosphere, galvanize parents into behavior change, and increase weight gain. The second session is for parents only and is designed to explore barriers to treatment and difficulties with renourishment. Finally, a second family meal is conducted and the family is directly coached on how to address barriers identified in the prior session. Although preliminary, data on the adaptive form of FBT is promising and may lead to greater weight gain in adolescents who struggle earlier in treatment than FBT alone.[76]

Finally, one trial examined FBT compared with a parent-only FBT (PFT). PFT follows the same phases and session content of FBT but does not include the adolescent or siblings. At the start of each session, the adolescent's medical stability and weight are assessed by a nurse practitioner. The nurse updates the therapists and provides supportive counseling to the adolescent for 15 min. The parents meet with the therapist and focus on issues related to renourishment and transitioning of responsibility back to the adolescent (when appropriate).[70,77,78] In an randomized controlled trial (RCT) comparing FBT to PFT, adolescents

were more likely to reach remission in PFT at the end of treatment, and there was no difference between groups at follow-up. Adolescents with eating disorder–related obsessionality did better in FBT; those with less obsessionality did better in PFT.[70]

Although FBT and its variants have received the most empirical support, systems-based family therapy (SB-FT) does have limited support.[79,80] SB-FT focuses more on family dynamics and their possible role in the etiology or maintenance of AN. Adding systems-based treatment to treatment as usual improved patient outcomes compared with a treatment as usual alone. Compared with FBT, a systems-based approach has a comparable outcome. However, patients receiving FBT gain weight more rapidly and have fewer hospitalizations, thus FBT is more acceptable to parents than SB-FT.[80]

There is also limited support for an individual approach to treatment—adolescent-focused therapy (AFT, also referred to as ego-oriented individual therapy). In a trial comparing FBT with AFT, both do equally well in terms of recovery rate by the end of treatment. However, patients in AFT were more likely to be hospitalized and FBT had better long-term outcome.[81] AFT is a viable treatment option for families who opt not to do FBT.

In AFT, it is assumed that adolescents with anorexia confuse self-control with biologic needs—likely due to an ego deficit. Treatment is aimed to increase self-efficacy and autonomy. Adolescents are charged with accepting responsibility for their food-related issues as opposed to their parents. They learn to identify and regulate emotions in treatment. AFT consists of 32 sessions with up to 8 sessions for meetings with parents. Like FBT, it has three phases. Phase 1 focuses on establishing rapport, assessing motivation of the adolescent to change behavior, and setting weight goals. In Phase 2 adolescents learn to increase their tolerance of distressing emotions, and there is a focus on separation and individuation from their parents. Finally, Phase 3 focuses on termination.[81]

Psychopharmacology

The common comorbid features of anxiety and depression observed in the acute phase of AN combined with the intense anxiety/distress that is seen clinically when a patient with an eating disorder is faced with the task of eating indicate antidepressant agents as hopeful candidates for ameliorating the core feature of the illness, i.e., the inability to recover and maintain sufficient body weight. Results of multiple medication trials of serotonergic/noradrenergic agents in adults (e.g., tricyclic antidepressants [TCAs] and selective serotonergic reuptake inhibitors [SSRIs]) for the treatment of AN reveal a paucity of evidence that these agents result in weight gain.[64,82] They do not appear to reduce time to relapse when used after weight restoration in adults with AN.[83] The use of TCAs has fallen out of favor of use in children and adolescents because of concern about side effects, particularly cardiac arrhythmias, with resultant increased use of SSRIs. No randomized trials of SSRIs for the treatment of AN in children and adolescents exist. SSRIs may be frequently prescribed by first-line providers in the community as early-onset AN can mimic an anxiety disorder, but in our clinical opinion, use of these medications seems to do little to change the trajectory of the core features of this illness.

Other medications have been examined in the treatment of adults with AN. There is some limited evidence for the use of typical antipsychotics, atypical antipsychotics, cyproheptadine, zinc supplementation, lithium, naltrexone, and nasogastric tube feeding.[82] δ-9-Tetrahydrocannabinol was not effective, and there was evidence that it produced undesirable side effects.[5] Although there is some evidence for utility of medications for treating the core features of AN in adults, the evidence level is weak.[70] Currently, clinical practice parameters for children with eating disorders reserve medications, in general, for treating comorbidities after some amount of weight restoration.[51]

A key concern in the use of medications in the treatment of AN is the malnourished state that mimics the signs and symptoms of a primary anxiety or depressive state. Much of what we know about the psychiatric side effects of a malnourished state comes from the Minnesota Starvation Study by Ancel Keys,[48] dating to the 1940s and clinical experience since that time. In summary, there is an increase in psychiatric symptoms, including anxiety and depression that is seen in a malnourished state. These resolve with the resolution of the malnutrition absent any other interventions. A careful assessment of the magnitude of the anxiety and/or depressive disorder that was present before the onset of weight loss should be performed to rule out that the clinical symptoms observed are not solely due to malnutrition. With a careful history and timeline, the clinician should ascertain which symptoms were present before the onset of the eating disorder and which paralleled the onset of a low weight state. If symptoms of the mood or anxiety disorder began at the same time as restriction, weight restoration is likely the only "medication" needed, barring severe symptoms.

A second key concern is perturbed brain protein metabolism in a low weight state, with presumed effects on serotonin and serotonin receptors.[84] As medications are hypothesized to work through effects on brain neurotransmitters such as monoamines and their receptors, effects and side effects may be altered. SSRIs have been looked at for their efficacy for treatment of anxiety and depression symptoms in low weight adults and adolescents with mixed results.[84–86]

Although SSRIs are often the initial medication choice in the treatment of anxiety and depression in children, these medications have not been tested for safety in low weight children and adolescents. Practice guidelines urge caution when using medications in a low weight state, as cardiac function may be compromised and medications can have side effects of affecting cardiac function.[64]

Atypical antipsychotics have interested clinicians for their potential in the use in the treatment of AN due to their side effect of weight gain in children and adolescents without AN[87] and use as augmenting agents for adults with other disorders, such as OCD.[88–90] Studies with atypical antipsychotics in adults have shown some potential for decreasing anxiety in the course of AN, although other studies have been equivocal.[82] A systematic review and metaanalysis compared eight studies where patients with AN were compared on and off atypical antipsychotics and found no differences in body weight, body mass index, psychopathology related to AN, depression symptoms, or anxiety symptoms. Patients on atypical antipsychotics experienced more sedation but not more of other side effects such as rapid weight gain or diabetes mellitus.[91]

There have been two double-blind, placebo-controlled trials of the use of the atypical antipsychotics risperidone and olanzapine, respectively, in adolescents up to 21 years of age with eating disorders.[92,93] Positive weight gain was not seen in either of these studies, and there was no measured improvement in psychologic functioning in the olanzapine study.[92] In the risperidone study, a secondary measure of eating disorder pathology (interpersonal distrust) was improved in the group that used risperidone.[93] A recent retrospective chart review showed that the use of Abilify in a continuum of care setting in adolescents with AN resulted in an increase in weight gain in the adolescents.[94] Generally, the symptom of compulsive exercise in AN is a risk factor for a poorer outcome[95] and can be difficult to manage in the outpatient setting. Administration of low-dose olanzapine to 13 adolescent patients undergoing multimodal therapy for restricting AN significantly decreased levels of hyperactivity.[96]

In our experience, the use of olanzapine may be helpful to children and adolescents during the course of FBT. Children and adolescents can exhibit externalizing behavior during the course of refeeding, and this behavior confers a high risk for illness.[97] The use of atypical antipsychotics are part of the evidence-based treatment algorithm for the treatment of aggression in children and adolescents.[98] Used cautiously, benefit may be seen in levels of aggression and impulsivity[99] that may make treatment of eating disorders with FBT in the outpatient realm feasible, which is significant as outpatient treatment may be more beneficial than inpatient treatment.

TREATMENT OF BULIMIA NERVOSA

Behavioral Treatments

Research in the treatment of adolescent BN lags behind that for anorexia. There are no empirically supported treatments for the treatment of adolescent BN. FBT that has been modified to treat bulimia has been shown to be effective; it is probably efficacious.[100,101] FBT for adolescent bulimia is very similar to FBT for AN. It differs in the fact that the secrecy and shame that often accompany bulimia are believed to confuse and disempower parents. Adolescent's development can also be negatively affected. Parents and adolescents are encouraged to work together to change behavior. Adolescents who received FBT had significantly higher rates of abstinence from binge/purge cycles than those who received cognitive behavioral therapy[101] or supportive psychotherapy.[100] There is Limited evidence for the use of a guided self-help version of cognitive behavioral therapy for adolescents with bulimia. More recent research has focused on the combination of dialectical behavior therapy, FBT,[102,103] and the development of multifamily groups.[104]

Psychopharmacology

Similar to AN, data for the medication treatment of bulimia come from studies in adults of typically short-term duration. Because of frequently comorbid anxiety and depression, serotonergic/noradrenergic medications have again seemed to be likely candidates for use in this disorder. Historically, there is some evidence for older antidepressants (TCAs as well as monoamine oxidase inhibitor (MAOIs)) for reducing bingeing and purging in adults with BN.[82] SSRIs have largely replaced the use of TCAs in children and adolescents, and thus studies of SSRI use in adults are of interest when considering medication management in children and adolescents with BN. Fluoxetine

is approved by the US Federal Drug Administration for the treatment of BN in adults and has the most evidence among medications for reduction of binge/purge behavior in BN.[82] Dosage at 60 mg is thought be superior to the dosage of 20 mg in adults. Other SSRIs, such as fluvoxamine, may also be effective in decrease of bingeing and purging behavior in adults.[82]

Other agents outside of antidepressants have been studied as having potential positive effects for adults with BN, such as topiramate and ondansetron.[105] It is unclear whether adding medication to effective psychologic treatment is more helpful above what the psychologic treatment itself offers,[105] although medication may be helpful with treating comorbid depressive symptoms, which may commonly be comorbid with BN.[106] Controlled trials of medications for BN have not been completed in children and adolescents. However, inferring from adult trials, use of SSRIs to reduce frequency of bingeing and purging in children and adolescents may be appropriate, although SSRIs should be offered in conjunction with excellent psychologic treatment when possible.

Since the approval of lisdexamfetamine (Vyvanse) for BED in adults, we have received questions about the use of this medication in BN. It should be noted that there is no evidence to support the use of this medication in BN. Given the high comorbidity of BN with drug and alcohol use disorders,[107] we encourage strong caution concerning use of any medication that may have potential risk for addiction.

TREATMENT OF AVOIDANT-RESTRICTIVE FOOD INTAKE DISORDER

No controlled trials exist for behavioral or psychopharmacologic interventions for ARFID. As with AN, children with ARFID who are malnourished exhibit many symptoms that appear to be anxiety but are in reality a side effect of malnutrition. As in AN, weight gain will often help the rigidity and inflexibility that accompanies malnutrition and will increase flexibility in eating behaviors such as consumption of adequate calories.[108] In our experience, weight gain promotes more varied and flexible food choices. Thus, a main intervention in malnourished children with ARFID should be full weight restoration to goal weights outlined in practice guidelines.[49,109] To achieve this goal, behavioral family interventions may be helpful. Frequently, families will use preferred foods to achieve weight gain. Once full weight restoration is achieved, then exposure is used to increase variety.

In our clinical experience, despite aggressive family and behavioral interventions, weight gain can be difficult in ARFID because of the extreme levels of anxiety that may accompany acute malnutrition (regardless if it was premorbid). In these instances, children may experience total food refusal and may have to undergo enteral nutrition initiation in the hospital for medical stabilization. In these situations, short-term use of an atypical antipsychotic may be the appropriate intervention, given the desirability of quick resolution of enteral feeds and resolution of the extreme distress experienced by these children. Short-term use of atypical antipsychotics, coupled with behavior therapy to resolve the use of enteral nutrition, avoids or lessens the need for residential treatment. The use of the atypical antipsychotic is curtailed to 3–6 months or until no longer needed because resolution of malnutrition may diminish feeding difficulties as well as anxiety. Once the total food refusal crisis is resolved, and the child or adolescent is weight-restored, consideration of transition to SSRI use at that time can be made. Atypical antipsychotics should be tapered slowly, as quicker tapers may adversely affect appetite and mood, and parents should be warned that they may have to be more vigilant about calorie intake as the atypical is being weaned, as appetite may diminish.

Behavioral Treatment

Case studies for severe picky and/or selective eating (predating categorization into DSM-5 criteria) show positive effects of behavior therapy in children, adolescents, and adults.[110-112] FBT has been adapted for ARFID, and there are currently ongoing trials.[113] For picky eating, reward systems are effective in increasing the intake of avoided foods. The full range of behavioral contingencies often must be employed, including positive rewards and response cost contingencies.[114]

Psychopharmacology

Case reports with patients with ARFID are emerging in the literature. Two pediatric patients with ARFID recovered with a combination of behavior therapy and risperidone.[115] Behavior therapy plus fluoxetine for anxiety was helpful in the successful treatment of another pediatric patient with ARFID.[22] Given the different subtypes of ARFID, it is likely that treatment will vary depending on the subtype. One major subtype of ARFID involves a phobic avoidance of food relating to phobias such as emetophobia, choking phobia, anaphylaxis phobia, or OCD. Given that this subtype of ARFID is coupled with a primary anxiety disorder, a sensible strategy

might couple behavior therapy with medication management, targeting the phobia. Although data for the treatment of phobias with SSRIs in children are sparse as behavior therapy works well,[88] a reasonable strategy for an anxious child who is not eating well would be to trial an SSRI.

TREATMENT OF BINGE EATING DISORDER

There are no empirically supported treatments for adolescents with BED. In adults, the starting treatment of choice is psychotherapy, with evidence for cognitive behavioral therapy and interpersonal therapy (IPT).[116] These treatments have been adapted for adolescents, and there is limited support for the use of IPT or cognitive behavioral therapy in adolescents with BED.[117,118]

Psychopharmacology

When considering medication management, in adults there is moderate evidence for the use of SSRIs[116] and lisdexamfetamine, which is FDA-approved in adults for the treatment of BED. Topiramate and atomoxetine also have some reported efficacy.[119] Currently medication is not thought to be the first-line intervention in adolescents; however, it is common clinical practice to use fluoxetine as an adjunctive treatment to psychotherapy for children and adolescents based on adult trials. Furthermore, treatment with a medication that might address comorbid conditions such as depression or attention deficit hyperactivity disorder, if they are present, may be a reasonable choice.

CONCLUSION

Eating disorders are severe psychiatric illnesses with significant morbidity and mortality. Early identification and swift intervention is necessary. Although comorbidities are common, apparent symptoms of a given syndrome may be side effects of malnutrition. Treatment should focus on increasing weight to a developmentally appropriate level and then reevaluate for comorbid conditions. The exception is when symptoms are interfering in treatment of the primary eating disorder. In this case, psychosocial or pharmacologic interventions to treat the comorbid symptoms may be necessary. In the treatment of eating disorders, physical recovery happens before behavioral recovery. The latter must occur before the patient can experience full psychologic (cognitive and emotional) recovery. Full recovery should be sought because it is associated with full return to functioning. Adults who meet stringent criteria for full recovery are indistinguishable from healthy controls.[120] Overall, FBTs have the most empirical support; however, they are not effective for every family. More research is needed on treatment of bulimia, BED, and ARFID in children and adolescents.

REFERENCES

1. Hoek HW. Classification, epidemiology and treatment of DSM-5 feeding and eating disorders. *Curr Opin Psychiatry*. 2013;26(6):529–531.
2. Roberts RE, Roberts CR, Xing Y. Rates of DSM-IV psychiatric disorders among adolescents in a large metropolitan area. *J Psychiatr Res*. 2007;41(11):959–967.
3. Swanson SA, Crow SJ, Le Grange D, Swendsen J, Merikangas KR. Prevalence and correlates of eating disorders in adolescents. Results from the national comorbidity survey replication adolescent supplement. *Arch Gen Psychiatry*. 2011;68(7):714–723.
4. Merikangas KR, He J-P, Brody D, Fisher PW, Bourdon K, Koretz DS. Prevalence and treatment of mental disorders among US children in the 2001–2004 NHANES. *Pediatrics*. 2010;125(1):75–81.
5. Nagl M, Jacobi C, Paul M, et al. Prevalence, incidence, and natural course of anorexia and bulimia nervosa among adolescents and young adults. *Eur Child Adolesc Psychiatry*. 2016;25(8):903–918.
6. Smink FR, Hoeken D, Oldehinkel AJ, Hoek HW. Prevalence and severity of DSM-5 eating disorders in a community cohort of adolescents. *Int J Eat Disord*. 2014;47(6):610–619.
7. Ornstein RM, Rosen DS, Mammel KA, et al. Distribution of eating disorders in children and adolescents using the proposed DSM-5 criteria for feeding and eating disorders. *J Adolesc Health*. 2013;53(2):303–305.
8. Norris ML, Apsimon M, Harrison M, et al. An examination of medical and psychological morbidity in adolescent males with eating disorders. *Eat Disord*. 2012;20(5):405–415.
9. Croll J, Neumark-Sztainer D, Story M, Ireland M. Prevalence and risk and protective factors related to disordered eating behaviors among adolescents: relationship to gender and ethnicity. *J Adolesc Health*. 2002;31(2):166–175.
10. Touchette E, Henegar A, Godart NT, et al. Subclinical eating disorders and their comorbidity with mood and anxiety disorders in adolescent girls. *Psychiatry Res*. 2011;185(1):185–192.
11. Casper RC. Depression and eating disorders. *Depress Anxiety*. 1998;8(S1):96–104.
12. Jaite C, Hoffmann F, Glaeske G, Bachmann CJ. Prevalence, comorbidities and outpatient treatment of anorexia and bulimia nervosa in German children and adolescents. *Eat Weight Disord Stud Anorexia Bulimia Obes*. 2013;18(2):157–165.
13. Campbell K, Peebles R. Eating disorders in children and adolescents: state of the art review. *Pediatrics*. 2014;134(3):582–592.
14. Binford RB, le Grange D. Adolescents with bulimia nervosa and eating disorder not otherwise specified-purging only. *Int J Eat Disord*. 2005;38(2):157–161.
15. Dakanalis A, Timko CA, Clerici M, Zanetti MA, Riva G. Comprehensive examination of the trans-diagnostic cognitive behavioral model of eating disorders in males. *Eat Behav*. 2014;15(1):63–67.
16. Herpertz-Dahlmann B. Adolescent eating disorders: definitions, symptomatology, epidemiology and comorbidity. *Child Adolesc Psychiatr Clin North Am*. 2009;18(1):31–47.
17. Peebles R, Wilson JL, Lock JD. Self-injury in adolescents with eating disorders: correlates and provider bias. *J Adolesc Health*. 2011;48(3):310–313.
18. Crow SJ, Swanson SA, le Grange D, Feig EH, Merikangas KR. Suicidal behavior in adolescents and adults with bulimia nervosa. *Compr Psychiatry*. 2014;55(7):1534–1539.
19. Sonneville KR, Horton NJ, Micali N, et al. Longitudinal associations between binge eating and overeating and adverse outcomes among adolescents and young adults: does loss of control matter? *JAMA Pediatr*. 2013;167(2):149–155.
20. Tozzi F, Thornton LM, Klump KL, et al. Symptom fluctuation in eating disorders: correlates of diagnostic crossover. *Am J Psychiatry*. 2005;162:732–740.
21. Kessler RC, Berglund PA, Chiu WT, et al. The prevalence and correlates of binge eating disorder in the World Health Organization World Mental Health Surveys. *Biol Psychiatry*. 2013;73(9):904–914.
22. Norris ML, Spettigue WJ, Katzman DK. Update on eating disorders: current perspectives on avoidant/restrictive food intake disorder in children and youth. *Neuropsychiatr Dis Treat*. 2016;12:213.
23. Strandjord SE, Sieke EH, Richmond M, Rome ES. Avoidant/restrictive food intake disorder: illness and hospital course in patients hospitalized for nutritional insufficiency. *J Adolesc Health*. 2015;57(6):673–678.
24. Sieke EH, Strandjord SE, Richmond M, Rome ES, Khadilkar AC. Avoidant/restrictive food intake disorder and anorexia nervosa subtypes: how do they compare? *J Adolesc Health*. 2016;58(2):S26–S27.
25. Pinhas L, Morris A, Crosby RD, Katzman DK. Incidence and age-specific presentation of restrictive eating disorders in children: a Canadian Paediatric Surveillance Program study. *Arch Pediatr Adolesc Med*. 2011;165(10):895–899.
26. Eddy KT, Dorer DJ, Franko DL, Tahilani K, Thompson-Brenner H, Herzog DB. Diagnostic crossover in anorexia nervosa and bulimia nervosa: implication for DSM-V. *Am J Psychiatry*. 2008;165:245–250.
27. Bulik CM, Sullivan PF, Fear J, Pickering A. Predictors of the development of bulimia nervosa in women with anorexia nervosa. *J Nerv Ment Dis*. 1997;185:704–707.
28. Eckert ED, Halmi KA, Marchi P, Grove W, Croshy R. Ten-year follow-up of anorexia nervosa: clinical course and outcome. *Psychol Med*. 1995;25:143–156.

29. Strober M, Freeman R, Morrell W. The long-term course of severe anorexia nervosa in adolescents: survival analysis of recovery, relapse, and outcome predictors over 10–15 years in a prospective study. *Int J Eat Disord.* 1997;22:339–360.

30. Keel PK, Mitchell JE. Outcome in bulimia nervosa. *Am J Psychiatry.* 1997;154:313–321.

31. Eddy KT, Keel PK, Dorer DJ, Delinksy S, Franko DL, Herzog DB. Longitudinal comparison of anorexia nervosa subtypes. *Int J Eat Disord.* 2002;31:191–201.

32. McElroy SL, Phillips KA, Keck Jr PE. Obsessive compulsive spectrum disorder. *J Clin Psychiatry.* 1994;55:33–51. discussion 52–33.

33. Cederlöf M, Thornton LM, Baker J, et al. Etiological overlap between obsessive-compulsive disorder and anorexia nervosa: a longitudinal cohort, multigenerational family and twin study. *World Psychiatry.* 2015;14(3): 333–338.

34. Meier SM, Bulik CM, Thornton LM, Mattheisen M, Mortensen PB, Petersen L. Diagnosed anxiety disorders and the risk of subsequent anorexia nervosa: a Danish population register study. *Eur Eat Disord Rev.* 2015;23(6):524–530.

35. Degortes D, Zanetti T, Tenconi E, Santonastaso P, Favaro A. Childhood obsessive–compulsive traits in anorexia nervosa patients, their unaffected sisters and healthy controls: a retrospective study. *Eur Eat Disord Rev.* 2014;22(4):237–242.

36. Sallet PC, de Alvarenga PG, Ferrão Y, et al. Eating disorders in patients with obsessive–compulsive disorder: prevalence and clinical correlates. *Int J Eat Disord.* 2010;43(4):315–325.

37. Yackobovitch-Gavan M, Golan M, Valevski A, et al. An integrative quantitative model of factors influencing the course of anorexia nervosa over time. *Int J Eat Disord.* 2009;42(4):306–317.

38. Hirani V, Serpell L, Willoughby K, Neiderman M, Lask B. Typology of obsessive-compulsive symptoms in children and adolescents with anorexia nervosa. *Eat Weight Disord Stud Anorexia Bulimia Obes.* 2010;15(1–2): 86–89.

39. Serpell L, Livingstone A, Neiderman M, Lask B. Anorexia nervosa: obsessive–compulsive disorder, obsessive–compulsive personality disorder, or neither? *Clin Psychol Rev.* 2002;22(5):647–669.

40. Le Grange D, Lock J, Agras WS, et al. Moderators and mediators of remission in family-based treatment and adolescent focused therapy for anorexia nervosa. *Behav Res Ther.* 2012;50(2):85–92.

41. Lock J, Agras WS, Bryson S, Kraemer HC. A comparison of short versus long term family therapy for adolescent anorexia nervosa. *J Am Acad Child Adolesc Psychiatry.* 2005;44:632–639.

42. Jassi A, Patel N, Lang K, Heyman I, Krebs G. Ritualised eating in young people with obsessive compulsive disorder; clinical characteristics and treatment outcomes. *J Obsess Compuls Relat Disord.* 2016;8:1–8.

43. Merikangas KR, He J-P, Burstein M, et al. Lifetime prevalence of mental disorders in US adolescents: results from the national comorbidity survey replication–adolescent supplement (NCS-A). *J Am Acad Child Adolesc Psychiatry.* 2010;49(10):980–989.

44. Adenzato M, Todisco P, Ardito RB. Social cognition in anorexia nervosa: evidence of preserved theory of mind and impaired emotional functioning. *PLoS One.* 2012;7(8):e44414.

45. Zucker NL, Losh M, Bulik CM, LaBar KS, Piven J, Pelphrey KA. Anorexia nervosa and autism spectrum disorders: guided investigation of social cognitive endophenotypes. *Psychol Bull.* 2007;133(6):976–1006.

46. Godart NT, Flament MF, Lecrubier Y, Jeammet P. Anxiety disorders in anorexia nervosa and bulimia nervosa: co-morbidity and chronology of appearance. *Eur Psychiatry.* 2000;15(1):38–45.

47. Herpertz-Dahlmann B, Müller B, Herpertz S, Heussen N, Hebebrand J, Remschmidt H. Prospective 10-year follow-up in adolescent anorexia nervosa—course, outcome, psychiatric comorbidity, and psychosocial adaptation. *J Child Psychol Psychiatry.* 2001;42(5):603–612.

48. Keys A, Brožek J, Henschel A, Mickelsen O, Taylor HL. The Biology of Human Starvation. 2 Vols. Oxford, England: Univ. of Minnesota Press; 1950.

49. Golden NH, Katzman DK, Kreipe RE, et al. Eating disorders in adolescents: position paper of the society for adolescent medicine. *J Adolesc Health.* 2003;33(6):496–503.

50. Stice E, Gau JM, Rohde P, Shaw H. Risk factors that predict future onset of each DSM–5 eating disorder: predictive specificity in high-risk adolescent females. *J Abnorm Psychol.* 2017;126(1):38.

51. Lock J, La Via MC. Practice parameter for the assessment and treatment of children and adolescents with eating disorders. *J Am Acad Child Adolesc Psychiatry.* 2015;54(5):412–425.

52. Garrido BJ, Lobera IJ. *Cardiovascular Complications in Eating Disorders.* INTECH Open Access Publisher; 2012.

53. Sullivan PF. Mortality in anorexia nervosa. *Am J Psychiatry.* 1995;152(7):1073–1074.

54. Misra M, Klibanski A. Bone health in anorexia nervosa. *Curr Opin Endocrinol Diabetes Obes.* 2011;18(6):376.

55. Eynde F, Suda M, Broadbent H, et al. Structural magnetic resonance imaging in eating disorders: a systematic review of voxel-based morphometry studies. *Eur Eat Disord Rev.* 2012;20(2):94–105.

56. Golden NH, Ashtari M, Kohn MR, et al. Reversibility of cerebral ventricular enlargement in anorexia nervosa, demonstrated by quantitative magnetic resonance imaging. *J Pediatr.* 1996;128(2):296–301.

57. Lock J, le Grange D. *Treatment Manual for Anorexia Nervosa: A Family-Based Approach.* 2nd ed. New York: Guildford Press; 2012.

58. Strumia R. Dermatologic signs in patients with eating disorders. *Am J Clin Dermatol.* 2005;6(3):165–173.

59. Le Grange D, Lock J, Loeb K, Nicholls D. Academy for eating disorders position paper: the role of the family in eating disorders. *Int J Eat Disord.* 2010;43(1):1–5.

60. Hay P, Chinn D, Forbes D, et al. Royal Australian and New Zealand College of Psychiatrists clinical practice guidelines for the treatment of eating disorders. *Aust N Zeal J Psychiatry.* 2014;48(11):977–1008.

61. Yager J, Devlin MJ, Halmi KA, et al. Guideline watch: practice guideline for the treatment of patients with eating disorders. *Focus.* 2005;3(4):546–551.

62. Peterson CB, Becker CB, Treasure J, Shafran R, Bryant-Waugh R. The three-legged stool of evidence-based practice in eating disorder treatment: research, clinical, and patient perspectives. *BMC Med.* 2016;14(1):69.

63. Monge MC, Forman SF, McKenzie NM, et al. Use of psychopharmacologic medications in adolescents with restrictive eating disorders: analysis of data from the National Eating Disorder Quality Improvement Collaborative. *J Adolesc Health.* 2015;57(1):66–72.

64. *Eating Disorders: Core Interventions in the Treatment and Management of Anorexia Nervosa, Bulimia Nervosa, and Related Eating Disorders.* National Collaborating Center for Mental Health; 2004.

65. Keel PK, Haedt A. Evidence-based psychosocial treatments for eating problems and eating disorders. *J Clin Child Adolesc Psychol.* 2008;37(1):39–61.

66. Liebman R, Minuchin S, Baker L. An integrated treatment program for anorexia nervosa. *Am J Psychiatry.* 1974;131(4):432–436.

67. Lock J. An update on evidence-based psychosocial treatments for eating disorders in children and adolescents. *J Clin Child Adolesc Psychol.* 2015;44(5):707–721.

68. Loeb KL, Lock J, Greif R, le Grange D. Transdiagnostic theory and application of family-based treatment for youth with eating disorders. *Cognit Behav Pract.* 2012;19(1):17–30.

69. Doyle PM, le Grange D, Loeb K, Doyle AC, Crosby RD. Early response to family-based treatment for adolescent anorexia nervosa. *Int J Eat Disord.* 2010;43(7):659–662.

70. Le Grange D, Hughes EK, Court A, Yeo M, Crosby RD, Sawyer SM. Randomized clinical trial of parent-focused treatment and family-based treatment for adolescent anorexia nervosa. *J Am Acad Child Adolesc Psychiatry.* 2016;55(8):683–692.

71. Eisler I, Dare C, Hodes M, Russell G, Dodge E, Le Grange D. Family therapy for adolescent anorexia nervosa: the results of a controlled comparison of two family interventions. *J Child Psychol Psychiatry.* 2000;41(6):727–736.

72. Eisler I, Simic M, Russell GFM, Dare C. A randomised controlled treatment trial of two forms of family therapy in adolescent anorexia nervosa: a five year follow-up. *J Child Psychol Psychiatry.* 2007;48(6):552–560.

73. Le Grange D, Eisler I, Dare C, Russell GFM. Evaluation of family therapy in anorexia nervosa: a pilot study. *Int J Eat Disord.* 1992;12:347–357.

74. Loeb KL, le Grange D. Family-based treatment for adolescent eating disorders: current status, new applications and future directions. *Int J Child Adolesc Health.* 2009;2(2):243.

75. Couturier JL, Kimber MS. Dissemination and implementation of manualized family-based treatment: a systematic review. *Eat Disord.* 2015;23(4):281–290.

76. Lock J, Le Grange D, Agras WS, et al. Can adaptive treatment improve outcomes in family-based therapy for adolescents with anorexia nervosa? Feasibility and treatment effects of a multi-site treatment study. *Behav Res Ther.* 2015;73:90–95.

77. Hughes EK, Le Grange D, Yeo MS, et al. Parent-focused treatment for adolescent anorexia nervosa: a study protocol of a randomised controlled trial. *BMC Psychiatry.* 2014;14(1):105.

78. Hughes EK, Sawyer SM, Loeb KL, Le Grange D. Parent-focused treatment. In: *Family Therapy for Adolescent Eating and Weight Disorders: New Applications;* 2015:59–71.

79. Godart N, Berthoz S, Curt F, et al. A randomized controlled trial of adjunctive family therapy and treatment as usual following inpatient treatment for anorexia nervosa adolescents. *PLoS One.* 2012;7(1):e28249.

80. Agras WS, Lock J, Brandt H, et al. Comparison of 2 family therapies for adolescent anorexia nervosa: a randomized parallel trial. *JAMA Psychiatry.* 2014;71(11):1279–1286.

81. Lock J, Le Grange D, Agras WS, Moye A, Bryson SW, Jo B. Randomized clinical trial comparing family-based treatment with adolescent-focused individual therapy for adolescents with anorexia nervosa. *Arch Gen Psychiatry.* 2010;67(10):1025–1032.

82. Aigner M, Treasure J, Kaye W, Kasper S. World Federation of Societies of Biological Psychiatry (WFSBP) guidelines for the pharmacological treatment of eating disorders. *World J Biol Psychiatry.* 2011;12(6):400–443.

83. Walsh BT, Kaplan AS, Attia E, et al. Fluoxetine after weight restoration in anorexia nervosa: a randomized controlled trial. *JAMA.* 2006;295(22):2605–2612.

84. Sebaaly JC, Cox S, Hughes CM, Kennedy MLH, Garris SS. Use of fluoxetine in anorexia nervosa before and after weight restoration. *Ann Pharmacother.* 2013;47(9):1201–1205.

85. Ferguson CP, La Via MC, Crossan PJ, Kaye WH. Are serotonin selective reuptake inhibitors effective in underweight anorexia nervosa? *Int J Eat Disord.* 1999;25(1):11–17.

86. Holtkamp K, Hebebrand J, Mika C, Heer M, Heussen N, Herpertz-Dahlmann B. High serum leptin levels subsequent to weight gain predict renewed weight loss in patients with anorexia nervosa. *Psychoneuroendocrinology.* 2004;29(6):791–797.

87. Caccia S. Safety and pharmacokinetics of atypical antipsychotics in children and adolescents. *Pediatr Drugs.* 2013;15(3):217–233.

88. Reinblatt SP, Walkup JT. Psychopharmacologic treatment of pediatric anxiety disorders. *Child Adolesc Psychiatr Clin North Am.* 2005;14(4):877–908.

89. Veale D, Miles S, Smallcombe N, Ghezai H, Goldacre B, Hodsoll J. Atypical antipsychotic augmentation in SSRI treatment refractory obsessive-compulsive disorder: a systematic review and meta-analysis. *BMC Psychiatry.* 2014;14(1):317.

90. Jensen KG, Juul K, Fink-Jensen A, Correll CU, Pagsberg AK. Corrected QT changes during antipsychotic treatment of children and adolescents: a systematic review and meta-analysis of clinical trials. *J Am Acad Child Adolesc Psychiatry.* 2015;54(1):25–36.

91. Kishi T, Kafantaris V, Sunday S, Sheridan EM, Correll CU. Are antipsychotics effective for the treatment of anorexia nervosa? Results from a systematic review and meta-analysis. *J Clin Psychiatry.* 2012;73(6):e757–e766.

92. Kafantaris V, Leigh E, Hertz S, et al. A placebo-controlled pilot study of adjunctive olanzapine for adolescents with anorexia nervosa. *J Child Adolesc Psychopharmacol.* 2011;21(3):207–212.

93. Hagman J, Gralla J, Sigel E, et al. A double-blind, placebo-controlled study of risperidone for the treatment of adolescents and young adults with anorexia nervosa: a pilot study. *J Am Acad Child Adolesc Psychiatry.* 2011;50(9):915–924.

94. Frank GK, Shott ME, Hagman JO, Schiel MA, DeGuzman MC, Rossi B. The partial dopamine D2 receptor agonist aripiprazole is associated with weight gain in adolescent anorexia nervosa. *Int J Eat Disord.* 2017;50(4):447–450.

95. Grave RD. Features and management of compulsive exercising in eating disorders. *Phys Sportsmed.* 2009;37(3):20–28.

96. Leggero C, Masi G, Brunori E, et al. Low-dose olanzapine monotherapy in girls with anorexia nervosa, restricting subtype: focus on hyperactivity. *J Child Adolesc Psychopharmacol.* 2010;20(2):127–133.

97. Marikar D, Reynolds S, Moghraby OS. Junior MARSIPAN (management of really Sick patients with anorexia nervosa). *Arch Dis Child Educ Pract.* 2016;101(3):140–143.

98. Rosato NS, Correll CU, Pappadopulos E, et al. Treatment of maladaptive aggression in youth: CERT guidelines II. Treatments and ongoing management. *Pediatrics.* 2012;129(6):e1577–e1586.

99. Masi G, Milone A, Canepa G, Millepiedi S, Mucci M, Muratori F. Olanzapine treatment in adolescents with severe conduct disorder. *Eur Psychiatry.* 2006;21(1):51–57.

100. Le Grange D, Crosby RD, Rathouz PJ, Leventhal BL. A randomized controlled comparison of family-based treatment and supportive psychotherapy for adolescent bulimia nervosa. *Arch Gen Psychiatry.* 2007;64(9):1049–1056.

101. Le Grange D, Lock J, Agras WS, Bryson SW, Jo B. Randomized clinical trial of family-based treatment and cognitive-behavioral therapy for adolescent bulimia nervosa. *J Am Acad Child Adolesc Psychiatry.* 2015;54(11):886–894. e882.

102. Murray SB, Anderson LK, Cusack A, et al. Integrating family-based treatment and dialectical behavior therapy for adolescent bulimia nervosa: preliminary outcomes of an open pilot trial. *Eat Disord.* 2015;23(4):336–344.

103. Anderson LK, Murray SB, Ramirez AL, Rockwell R, Le Grange D, Kaye WH. The integration of family-based treatment and dialectical behavior therapy for adolescent bulimia nervosa: philosophical and practical considerations. *Eat Disord.* 2015;23(4):325–335.

104. Stewart C, Voulgari S, Eisler I, Hunt K, Simic M. Multi-family therapy for bulimia nervosa in adolescence. *Eat Disord.* 2015;23(4):345–355.

105. Zhu AJ, Walsh BT. Pharmacologic treatment of eating disorders. *Can J Psychiatry.* 2002;47(3):227–234.

106. Walsh BT, Wilson GT, Loeb KL, et al. Medication and psychotherapy in the treatment of bulimia nervosa. *Am J Psychiatry.* 1997;154(4):523–531.

107. Gadalla T, Piran N. Co-occurrence of eating disorders and alcohol use disorders in women: a meta analysis. *Arch Women's Ment Health.* 2007;10(4):133–140.

108. Accurso EC, Ciao AC, Fitzsimmons-Craft EE, Lock JD, Le Grange D. Is weight gain really a catalyst for broader recovery?: the impact of weight gain on psychological symptoms in the treatment of adolescent anorexia nervosa. *Behav Res Ther.* 2014;56:1–6.

109. Katzman DK, Peebles R, Sawyer SM, Lock J, Le Grange D. The role of the pediatrician in family-based treatment for adolescent eating disorders: opportunities and challenges. *J Adolesc Health.* 2013;53(4):433–440.

110. Ahearn WH, Kerwin ME, Eicher PS, Lukens CT. An ABAC comparison of two intensive interventions for food refusal. *Behav Modif.* 2001;25(3):385–405.

111. Anderson CM, McMillan K. Parental use of escape extinction and differential reinforcement to treat food selectivity. *J Appl Behav Anal.* 2001;34(4):511–515.

112. Luiselli JK. Cueing, demand fading, and positive reinforcement to establish self-feeding and oral consumption in a child with chronic food refusal. *Behav Modif.* 2000;24(3):348–358.

113. Fitzpatrick KK, Forsberg SE, Colborn D. Family-based therapy for avoidant restrictive food intake disorder: families facing food neophobias. In: Loeb KL, Le Grange D, Lock J, eds. *Family Therapy for Adolescent Eating and Weight Disorders: New Applications.* New York: Routledge; 2015:256–276.

114. Dahlsgaard KK. *Manual for Brief, Group-Based, Parent Management Training for Extreme Picky Eating. Unpublished Treatment Manual;* 2017.

115. Pennell A, Couturier J, Grant C, Johnson N. Severe avoidant/restrictive food intake disorder and coexisting stimulant treated attention deficit hyperactivity disorder. *Int J Eat Disord.* 2016;49(11):1036–1039.

116. Tsappis M, Freizinger M, Forman SF. Binge-eating disorder: emerging treatments for a new diagnosis. *Curr Opin Pediatr.* 2016;28(4):415–420.

117. Tanofsky-Kraff M, Wilfley DE, Young JF, et al. Preventing excessive weight gain in adolescents: interpersonal psychotherapy for binge eating. *Obesity.* 2007;15(6):1345–1355.

118. Tanofsky-Kraff M, Wilfley DE, Young JF, et al. A pilot study of interpersonal psychotherapy for preventing excess weight gain in adolescent girls at-risk for obesity. *Int J Eat Disord.* 2010;43(8):701–706.

119. Brownley KA, Peat CM, La Via M, Bulik CM. Pharmacological approaches to the management of binge eating disorder. *Drugs.* 2015;75(1):9–32.

120. Bardone-Cone AM, Harney MB, Maldonado CR, et al. Defining recovery from an eating disorder: conceptualization, validation, and examination of psychosocial functioning and psychiatric comorbidity. *Behav Res Ther.* 2010;48(3):194–202.

CHAPTER 8

Childhood Stress and Trauma

STEPHEN DIDONATO, PHD, LPC • STEVEN J. BERKOWITZ, MD

INTRODUCTION

Many children presenting with mental health challenges have or are subject to childhood stress and traumatic (CST) experiences. CST increases the risk of developing a range of issues across the life span that affect functioning.[1,2] The most common reasons that children and adolescents are referred to treatment are for disruptive behaviors and attention deficit hyperactivity disorder (ADHD)[3]; in both cases it is highly likely that the problematic behaviors have been caused or exacerbated by CST.[4]

Over the last 20 years and, in part, because of the catastrophe of 9/11, the importance of "trauma" has been recognized as a key factor in the development of psychopathology.[4] More recently, the role of early life stress in the etiology of both mental and physical health issues, as well as the associated biologic mechanisms and related brain changes, has been elucidated.[5,6] The term "trauma" has now become part of our daily language. Systems and organizations are implementing "trauma-informed" models and, in popular parlance, "traumatizing" and "upsetting" have become interchangeable. Although the increased recognition of trauma and stress and its ubiquity is undoubtedly a positive development, there are inherent dilemmas for the field in integrating new knowledge and concepts into practice.

This chapter offers providers across child-serving disciplines with a comprehensive framework that, we think, supports more effective assessment and treatment of childhood psychiatric disorders. Its goals are to (1) elaborate and clarify the meaning of CST, (2) establish a common language, (3) enhance providers' understanding of the association between CST and psychopathology, and (4) provide current best practices on assessment and treatment of CST.

CLARIFICATIONS

As the correlation between various negative childhood experiences and changes in neurophysiology, brain structure and related psychiatric issues are clarified; the meaning of "Trauma" requires a corresponding clarification. Our growing understanding has led to disparate and confusing language. Perhaps the first confusion is the shorthand use of a "Trauma" to signify an upsetting event rather than the symptomatic reaction to an event. In an attempt to alleviate some of this confusion, we will refer to the traumatic event as trauma and the symptomatic response to the event as TRAUMA. Further inadvertent confusion has been caused by terminology used to distinguish CST from a single-event TRAUMA. Terms such as adverse childhood experiences (ACEs), toxic stress, and early life stress are used both interchangeably with trauma and as an attempt to be more precise in discussing CST. Unfortunately, the manner in which these terms are used further confuses our communications. Youth exposed to CST may not only develop traumatic stress symptoms and post-traumatic stress disorder (PTSD) but also present with a range of emotional and behavioral issues; diagnoses such as complex PTSD, complex trauma, and developmental trauma disorder[7,8] were proposed in an attempt to capture individuals' heterogeneous symptom presentations. The complexity of CST-induced symptomatology makes it imperative that the field clarifies its terminology to avoid continued confusion and miscommunication.

PATHOPHYSIOLOGY: THE INJURY PARADIGM

TRAUMA is an ancient Greek word for wound or injury; injuries may be caused by a single event or by repetitive insults to one's body. Injuries are on a spectrum from minor with minimal or no impact and of brief duration (even minutes) to severe and causing profound functional problems and lifelong duration. Conceiving of TRAUMA as injury allows us to understand psychologic TRAUMA as caused by a range of negative experiences with a range of outcomes. With this in mind, psychologic TRAUMA may be best defined as an experience or a series of experiences that cause changes (injury) to neurophysiology and potentially to brain structure, resulting in dysregulation of psychologic, cognitive, and behavioral functioning.

An injury model incorporates the notion that most injuries do not cause lasting damage and physical dysfunction and that most people return to baseline functioning while recognizing that they suffered some form of injury. Similarly, in most cases of psychologic TRAUMA, individuals, after brief symptomatology, return to baseline functioning after a stressful event. Yet despite transient symptoms, we disregard that any injury, however minor, has occurred. Conceptualizing TRAUMA as an injury places natural recovery into a dimensional and consistent framework.

In medicine, an injury or illness demonstrates a change to a specific structure(s) in the human body that may be considered damaging or benign. These changes may occur in an individual's molecular structure (e.g., epigenetic methylation, DNA mutations), musculoskeletal system (e.g., fractures, changes in bone density, muscle tone), integumentary system (e.g., melanoma, hives), or central nervous system (e.g., head trauma, stroke, cortical thinning).

By viewing CST within an injury paradigm, the various terms to describe experiences that cause symptoms and impairment may all be considered TRAUMA. This conceptualization ameliorates the current confusion and unifies the varied methodologies used to describe the multitude of stressful experiences and resulting symptoms and impairment. Neuroscience research has now confirmed through molecular investigation and brain imaging that the CST leading to psychopathology or a single-incident event leading to PTSD is caused by injury to neurophysiology such as hypothalamic-pituitary-adrenal axis dysregulation, genes via epigenetic mechanisms (e.g., methylation/demethylation, telomeric shortening), and brain structure through multiple pathways.[9,10]

Tables 8.1 and 8.2 explicate our trauma paradigm along a spectrum by comparing physical injuries to psychologic injuries and offer examples to illustrate the similarities between these injuries, which support the injury model for psychologic TRAUMA. The comparison between a single-incident physical injury and a psychologic injury such as a motor vehicle crash (MVC) should be fairly evident. After an MVC, one can have a range of physical symptomatic responses from a minor (abrasion) requiring no intervention to a severe (internal bleeding) injury requiring intensive and multiple interventions. Similarly the time course can be brief to lifelong in some instances.

Chronic physical injuries are more complex. Perhaps the best example of a chronic injury is a stress fracture where the individual does an activity that puts continuous physical strain on bone, resulting in a fracture.

TABLE 8.1
Single-Incident Trauma: Motor Vehicle Crash

Injury Type	Intervention/Treatment	Period to Recovery
Abrasion	Natural recovery	Days
Knee sprain	Ice, brace, analgesia	Several weeks
Simple fracture	Casting, analgesia	Many weeks/months
Organ laceration/internal bleeding	Surgery, rehabilitation, analgesia	Months or longer
Psychologic Injury	**Intervention/Treatment**	**Period to Recovery**
Irritability, anxiety	None	Days
Above and hypervigilance, intrusive thoughts	Support from family/friends	Several weeks
Partial PTSD	Brief counseling	Many weeks/months
DSM-5 PTSD	Psychotherapy, medications, possible inpatient hospitalization	Months or longer

DSM, Diagnostic and Statistical Manual of Mental Disorder; *PTSD*, posttraumatic stress disorder.

However, CST rarely involves one type of negative experience, but typically there are multiple types that covary with experiences as described in Table 8.2. The potentially injurious physical experiences mentioned in the table are more analogous to CST and frequently covary and may cause damage at the genetic, physiologic, and, ultimately, structural level. Again, a minor injury in which there may be no obvious sequelae may heal without intervention for both physical and psychologic issues but may ultimately result in a range of injury severity, intervention need, and time course.

STRESS-RELATED DIAGNOSES
Posttraumatic Stress Disorder Changes in *Diagnostic and Statistical Manual of Mental Disorder-5*

Perhaps most important to the changes in the diagnosis of PTSD from the *Diagnostic and Statistical Manual of Mental Disorder* (*DSM-IV*) to *DSM-5* was the addition of the *TRAUMA and Stress-Related Disorders* to the *DSM*. The *DSM-5* became more child sensitive with the addition of criteria for *Preschool Children, 6 years old*

TABLE 8.2
Chronic Stress and Trauma

Injury Type: Multiple (e.g., Smoking, SUD, Little Exercise)	Intervention/ Treatment	Period to Recovery
No negative effects	Natural recovery	None
Pneumonia	Medications, antibiotics	Several weeks
Obesity, lung disease	Diet, exercise, medication, oxygen	Months/ years
Cancer, CVD	Surgery, chemo-therapy, rehabilita-tion, analgesia, medications	Years
Psychologic Injury: Multiple (e.g., Sexual Abuse, IPV, Poverty, Physical Abuse)	**Intervention/ Treatment**	**Period to Recovery**
Irritability, anxiety, moodiness	Natural recovery	Days, weeks
Above and hyper-vigilance, intrusive thoughts, depressed mood, irritability, substance use, oppositionality	Support from family/friends, child protective services, counseling	Months
Above, partial PTSD, antisocial behavior, obesity, learning disorders, SUD	Counseling, medication	Months, years
PTSD, self-injurious behavior, promiscu-ity, suicide attempts, CVD, lung disease	Psychotherapy, medications, possible inpatient hospitalization	Years, decades

CVD, cardiovascular disease; IPV, intimate partner violence; PTSD, posttraumatic stress symptoms; SUD, substance use disorder.

or younger, based on the research demonstrating that PTSD in children can occur as early as 1 year old. Parental (caregiver) and child-related losses were added as a primary type of trauma that may lead to symptoms of PTSD.[11] In addition, the type and number of symptoms required have been modified consistent with greater focus on behavioral manifestations that are commonly seen in traumatized children.[12] *See the DSM-5 for a full set of the PTSD criterion.*[11]

Clinical research indicated that a change was needed in the *DSM* to Criterion A of the diagnosis of PTSD in young children to better account for the types of trauma children are exposed to and the responses seen in young children. Studies have shown that an alternative algorithm to account for the diagnosis of PTSD in young children exposed to trauma showed an increase of 10%–26%.[13,14] Proposals were made for the inclusion of diagnoses in the *DSM-5* to address the broad range symptoms caused by CST in childhood (e.g., developmental trauma disorder [DTD]),[15] which expand traumatic disorders to include more than PTSD. Although these proposed diagnoses were not included in the *DSM-5*, the *DSM-5* includes a greater emphasis on cognitive and mood issues in Criterion D, as well as the preschool and dissociative subtype.[11] Although the *DSM-5* has specific considerations for preschool children, many of which may be present in older children, it does not account for the complexity of presentations resulting from the interaction of development with CST in children, adolescents, and adults.[15]

Diagnostic Dilemmas—Trauma Syndrome Continuum

When children are exposed to CST, posttraumatic stress symptoms (PTSSs) are a common response; however, these symptoms do not necessarily lead to acute stress disorder or PTSD diagnosis. Children exposed to CST are often diagnosed with other DSM diagnoses.[4] There are numerous factors that contribute to missing the impact of CST when evaluating children, including (1) obstacles to obtaining child CST history, (2) lack of recognition of these experiences by the caregiver/adults (e.g., parents, teachers, healthcare providers) and the deleterious effects of negative experience in the etiology of emotional disturbances, (3) cultural factors, and (4) limitations of the *DSM*.

When children are exposed to overwhelming stress, both the sympathetic nervous system (SNS) (hyperarousal—anxiety, panic, restlessness, hostility) and parasympathetic nervous system (PNS) (hypoarousal—depression, lethargy, chronic fatigue, poor digestion) may be dysregulated. Depending on the most prominent symptomatology, one might see the SNS or PNS as being predominantly dysregulated. This has been referred to as the *Window of Tolerance* model.[16]

The Window of Tolerance model is consistent with the findings that disorders related to CST manifest not only as PTSD but also as diagnoses consistent with disruptive behaviors (e.g., disruptive mood dysregulation disorder [DMDD], ADHD, and oppositional defiant disorder [ODD]), mood issues (e.g., depression and anxiety), learning disorders, and other common childhood psychiatric disorders.[4,16] This approach provides a conceptual foundation for the recognition that a significant percentage of common childhood psychiatric disorders may be caused by and/or greatly exacerbated by exposure to CST. For example, ADHD symptomatology may be the consequence of exposure to CST as hyperarousal, whereas depression symptomatology may be understood as hypoarousal. Temper outbursts and mood lability or irritability in a child may be diagnosed as DMDD, but the etiology may be due to exposure to CST.[12] Identifying and recognizing the impact of CST and incorporating it into formulations of children exposed to CST can be quite intricate and take significant time. But recognizing that CST can cause or contribute to multiple psychiatric symptoms and DSM disorders will aid clinicians in developing more comprehensive, effective, and accurate treatment plans.

Complex Trauma

Complex trauma has become a designation to describe people who have endured CST and have heterogeneous symptoms as a result.[8] The term complex trauma is used to describe the "dual problem" of children's exposure to multiple traumatic events (trauma) and the impact of this exposure (TRAUMA) on immediate and long-term outcomes, generating multiple sequelae that add to the diagnostic complexity previously discussed.[17]

Utilizing complex trauma as a framework allows providers to fully understand the origin and maintenance factors of a child's clinical concerns: for example, a child who has witnessed his/her father abusing his/her mother for a prolonged period and has endured cooccurring exposures such as emotional and physical abuse and parental substance abuse. Additionally, the same child is likely to have additional external stressors in his/her life such as poverty and community violence. Many children referred for treatment are subjected to these stressors and/or are currently experiencing stressors that may not be identified as the "index" event that affect the child's physical, emotional, relational, and academic well-being.[4,18] Taking these stressors into account is essential to making appropriate treatment/care decisions.

Complex TRAUMA helps to explain those children who are frequently diagnosed with multiple disorders as the affected domains manifest as symptom criteria and related features that overlap. Table 8.3 displays examples of the various domains and potential sequelae associated with complex TRAUMA exposure.[7,18–25]

TABLE 8.3
Complex TRAUMA Sequelae

Domain	Sequelae
Development	Language delays
Attachment	Disorganized or ambivalent attachment; uncertainty about the world; difficulty attuning to other people's emotional states
Relational	Development and maintenance of relationships
Biologic	Neurologic delays; inability to regulate ANS; sensorimotor developmental problems
Cognitive	Attention and executive functioning difficulties; learning difficulties; and difficulty planning and anticipating
Behavioral	Externalized behaviors (i.e., physical aggression, oppositional behaviors) and internalized behaviors (i.e., isolation); and sleep disturbances
Emotional	Attuning to other's emotional state
Behavioral	Increase in juvenile justice encounters
Psychopathology	Depression, anxiety, PTSD, substance use, suicide
Affect regulation	Difficulty with self-regulation; difficulty labeling, and expressing feelings
Self-concept	Disturbances of body image; low self-esteem

ANS, autonomic nervous system; *PTSD*, posttraumatic stress disorder.

PREVALENCE AND EPIDEMIOLOGY

The ACE Study demonstrated that CST has negative impacts on health and importantly showed that CST is common during childhood. The study was conducted in a predominantly white and economically secure sample, but 26% of the sample experienced one ACE and 12.5% experienced four or more ACEs (see CDC website for more information).[1] The Urban ACE Study in Philadelphia expanded on the original study to add indicators that are prevalent in urban communities (being bullied, witnessing violence, experiencing racism, feeling unsafe in one's neighborhood, and lived in foster care). In the Philadelphia Urban ACE Study, 37.5% of the sample experienced four or more ACEs, a significant increase from the original study (see http://

TABLE 8.4
Original ACE Study Versus Philadelphia Urban ACE Survey

ACE Indicator	Original ACE Study (%)	Philadelphia Urban ACE Study (%)
Emotional abuse	10.6	33.2
Physical abuse	28.3	35.0
Sexual abuse	20.7	16.2
Physical neglect	14.8	19.1
Emotional neglect	9.9	7.7
Substance-abusing household member	26.9	34.8
Mentally ill household member	19.4	24.1
Witnessing domestic violence	12.7	17.9
Household member in prison	4.7	12.9

Philadelphia Urban ACE Indicator	Prevalence (%)
Witnessed violence	40.5
Felt discrimination	34.5
Felt unsafe in neighborhood	27.3
Bullied	7.9
Lived in foster care	2.5

ACE, adverse childhood experience.

TABLE 8.5
Childhood Prevalence of Mental Health Disorders

Diagnosis	Specifier	Prevalence (%)
PTSD	Adolescents[a]	5
ADHD	Youth aged 4–17 years[a]	11
Mood disorders (any type)	Children[a]	3.7
Depression	Adolescents[b]	12.5
Any anxiety disorder	Adolescents[a]	25.1
ODD	Children and adolescents[a]	Range of 1–16
Conduct disorder	Children and adolescents[a]	3.5
Separation anxiety	Children	4.1

[a]Lifetime.
[b]Past month.
ADHD, attention deficit hyperactivity disorder; *ODD*, oppositional defiant disorder; *PTSD*, posttraumatic stress disorder.

www.instituteforsafefamilies.org/philadelphia-urban-ace-study).[1,2] Table 8.4 compares the prevalence between the original ACE and Philadelphia Urban ACE Studies and data of the additional adverse experiences from the Philadelphia study.[1,2]

In a study in North Carolina, more than 68% of children and adolescents had experienced a potentially traumatic event by the age of 16 years.[26] Finkelhor and colleagues[27] found in a national survey that 80% of youth aged 2–17 years experienced at least 1 type of trauma during their lifetime, with a lifetime exposure average of 3.7 types of trauma. Within a single year, 22% of youth (2–17 years old) were exposed to four or more types of trauma and 10% of youth suffered seven or more types of trauma.[27] Typical contextual factors that lead to increased trauma are unsafe neighborhoods, distressed and/or chaotic families, preexisting personal or family

psychologic conditions, and living within a violent family.[28] One needs to consider early life stressors within the conceptualization of TRAUMA in children and adolescents.

This chapter has discussed the diagnostic dilemmas when incorporating CST as a factor using our current nosology. Although some children who experience CST meet the criterion for PTSD, even with the current *Preschool Children, 6 years old or younger*, this conceptualization is narrow, as PTSD, as it stands, does not necessarily capture the inherently complex nature of TRAUMA in children.[18,29] As previously discussed, when children experience CST, their responses may fall at varying places on a "trauma syndrome continuum." Table 8.5 represents prevalence rates for some of the mental health diagnosis that have been correlated with childhood trauma exposure.[3,30–36]

PREVENTION

To address the prevention of trauma and TRAUMA, providers must engage in a multilevel prevention effort to support the child such as primary prevention efforts such as effective parenting education or the need for early identification to apply secondary prevention.

There are also community-level strategies for primary prevention such as increasing connectedness or increasing employment opportunities or primary prevention in schools such as improving school climate with trauma-sensitive approaches.[37]

Engaging caregivers in parenting and family programs to increase caregiver self-efficacy and capacity to support their child's TRAUMA (e.g., Triple-P, Incredible Years)[38,39] is one primary prevention strategy. Other primary prevention strategies include nurse-family partnerships, to increase the mother's attachment to the child and the mother's (and child's) healthy behaviors.[40] Secondary prevention efforts have been shown efficacious in reducing the child's symptoms posttrauma. An example is the Child and Family Traumatic Stress Intervention (CFTSI),[41] which is a secondary prevention intervention that aims to reduce the development of PTSD posttrauma. CFTSI, conducted within the first month posttrauma, improved family support through enhancing the communication between the child and primary caregiver and also increased the awareness of the caregiver to better understand the child's TRAUMA.[41] Sustaining prevention programs is contingent on communities and schools having the resources needed to support their children and families through increased access to care, employment, and social services, as well as the awareness of the impact of trauma on how children develop, learn, and socialize (i.e., trauma-informed training).[42]

CONCEPTUALIZING TRAUMA AND THE CLINICAL WORKUP

CST plays a pivotal role not only in understanding of the etiology and epidemiology of medical, behavioral, emotional, academic, and other concerns but also in the treatment process. Any diagnostic assessment should include an assessment of TRAUMA and a comprehensive developmental history, including a psychosocial evaluation of stress and trauma exposure. Assessing a child's (and family's) functioning is useful to assess a child's prognosis. This may be accomplished by evaluating his/her current and previous coping skills and strengths, as well as his/her current supports. Understanding a child's (and family's) capacity to deal with stressful situations is a way to immediately engage in a strength-based approach that empowers him/her (and families) and builds rapport to increase the efficacy of more formalized processes.

Trauma Assessment

Formalized trauma assessments should begin with structured screening processes, which allow for a broad range understanding of the child's current functioning, behaviors, and presenting TRAUMA symptoms. Initial attention should be paid to symptoms that the child is currently exhibiting, such as nightmares ("Do you have bad dreams?"), intrusive thoughts ("Do you have thoughts or pictures come into your head that you don't like?"), changes in mood ("Do you feel alone and not close to people?"), and other changes in social functioning. When providers have evidence that a child is dealing CST and the child is avoiding, providers should be transparent in what has been learned from the referral (or other) sources.

At the core of all evidence-based trauma practices are (1) engagement with the child (and family), (2) risk screening, (3) triage to a determined level of care, and (4) a tailored assessment(s).[43–45] Scales to assess children should assess more than trauma history and/or TRAUMA symptoms, looking to see if children meet the criterion of PTSD, but should include an assessment of complex TRAUMA domains (as per Complex Trauma section).[7]

The clinician-administered PTSD Scale (CAPS)[46] continues to be the gold standard of PTSD assessments in the field of trauma. A child and adolescent version of the CAPS (CAPS-CA-5) has been developed for the criterion of PTSD in the *DSM-5*.[47] Table 8.6 identifies additional assessment measures for trauma history and TRAUMA symptoms, and other domains and contextual factors identified throughout this chapter.

TREATMENT

Treatment of traumatized children requires a multimodal approach that goes beyond evidence-based practices (EBPs) for PTSD. The National Child Traumatic Stress Network identified the following core components to evidence-based trauma treatments: (1) engagement, (2) psychoeducation, (3) emotional regulation, (4) promoting positive adjustment, (5) parenting skills, (6) trauma narrative, and (7) promoting safety.[43] In addition, a 2013 review of the core components to childhood trauma treatments found other areas of focus: (1) attachment and strengthening relationships, (2) attention to social context, and (3) posttrauma growth.[44] These components are at the core of effective treatments for a wide range of children who have experienced CST.

TABLE 8.6
CST Assessment Measures

Domain	Measure	Target
Trauma symptoms	Clinician-Administered PTSD Scale for *DSM-5*—Child/Adolescent Version[47]	≥7 years old
	Child PTSD Symptom Scale-Interview for *DSM-5*[48,49]	
	Trauma Symptom Checklist for Children[50]	8–16 years old
	Trauma Symptom Checklist for Young Children[51]	3–12 years old
	UCLA PTSD Reaction Index[52,53]	7–17 years old; Parent version
Trauma history	Traumatic Events Screening Inventory—Self-Report Revised[54] Traumatic Events Screening Inventory—Parent Report Revised[55]	3–17 years old
	Childhood Trauma Questionnaire—Short Form[56]	>12 years old
Bereavement	Persistent Complex Bereavement Disorder Checklist[57]	8–18 years old
Dissociation	Child Dissociative Checklist[58]	5–12 years old
	Adolescent Dissociative Experiences Scale[59]	11–18 years old
General/broad overview	Behavior Assessment System for Children (teacher, parent, self-report)[60]	Child, adolescent versions
	Ages and Stages Questionnaire[61]	6–60 months
Developmental milestones and profiles	CARE Index Infancy CARE Index Toddler[62]	From birth to ~16 months ~16 months–6 years old
Attachment	School-Aged Assessment of Attachment[63]	6–13 years old
	Attachment Interview for Children and Adolescents[64]	10–16 years old

The authors of this chapter do not endorse any specific assessment measures listed above. *PTSD*, posttraumatic stress disorder; *UCLA PTSD*, the University of California at Los Angeles posttraumatic stress disorder.

Making the decision on the "best" EBP for a child should be developed through trauma-informed assessments, review of appropriate EBPs (see http://nctsn.org/training-guidelines for EBP fact sheets),[43] and providers' clinical acumen. In addition, throughout treatment, therapists should monitor the child's (and family's) progress and ensure the chosen treatment is most efficacious for the child (and family).[43] Although Trauma-Focused Cognitive Behavior Therapy has the strongest empiric base among child trauma–focused EBPs,[65] other child trauma treatments that have shown efficacy in treating TRAUMA domains, such as affective, behavioral, cognitive, and relational dysregulation, include Cognitive Behavioral Interventions for Trauma in Schools, Structured Psychotherapy for Adolescents Responding to Chronic Stress, and Child-Parent Psychotherapy.[65] Flexible treatment models that are highly tailored to the child (and family) are called for to effectively treat complex TRAUMA.[45,66,67] For example, the Attachment, Regulation and Competency (ARC) framework aims to enhance/secure the child's *attachment*, help to develop and nurture *self-regulation* skills, and increase *competencies* across the child's lived domains.[66] An aspect that is not always part of the core components to treating children (and families) who have endured CST is therapist self-care. Ensuring that self-care is in place for clinicians and providers working with this population is imperative to increasing treatment efficacy.[44]

Pharmacology

The pharmacologic treatment of trauma and stress-related disorders require a symptom-based approach, as there is no one medication that effectively treats PTSD, PTSS, or complex TRAUMA. However, in all cases, medication should only be used in conjunction with psychosocial treatments. At present, medications should be used to treat the impairing symptoms whether alone or in combination. For instance, selective serotonin reuptake inhibitors such as fluoxetine are the first line for depression and anxiety symptomology; however, there is some evidence that suggests they tend to be less effective in TRAUMA-induced symptoms than in classic depression and anxiety disorders.[68]

There is some evidence for the use of second-generation antipsychotics for hyperarousal symptoms. They have often used in cases of aggressive behavior and extreme mood dysregulation; however, given the side effects of obesity and metabolic syndrome, they should be used rarely and only for short term if deemed necessary.[69]

A safer and perhaps more effective option for hyperarousal symptoms are α-1 agonists such as prazosin and clonidine and the α-2 agonist guanfacine. Clonidine is especially sedating, but both α-1 agonists are excellent at decreasing nightmares and have shown positive effects on other hyperarousal symptoms and anxiety.[70–72] Treating nightmares may be especially important as they may a key symptom in the maintenance of other TRAUMA symptomatology and impairment.[73] Guanfacine has demonstrated effectiveness in the treatment of ADHD-related behaviors and may help with irritability, aggression, and impulsivity associated with TRAUMA.[70]

Lastly, the mood stabilizers carbamazepine and divalproex have demonstrated efficacy in PTSS in a few studies.[70] However, the difficulty of maintaining a therapeutic window with the need for frequent blood work during initiation makes the use of these medications difficult in highly impaired population.[74]

CONCLUDING CLINICAL PEARLS

In concluding this chapter, clinical pearls are offered for providers to consider when engaging with children and families in their practice. These clinical pearls are intended to provide clinicians with a short list of points to refer to when conceptualizing and treating CST.

- Consider CST and traumatic reactions when there has been a sudden change in behavior, disruptive behaviors, anxious and depressive symptoms especially in prepubescents, and when children present with vague and chronic pain.
- Conceptualizing CST through an injury model allows clinicians to make informed treatment decisions based on injury severity and also potential time course to healing (see Tables 8.1 and 8.2).
- Providers must engage in multilevel prevention efforts:
  - Primary—effective parenting education (Triple-P) or community-level strategies (improving school climate with trauma-sensitive approaches);
  - Secondary–reduction of the development of PTSD (e.g., CFTSI).
- Formalized assessment should begin with structured screening process—broad range understanding of current functioning, behaviors, and TRAUMA symptoms.
  - Ensuring that clinical conceptualizations are not limited to more overt psychopathology such as ADHD, ODD, and anxiety.
- Assessment should include assessment of TRAUMA, comprehensive developmental history, child and family functioning, child and family capacity to cope with stressful events (current and previous coping skills and strengths and current supports).
- Formalized trauma-informed assessments should be tailored to each child and family[43–45] (see Table 8.6 for a list of measures).
- Trauma-informed assessments should drive the decision-making for the optimal EBP for each child. All treatments should focus on (1) attachment and strengthening relationships, (2) attention to social context, and (3) posttrauma growth.[44]
  - See http://nctsn.org/training-guidelines for EBP fact sheets.
  - Similar to assessment, treatment models need to be flexible and tailored to the child and family to effectively treat the complexity of TRAUMA (e.g., ARC framework).
- When it comes to pharmacologic treatments, only prazosin and clonidine seem be useful, especially with sleep disturbances and nightmares. Other medications can be used to target specific symptoms. However, they are generally less effective for traumatized individuals.

REFERENCES

1. Felitti VJ, Anda RF, Nordenberg D, et al. Relationship of childhood abuse and household dysfunction to many of the leading causes of death in adults. *Am J Prev Med.* 1998;14(4):245–258. PMID:9635069.
2. Public Health Management Corporation. Findings from the Philadelphia Urban ACE Survey 2013. http://www.instituteforsafefamilies.org/sites/default/files/isfFiles/Philadelphia%20Urban%20ACE%20Report%202013.pdf.
3. Merikangas KR, He J, Burstein M, et al. Lifetime prevalence of mental disorders in the U.S. adolescent comorbidity survey replication-adolescent supplement. *J Am Acad Child Adolesc Psychiatry.* 2010;49(10):980–988. PMC2946114.
4. D'Andrea W, Ford J, Stolbach B, Spinazzola J, van der Kolk B. Understanding interpersonal trauma in children: why we need a developmentally appropriate trauma diagnosis. *Am J Orthopsychiatry.* 2012;82(2):187–200. https://doi.org/10.1111/j.1939-0025.2012.01154.x.

5. Heim C, Newport DJ, Mletzko T, Miller AH, Nemeroff CB. The link between childhood trauma and depression: insights from HPA axis studies in humans. *Psychoneuroendocrinology*. 2008;33:693–710. https://doi.org/10.1016/j.psyneuen.2008.03.008.

6. Faravelli C, Lo Sauro C, Lelli L, et al. The role of life events and HPA axis in anxiety disorders: a review. *Curr Pharm Des*. 2012;18(35). https://doi.org/10.2174/138161212803530907.

7. Cook A, Spinazzola J, Ford J, et al. Complex trauma in children and adolescents. *Psychiatr Ann*. 2005;35(5):390–398.

8. van der Kolk BA. Developmental trauma disorder: toward a rational diagnosis for children with complex trauma disorders. *Psychiatr Ann*. 2005;35(5):401–408.

9. Lucassen PJ, Pruessner J, Sousa N, et al. Neuropathology of stress. *Acta Neuropath*. 2014;127:109–135. https://doi.org/10.1007/s00401-013-1223-5.

10. Szyf M, Bick J. DNA methylation: a mechanism for embedding early life experiences in the genome. *Child Dev*. 2013;84(1):49–57. https://doi.org/10.1111/j.1467-8624.2012.01793.x.

11. American Psychiatric Association. *Diagnostic and Statistical Manual of Mental Disorders: DSM-5*. Washington, DC: American Psychiatric Association; 2013.

12. Substance Abuse and Mental Health Services Administration. *DSM 5 Changes: Implications for Child Serious Emotional Disturbance*; 2013. https://www.samhsa.gov/data/sites/default/files/NSDUH-DSM5ImpactChildSED-2016.pdf.

13. Scheeringa MS, Zeanah CH, Cohen JA. PTSD in children and adolescents: toward an empirically based algorithm. *Depress Anxiety*. 2011;28:770–782. https://doi.org/10.1002/da.20736.

14. Scheeringa MS, Zeanah CH, Myers L, Putnam FW. New findings on alternative criteria for PTSD in preschool children. *J Am Acad Child Adolesc Psychiatry*. 2003;42(5):561–570. https://doi.org/10.1097/01.CHI.0000046822.95464.14.

15. van der Kolk BA, Pynoos RS, et al. Proposal to Include a Developmental Trauma Disorder Diagnosis for Children and Adolescents in DSM-V. http://www.traumacenter.org/announcements/dtd_papers_oct_09.pdf.

16. Corrigan FM, Fisher JJ, Nutt DJ. Autonomic dysregulation and the Window of Tolerance model of the effects of complex emotional trauma. *J Psychopharmacol*. 2010:1–9. https://doi.org/10.1177/0269881109354930.

17. Complex Trauma. http://www.nctsn.org/trauma-types/complex-trauma.

18. Cook A, Blaustein M, Spinazzola J, van der Kolk BA. Complex Trauma in Children and Adolescents. http://www.nctsnet.org/nctsn_assets/pdfs/edu_materials/ComplexTrauma_All.pdf.

19. Substance Abuse and Mental Health Services Administration, U.S. Department of Health and Human Services. http://www.samhsa.gov/children/social_media_apr2011.asp.

20. Thomas D, Leicht C, Hughes C, Madigan A, Dowell K. Emerging practices in the prevention of child abuse and neglect. *Off Child Abuse Negl*. 2015. https://www.childwelfare.gov/pubPDFs/report.pdf.

21. Centers for Disease Control and Prevention, National Center for Injury Prevention and Control. Understanding Child Maltreatment: Fact Sheet 2014. https://www.cdc.gov/violenceprevention/pdf/understanding-cm-factsheet.pdf.

22. Perry BD. Neurobiological sequelae of childhood trauma: post traumatic stress disorders in children. In: Murburg M, ed. *Catecholamine Function in PostTraumatic Stress Disorder: Emerging Concepts*. Washington, DC: American Psychiatric Press; 1994:253–276.

23. Noll JG, Trickett PK, Putnam FW. A prospective investigation of the impact of child sexual abuse on the development of sexuality. *J Consult Clin Psychol*. 2003;71:575–586. PMID:12795580.

24. Broman-Fulks JJ, Ruggiero KJ, Hanson RF, et al. Sexual assault disclosure in relation to adolescent mental health: results from the National Survey of Adolescents. *J Clin Child Adolesc Psychol*. 2007;36:260–266. PMID:17484698.

25. Treisman T. *Working with Relational and Developmental Trauma in Children and Adolescents*. 1st ed. New York, NY: Routledge; 2017.

26. Copeland WE, Keeler G, Angold A, Costello EJ. Traumatic events and posttraumatic stress in childhood. *Arch Gen Psychiatry*. 2007;64(5):577–584. https://doi.org/10.1001/archpsyc.64.5.577.

27. Finkelhor D, Ormrod RK, Turner HA. Lifetime assessment of poly-victimization in a national sample of children and youth. *Child Abuse Negl*. 2009;33:403–411. https://doi.org/10.1016/j.chiabu.2008.09.012.

28. U.S. Department of Justice. 2015 National Crime Victims' Rights Week Resource Guide. https://www.ncjrs.gov/ovc_archives/ncvrw/2015/pdf/FullGuide.pdf.

29. NCTSN Core Curriculum on Childhood Trauma Task Force. The 12 Core Concepts: Concepts for Understanding Traumatic Stress Responses in Children and Families. Core Curriculum on Childhood Trauma 2012. Los Angeles, CA, and Durham, NC: UCLA-Duke University National Center for Child Traumatic Stress.

30. Center for Disease Control. Attention-Deficit Hyperactivity Disorder. https://www.cdc.gov/ncbddd/adhd/data.html. Updated July 18, 2017.

31. National Institute of Mental Health. Major Depression Among Adolescents. https://www.nimh.nih.gov/health/statistics/prevalence/major-depression-among-adolescents.shtml.

32. Loeber R, Burke JD, Lahey BB, Winters A, Zera M. Oppositional defiant and conduct disorder: a review of the past 10 years, part I. *J Am Acad Child Adolesc Psychiatry*. 2000;39:468–1484. https://doi.org/10.1097/00004583-200012000-00007.

33. Perou R, Bitsko RH, Blumberg SJ, et al. Mental health surveillance among children: United States 2005-2011. *Supplements*. 2013;62(02):1–35. https://www.cdc.gov/mmwr/preview/mmwrhtml/su6202a1.htm.

34. National Institute of Mental Health. Any Mood Disorder in Children 2015. https://www.nimh.nih.gov/health/statistics/prevalence/any-mood-disorder-in-children.shtml.

35. National Institute of Mental Health. Any Anxiety Disorder Among Children 2015. https://www.nimh.nih.gov/health/statistics/prevalence/any-anxiety-disorder-among-children.shtml.

36. Masi G, Mucci M, Millepiedi S. Separation anxiety disorder in children and adolescents: epidemiology, diagnosis and management. *CNS Drugs*. 2001;15:93–104. PMID:11460893.

37. Child Welfare Information Gateway. Framework for Prevention of Child Maltreatment. https://www.childwelfare.gov/topics/preventing/overview/framework/.

38. MacMillan HL, Wathers CN, Barlow J, et al. Interventions to prevent child maltreatment and associated impairment. *Lancet*. 2009;373:250–266. https://doi.org/10.1016/S0140-6736(08)61708-0.

39. Barth RP. Preventing child abuse and neglect with parent training: evidence and opportunities. *The Future Child*. 2009;19(2):95–118.

40. Olds DL. Preventing child maltreatment and crime with prenatal and infancy support of parents: the nurse-family partnership. *J Scand Stud Criminol Crime Prev*. 2008;9(S1): 2–24. https://doi.org/10.1080/14043850802450096.

41. Berkowitz SJ, Stover CS, Marans SR. The child and family traumatic stress intervention: secondary prevention for youth at risk for developing PTSD. *J Child Psychol Psychiatry*. 2011;52(6):676–685. https://doi.org/10.1111/j.1469-7610.2010.02321.x.

42. Ko SJ, Ford JD, Kassam-Adams N, et al. Creating trauma-informed systems: child welfare, education, first responders, health care, juvenile justice. *Prof Psychol Res Pr*. 2008;39(4):396–404. https://doi.org/10.1037/0735-7028.39.4.396.

43. National Child Traumatic Stress Network. National Child Traumatic Stress Network Empirically Supported Treatments and Promising Practices. http://nctsn.org/training-guidelines.

44. Strand VC, Hansen S, Courtney D. Common elements across evidence-based trauma treatment: discovery and implications. *Adv Social Work*. 2013;14(2):334–354. https://journals.iupui.edu/index.php/advancesinsocialwork/article/view/3052.

45. Cook JM, Newman E, The New Haven Trauma Competency Group. A consensus statement on trauma mental health: the new haven competency conference process and major findings. *Psychol Trauma*. 2014;6(4):300–307. https://doi.org/10.1037/a0036747.

46. Nader K, Kriegler JA, Blake DD, Pynoos RS, Newman E, Weathers FW. *Clinician-Administered PTSD Scale, Child and Adolescent Version*. White River Junction, VT: National Center for PTSD; 1996. https://www.ptsd.va.gov/professional/assessment/child/caps-ca.asp. Updated March 9, 2018.

47. Pynoos, RS, Weathers, FW, Steinberg, AM, et al. Clinician-Administered PTSD Scale for DSM-5-Child/Adolescent Version. Scale available from: the National Center for PTSD at: www.ptsd.va.go. Updated July 20, 2017.

48. Foa EB, Johnson KM, Feeny NC, Treadwell KRH. The Child PTSD Symptom Scale: a preliminary examination of its psychometric properties. *J Clin Child Adolesc Psychol*. 2001;30:376–384. https://doi.org/10.1207/S15374424JCCP3003_9.

49. Foa EB, Capaldi S. Manual for the Administration and Scoring of the Child Posttraumatic Stress Scale – Interview for DSM-5 (CPSS-I-5). https://www.div12.org/wp-content/uploads/2014/11/CPSS-I-5-Manual.doc.

50. Briere J. *Trauma Symptom Checklist for Children: Professional Manual*. Florida: Psychological Assessment Resources Inc.; 1996.

51. Briere J. *Trauma Symptom Checklist for Young Children: Professional Manual*. Florida: Psychological Assessment Resources Inc.; 2005.

52. Steinberg AM, Brymer MJ, Kim S, et al. Psychometric properties of the UCLA PTSD reaction index: Part 1. *J Trauma Stress*. 2013;26:1–9. https://doi.org/10.1002/jts.21780.

53. U.S. Department of Veterans Affairs. UCLA Child/Adolescent PTSD Reaction Index for DSM-5. https://www.ptsd.va.gov/professional/assessment/child/ucla_child_reaction_dsm-5.asp. Updated July 6, 2017.

54. Ippen CG, Ford J, Racusin R, et al. *Traumatic Events Screening Inventory - Parent Report Revised*; 2002.

55. Ribbe D. Psychometric review of traumatic event screening instrument for children (TESI-C). In: Stamm BH, ed. *Measurement of Stress, Trauma, and Adaptation*. Lutherville, MD: Sidran Press; 1996.

56. Bernstein DP, Stein JA, Newcomb MD, et al. Development and validation of a brief screening version of the childhood trauma questionnaire. *Child Abuse Negl*. 2003;27(2):169–190. PMID:12615092.

57. The Persistent Complex Bereavement Disorder (PCBD) Checklist – Youth Version. http://tdg.ucla.edu/sites/default/files/1-Pager_PCBD_Checklist.pdf.

58. Putnam FW, Helmers K. Development, reliability, and validity of a child dissociation scale. *Child Abuse Negl*. 1993;17(6):731–741. https://doi.org/10.1016/S0145-2134(08)80004-X.

59. Armstrong JG, Putnam FW, Carlson EB, Liebro DZ, Smith SR. Development and validation of a measure of adolescent dissociation: the adolescent dissociative experiences scale. *J Nerv Ment Dis*. 1997;185(8):491–497. PMID:9284862.

60. Reynolds, CR, Kamphaus, RW. *Behavior Assessment System for Children*. 2nd ed. (BASC-2). http://www.pearsonclinical.com/education/products/100000658/behavior-assessment-system-for-children-second-edition-basc-2.html.

61. Squires J, Bricker D, Twombly E. *Ages & Stages Questionnaires: Socio-emotional*. Baltimore, MD: Paul H. Brooks Publishing, Co; 2002. https://clas.uiowa.edu/nrcfcp/sites/clas.uiowa.edu.nrcfcp/files/Ages%20and%20Stages%20Questionnaires%20ASQSE.PDF.

62. Crittendan PM. Using the CARE-Index for Screening, Intervention, and Research. http://www.patcrittenden.com/include/docs/care_index.pdf.

63. Crittendan PW, Kozlowska K, Landini A. Assessing attachment in school-aged children. *Clin Child Psychol Psychiatry.* 2010;15(2). https://doi.org/10.1177/1359104509356741.

64. Ammaniti M, Van Ijzendoorn MH, Speranza AM, Tambelli R. Internal working models of attachment during late childhood and early adolescence: an exploration of stability and change. *Attach Hum Dev.* 2000;2(3):328–346. https://doi.org/10.1080/14616730010001587.

65. Schneider SJ, Grilli SF, Schneider JR. Evidence-based treatments for traumatized children and adolescents. *Curr Psychiatry Rep.* 2013;15:332. https://doi.org/10.1007/s11920-012-0332-5.

66. Ford JD, Blaustein ME, Habib M, Kagan R. Developmental trauma therapy models. In: Ford JD, Courtois CA, eds. *Treating Complex Traumatic Stress Disorders in Children and Adolescents: Scientific Foundations and Therapeutic Models.* New York, NY: The Guildford Press; 2013.

67. Saunders BE, Adams ZW. Epidemiology of traumatic experiences in childhood. *Child Adolesc Psychiatr Clin N Am.* 2014;23(2):167–184. https://doi.org/10.1016/j.chc.2013.12.003.

68. Nanni V, Uher R, Danese A. Childhood maltreatment predicts unfavorable course of illness and treatment outcome in depression: a meta-analysis. *Am J Psychiatry.* 2012;169(2):141–151. PMID:22420036.

69. Meighen KG, Hines LA, Lagges AM. Risperidone treatment of preschool children with thermal burns and acute stress disorder. *J Child Adolesc Psychopharmacol.* 2007;17(2):223–232. https://doi.org/10.1089/cap.2007.0121.

70. Strawn JR, Keeshin BR. Successful treatment of posttraumatic stress disorder with prazosin in a young child. *Ann Pharmacother.* 2011;45(12):1590–1591. https://doi.org/10.1345/aph.1Q548.

71. Boehnlein JK, Kinzie JD. Pharmacologic reduction of CNS noradrenergic activity in PTSD: the case for clonidine and prazosin. *J Psychiatr Pract.* 2007;13(2):72–78. https://doi.org/10.1097/01.pra.0000265763.79753.c1.

72. Strawn JR, DelBello MP, Geracioti Jr TD. Prazosin treatment of an adolescent with posttraumatic stress disorder. *J Child Adolesc Psychopharmacol.* 2009;19(5):599–600. https://doi.org/10.1089/cap.2009.0043.

73. Germain A, Buysse DJ, Nofzinger E. Sleep-specific mechanisms underlying posttraumatic stress disorder: integrative review and neurobiological hypotheses. *Sleep Med Rev.* 2008;12(3):185–195. https://doi.org/10.1016/j.smrv.2007.09.003.

74. Zito JM, Derivan AT, Kratochvil CJ, Safer DJ, Fegert JM, Greenhill LL. Off-label psychopharmacologic prescribing for children: history supports close clinical monitoring. *Child Adolesc Psychiatry Ment Health.* 2008;2(1):24. https://doi.org/10.1186/1753-2000-2-24.

FURTHER READING

1. Cohen JA, Mannarino AP. Psychotherapeutic options for traumatized children. *Curr Opin Pediatr.* 2010;22(5):605–609. https://doi.org/10.1097/MOP.0b013e32833e14a2.

CHAPTER 9

Factitious Disorder Imposed on Another

MICHAEL KELLY, MD • BRENDA BURSCH, PHD

INTRODUCTION

This chapter focuses on a form of psychopathology in a *caregiver* that can severely, sometimes fatally, affect a child. Given the low prevalence of some of the preceding diagnoses reviewed, it is important that professionals are aware that severe psychiatric disorders in childhood are sometimes falsified by their caregivers. Thus, the objectives of this chapter are to review the literature and provide recommendations related to the identification and management of factitious disorder imposed on another (FDIA).

DEFINITION/SYMPTOM CRITERIA

FDIA is a psychiatric diagnosis characterized by an individual using deceptive tactics to falsify illness or impairment in another without obvious external incentives to fully explain the behavior. FDIA is classified within the *somatic symptom and related disorders* category of the *Diagnostic and Statistical Manual of Mental Disorders, Fifth Edition* (*DSM-5*).[1] The actions of people who qualify for this diagnosis can cause substantial suffering, and even death, for their victims. The *DSM-5* describes FDIA as the "falsification of physical or psychological signs or symptoms, or induction of injury or disease, in another, associated with identified deception." To meet full criteria for the disorder, an individual must present "another individual (victim) to others as ill, impaired, or injured." In addition, the deceptive behavior must be "evident even in the absence of obvious external rewards." Furthermore, such behavior cannot be "better explained by another mental disorder, such as delusional disorder or another psychotic disorder." The *DSM-5* includes the specifiers "single episode" and "recurrent episodes," the latter applying to cases involving "two or more events of falsification of illness and/or induction of injury." It is important to note that this diagnosis applies only to the perpetrators of abuse, not their victims.

Abusive illness falsification was first described in the medical literature by the British pediatrician,

Dr Roy Meadow,[2] in his seminal paper entitled "Mu̇nchausen syndrome by proxy: The hinterland of child abuse." The introduction of Dr Meadow's paper includes the following excerpt that does a good job of describing the insidious nature of FDIA:

> *Doctors dealing with young children rely on the parents' recollection of the history. The doctor accepts that history, albeit sometimes with a pinch of salt, and it forms the cornerstone of subsequent investigation and management of the child.*

Although the word "syndrome" has been dropped for the term, Munchausen by proxy, which has never been a formal ICD or DSM diagnosis, remains the most commonly used term to describe abusive illness or condition falsification due to FDIA.[3]

There are several terms that are used to label the child abuse separately from the psychopathology of the abuser. In 1996, a task force created by American Professional Society on the Abuse of Children coined the term "pediatric condition (illness, impairment, or symptom) falsification" to label the child maltreatment in which a caregiver intentionally falsifies physical and/or psychological signs and/or symptoms in a child victim.[4] With a call for increased action and responsibility by pediatricians, Roesler and Jenny[5] advocated that pediatricians use the term "medical child abuse" to describe when a child receives unnecessary and harmful, or potentially harmful, medical care at the instigation of a caretaker. More recently, the American Academy of Pediatrics[6] proposed the term "caregiver-fabricated illness in a child" to describe this type of abuse/neglect of a child victim. Although there are some minor differences among these terms, they all generally refer to the same type of child abuse/neglect. Because it is the most comprehensive term, one that includes presentation of the child to professionals who are not pediatricians (such as mental health clinicians), we will use the term pediatric condition falsification (PCF) to label the abuse throughout this chapter.

EPIDEMIOLOGY

FDIA is often considered to be a rare diagnosis; however, reliable data regarding its incidence and prevalence are limited. This lack of data is due in large part to the deceptive practices that are inherent to FDIA. A 2-year prospective study by McClure and colleagues[7] yielded the estimation that at least 0.5 per 100,000 youths under 16 years of age in the United Kingdom are the victims of abusive condition falsification, nonaccidental poisoning, and/or nonaccidental suffocation, annually. The rate for children under 1 year of age was estimated to be at least 2.8/100,000. The mortality rate among the abused children was 6.25%, and the mother of the victim was the perpetrator in 85% of cases. A study from Italy by Ferrara and colleagues[8] discovered that abuse associated with FDIA was present in 4 out of 751 youth between the ages of 11 months and 16 years, yielding a prevalence of 0.53%. Similar to the studies listed above, the perpetrator of abuse was the child's mother in three out of four cases. Some have viewed FDIA as a problem of modernized Western cultures; however, a review of the literature by Feldman and Brown[9] yielded descriptions of PCF from 24 countries. Congruent with other reports, 86% of the identified cases from this review involved a mother who was the sole perpetrator of abuse.

Although the induction of illness in a victim, such as via poisoning or suffocation, is not a necessary requirement for the diagnosis of FDIA, such behavior is not unusual. In McClure's prospective study, of the 128 identified victims, ~57% included some form of induction.[7] A review of 451 published cases by Sheridan[10] also showed that perpetrators induced illness in roughly 57% of the cases. Furthermore, nearly half of the instances of illness induction occurred during hospital admissions, under the noses of the victims' treatment providers.

Any medical condition can be created, falsified, or exaggerated, and children with genuine medical or psychiatric problems are often targets.[11] Caregivers with FDIA might target all children in their care or serially focus on a subset or one child, such as the youngest child, the child with highest needs, the child with genuine medical or psychiatric problems, or the child with whom they have a disrupted attachment. Intergenerational abuse of this type can be a contributing factor.

ETIOLOGY

A common hypothesis regarding origins of FDIA is that it is born out of childhoods beset by abuse and/or neglect. Some have offered explanations based on psychodynamic thinking wherein abusers with factitious disorders attempt to reenact earlier forms of abuse or neglect, on themselves and/or others, as a means of reliving and correcting disruptions in childhood attachment. Such a perspective on the origin of factitious disorders is summarized succinctly by R.J. Carlson[12] who wrote, "The fabrication of symptoms may serve as a mechanism whereby these individuals can temporarily relate to others, overcome their isolation, obtain caring, have certainty of their needs being met, and possibly act out previous family dynamics." Although the above ideas may be quite useful for understanding and treating perpetrators of abuse with FDIA, there is no identified "cause" for this condition. As with all forms of child abuse and neglect, each story is unique. The current literature does not provide clear indicators of the genetic, epigenetic, or neuroanatomic correlates of FDIA.

SCREENING

FDIA always includes a caretaker knowingly giving or producing false information. The *DSM-5* characterizes of the types of actions constituting illness falsification as the exaggeration, fabrication, simulation, or induction of physical or psychologic impairments.[1] An example of illness exaggeration might involve a child with mild gastroenteritis being reported by a caregiver to have extreme symptoms (e.g., constant retching and vomiting with an inability to take fluids over many days along with explosive diarrhea). In this situation, genuine symptoms are exaggerated to suggest that they are more severe and dangerous than is objectively true. Supporting such a conclusion, clinicians might observe that the caregiver assertions are not supported by objective findings (e.g., physical and/or mental status examination, blood work, imaging). Illness fabrication is reporting symptoms that are not present at all. An example would be the case just described, except the child does not have a mild gastroenteritis at baseline. Illness simulation refers to behaviors that directly cause medical tests or records to appear pathological. Examples include altering urine samples, interfering with equipment involved in medical tests, and doctoring medical records. Finally, induction means directly causing symptoms, most commonly by poisoning, nonadherence to medical instructions, or suffocation.

Warning signs include caregivers who provide medical histories that are inconsistent, convoluted, odd, and/or incapable of being verified for unusual reasons (e.g., parents who refuse to provide a release of information despite repeated requests). Another red flag occurs when children provide verbal accounts of their illness that do not match their developmental level and/or the known course of a disease (e.g., a neurotypical and apparently normally developing toddler whose parents claim that the child tells them about vividly detailed auditory and visual hallucinations, or the same child who describes symptoms to a clinician with advanced language, suggestive of coaching). Even toddlers and teens can be effectively coached by their abusers to portray themselves as ill (e.g., walking with a limp, feigning seizures). A child may or may not be aware that the behavior request is deceptive. Some children have been known to adopt behaviors associated with an illness on their own in response to being portrayed to others as sick or impaired for a long time.[13]

It is important to note that underlying medical or psychiatric disorders in the child that are congruent with the symptoms being reported *do not need to be ruled out* for a conclusion of abusive condition falsification or neglect to be made. Examples include a child with epilepsy that the caregiver exacerbates by withholding antiseizure medication or a child with a benign mitochondrial defect that the parent falsely claims, causing an array of symptoms and impairment in the child.

DIFFERENTIAL DIAGNOSIS

It is important to note that there are many cases of suspected PCF that are not due to FDIA. Some examples include false allegations in the settling of a child custody dispute for purposes of winning custody, the presence of a genuine, rare medical condition that is being described accurately, and medical abuse or neglect driven by other factors (e.g., financial incentives for having a medically impaired child; untreated severe mental illness and/or substance use disorder in a parent). Although individuals with FDIA can have any type of cooccurring mental disorder, there are some diagnoses that can mimic the condition and/or commonly cooccur.

Additional Somatic Symptom and Related Disorders

As stated previously, FDIA is included within a chapter of the DSM-5 called *somatic symptoms and related disorders*.[1] Additional conditions within this section of the DSM-5 include "somatic symptom disorder," "illness anxiety disorder," "conversion disorder," "factitious disorder imposed on self (FDIS)," and "psychological factors affecting other medical conditions." Of note, an important factor distinguishing FDIA and FDIS from the other conditions within the somatic symptom and

related disorders section of the DSM-5 is that the factitious disorders require one to intentionally deceive others. The remaining diagnoses describe persons who believe that they are in need of frequent medical attention yet do not take steps to deceive care providers. A study by Bools and colleagues[14] examined the histories of 47 mothers who had engaged in Munchausen by proxy behaviors and discovered that over two-thirds of them also met criteria for comorbid diagnoses (from an earlier version of the DSM) that were akin to FDIS and/or somatic symptom disorder. All of the somatic symptom and related disorders involve the presence of apparent distress and/or impairments that are beyond rational explanation.

Malingering

The *DSM-5*[1] defines malingering as the "intentional production of false or grossly exaggerated physical or psychological symptoms, motivated by external incentives such as avoiding military duty, avoiding work, obtaining financial compensation, evading criminal prosecution, or obtaining drugs." Malingering is not considered to be a formal "mental disorder" within the *DSM-5*; however, it is an important consideration in forensic evaluations. The *DSM-5* explicitly recommends that the possibility of malingering be strongly suspected whenever more than one of the following circumstances is apparent:

1. Medicolegal context of presentation (e.g., the individual is referred by an attorney to the clinician for examination, or the individual self-refers while litigation or criminal charges are pending).
2. Marked discrepancy between the individual's claimed stress or disability and the objective lack of findings and observations.
3. Lack of cooperation during the diagnostic evaluation and in complying with the prescribed treatment regimen.
4. The presence of antisocial personality disorder.

In the context of suspected PCF, malingering may involve fabricating illness, with the intention of obtaining financial compensation, custody, prescription medications, and/or additional medical or social benefits, to name just a few possibilities. Of note, it is possible for both FDIA and malingering to cooccur in some circumstances. A possible distinguishing feature of FDIA in cases with concomitant malingering is the continuation of PCF even after all available external incentives have been obtained (e.g., a foster parent who continues to fabricate new forms of illness in a child despite having already maximized funds and/or other benefits from the state).

Schizophrenia Spectrum and Other Psychotic Disorders

The DSM-5[1] criteria for FDIA require that an individual's "behavior is not better explained by another mental disorder, such as delusional disorder or another psychotic disorder." It is important to determine if a care provider suspected of perpetrating PCF is basing his/her actions on delusions (i.e., fixed false beliefs despite credible evidence to the contrary) about a child's health. Indicators of a psychotic disorder (e.g., delusional disorder, schizophrenia) being a driving force behind the acts of PCF include reports of bizarre parasitic infections, melting body organs, or similarly strange or macabre phenomena.[15–17] A delusional parent without concomitant FDIA may seem genuinely mystified by care providers' lack of response to their child's perceived illness and is typically forthcoming about the incredulousness of previous treatment providers. They do not intentionally deceive or mislead clinicians.

Anxiety Disorders

Anxiety-prone caregivers may overestimate the severity of a child's medical problems or fear the worst possible outcomes in situations that are typically benign or unworthy of acute alarm (e.g., a parent who fears that his/her child has leukemia in response to a single nosebleed). Green and Solnit[18] describe a construct they called the "vulnerable child syndrome" in which a parent, because of some form or trauma (e.g., death of a previous child or early illness in the target child), becomes excessively concerned about his/her child becoming deathly ill or dying. Misdiagnosis and iatrogenic harm can occur when well-intentioned parents seek out excessive medical attention for their child. However, what distinguishes anxiety disorders from FDIA is that anxious parents who do not have FDIA do not use deception to make a child appear more ill than is objectively true.

Neurodevelopmental Disorders

Some caregivers with neurodevelopmental disorders such as *autism spectrum disorder* or *intellectual disability* have problems identifying the health needs of others and/or interacting with medical providers appropriately. Deficits in perspective taking, also referred to more broadly as "Theory of Mind" (i.e., how a person imagines and responds to the mental states of others), can lead to misinterpretations and poor communication with medical providers. Some individuals on the autistic spectrum may engage in perseverative behaviors related to a particular area of interest (e.g., medical terminology or technologies). The rigidity and perfectionistic tendencies of some people on the autistic spectrum may cause them to become upset over relatively small observed irregularities (e.g., a skin tag or birthmark) or indirectly observed (e.g., benign incidental findings on an MRI or blood test), leading them to seek unnecessary medical interventions. The presence of a neurodevelopmental disorder does not rule out a diagnosis of FDIA. An intellectually disabled and/or autistic individual who uses deceptive tactics to make a child under his/her care appear more ill or impaired than is true would still qualify for comorbid diagnosis of FDIA.

COMMON COMORBID DIAGNOSES

Identification of comorbid diagnoses is helpful for determining prognosis and for treatment planning purposes. It is important to carefully distinguish FDIA from the diagnoses listed above; however, FDIA may also be comorbid with somatic symptom disorders, FDIS, malingering, psychosis, anxiety, or neurodevelopmental disorders. Factitious disorders (both FDIA and FDIS) are also associated with personality disorders, substance use disorders, eating disorders, posttraumatic stress disorder, and learning disorders.[14,19–21]

A large body of literature shows that traumatic early-life experiences (e.g., child abuse and/or neglect) can foster the development of personality disorders.[22] Numerous case reports and case series suggest that histories of abuse and neglect are commonly reported by persons with factitious disorders (i.e., FDIA and FDIS) and that such individuals typically possess overlapping personality disorder traits, most commonly cluster B personality disorders (antisocial, borderline, histrionic, narcissistic).[14,23,19,21,24]

ASSESSMENT

Mental health professionals with expertise in factitious disorders can be valuable members of clinical or forensic multidisciplinary teams assessing whether suspected PCF has occurred. Such evaluations typically include a comprehensive record review and behavioral analysis, a clinical interview of the suspected abuser, observations from foster care providers if the alleged child victim has been removed from the home, and collateral accounts from other important figures in the alleged victim's life (e.g., teachers, extended family). Additionally, clinical evaluations may be informational if done in a closely observed and controlled setting. These procedures are described in the following sections.

The Record Review

A thorough and comprehensive record review and chronological summary, along with an analysis of the suspected abusers' behaviors, is the foundation on which assessment of suspected PCF and FDIA rests. Records, especially those that were recorded before allegations of abuse, are less likely to be influenced by recall bias or defensiveness from care providers. A variety of records should be obtained, which may include, but are not limited to, records from inpatient medical facilities, outpatient medical clinics, mental health providers, schools the child has attended, speech therapists, occupational therapists, and physical therapists; police reports; and documentation from child protective services and/or related agencies. Whenever possible, it can be helpful to obtain a record of a suspected abuser's online activity (e.g., posts on social media, blog posts, text messages, emails, online videos). Additional examples of the types of information to take note of during the record review are missed appointments, laboratory and other test results, pharmacy records, and discharges against medical advice.

In some cases, there may be a history of siblings with unusual medical problems or who have died. A foster parent who is suspected of FDIA may have had other children placed in their home in the past. Such records should be reviewed whenever possible, as they can identify past abuse that went undetected and/or patterns of behavior that are relevant to the current evaluation.

Suspected abusers may refrain from participating fully in the evaluation, thereby limiting access to their personal medical records. However, gaining access to such records can help the evaluator identify prescription substance use disorders, personality disorders, somatic symptom disorders, and/or FDIS. Other collateral contacts may prove helpful when the suspected abuser's medical records are not available.

A key element of the record review is the creation of a chronological table summarizing the information within the records.[20] Such a timeline makes it easier to keep track of the various hospitalizations, outpatient appointments, and meetings with other providers involved in a suspected victim's care. Tables such as the one provided here (Table 9.1) are also an important means of readily identifying inconsistencies in the story being presented to clinicians by the suspected abuser.

Elizabeth Loftus wrote in her seminal text, *Eyewitness Testimony*, "People's memories are fragile things. It is important to realize how easily information can be introduced into memory, to understand why this happens, and to avoid it when it is undesirable." Analysis of a suspected victim's medical record allows evaluators to obtain input from treatment providers while minimizing recall bias and/or guardedness regarding scrutiny of their clinical impressions. Although this approach may seem extremely detailed, research on another type of high-stakes forensic evaluation, cases of alleged child sexual abuse, suggests that "conducting comprehensive evaluations may be the single most effective strategy for improving the reliability and validity of case decisions."[25] In our view, conducting a thorough evaluation is an essential part of protecting abuse victims, safeguarding parental rights, and mitigating bias.

Pitfalls to avoid when conducting a record review include (1) failing to clearly identify and/or consider the sources of documented information, (2) not obtaining and reviewing primary data (e.g., reviewing actual test results, rather than relying solely on how they have been summarized by various providers), (3) failing to consider whether diagnoses match objective data, (4) neglecting to consider whether objective findings could have been falsified or induced, and (5) failing to consider whether the medical record makes clinical sense.[26] Existing literature can aid evaluators in distinguishing sudden infant death syndrome from suffocation,[27–30] chronic intestinal pseudoobstruction from PCF,[31] and genuine failure to thrive from that which is due to abuse or neglect.[32]

Mental Health Assessment

A comprehensive review of an alleged victim's records may be all that is required to make a well-informed opinion about whether or not PCF has occurred. However, a psychiatric interview of the suspected abuser is necessary to rule out potential mental disorders that could be responsible for deceptive behaviors uncovered in the records and to identify psychiatric comorbidities. As mentioned earlier, factitious disorders are associated with an array of mental illnesses that include personality disorders, substance use disorders, anxiety disorders, eating disorders, and posttraumatic stress disorder.[14,19,21]

The psychiatric interview should cover all the topics normally included in a clinical interview. Additionally, (1) forensic interviewers should be sure to explain the limits of confidentiality, making it clear that everything discussed may be included in a report or discussed in court; (2) examiners may wish to obtain the suspected abuser's perspective on the alleged victim's medical problems and/or the allegations of abuse; (3) evaluators should ask questions designed to assess the abuser's level of insight into how his/her behaviors have affected the alleged victim and/or raised suspicious for

TABLE 9.1
Sample Timeline

Date	Patient	Location	Subjective/Reported Problems	Objective Observations	Diagnosis/Plan/Treatment	Other Information to Track
01/05/2015	Pete	University Hospital	A 5-year-old girl presents to emergency room with report by her mother of reduced need for sleep, irritable mania, and command auditory hallucinations. Per mother, child was provided risperidone 0.5 mg 30 minutes before arrival in emergency room.	**Mental status examination:** Calm, making good eye contact, watching children's video, denies auditory hallucinations, states that she was "mad at mommy" because she did not want to go to bed. **Physical examination:** Unremarkable.	**Diagnosis:** Pediatric bipolar disorder, per mother. Mania resolved with home dose of risperidone. **Plan:** Discharge home with plan to follow up with psychiatrist in 3 days. Will check TSH and NMDA receptor antibodies per mother's request. Mom also requesting MRI of the brain.	Nursing staff observed patient drinking apple juice and eating crackers in ED without complaint.
01/08/2015	Pete	Healthy Kids Primary Care Clinic	Mother reports that her daughter has experienced reduced need for sleep, irritability, increased goal-directed activity, and intermittent command auditory hallucinations instructing her to hurt her younger brother for the past 3 days. Mom reports that her daughter was prescribed risperidone in the ED with good result; however, the symptoms returned. Requesting prescription.	**Mental status examination:** Limited eye contact, yawning, brief one- to two-word responses to questions. **Physical examination:** Unremarkable.	**Diagnosis:** Rule out Bipolar I disorder versus pediatric-onset schizophrenia versus encephalitis. **Plan:** Referral to child psychiatry and pediatric neurology. Provided prescription: Risperidone 0.5 mg at bedtime.	Mother reports strong family history of bipolar disorder.
01/11/2015	Pete	University Hospital	A 5-year-old girl with history of bipolar disorder versus autoimmune encephalitis presenting with reduced need for sleep, violent behavior, and command auditory hallucinations at bedtime, after receiving one dose of risperidone 1 mg per mother.	**Mental status examination:** Sleeping in emergency room. Pleasant and calm on waking. States she became mad at mom at bedtime. Says she hears voices telling her that her mom is "bad." **Physical examination:** Unremarkable.	**Diagnosis:** Bipolar I disorder versus autoimmune encephalitis. **Plan:** Admit to psychiatric unit. Mom requests MRI of the brain. Consult peds neurology.	Nursing staff comments that child is calm and pleasant. Nursing staff adds that patient falls asleep while watching video in ED.

ED, emergency department; *h/o*, history of.

abuse, (4) given the high stakes associated with evaluations of PCF and high rates of psychiatric comorbidities among persons with factitious disorders, it is important to ask questions pertaining to the suspected abuser's risk of self-harm and suicide; and (5) interviewers should inquire about the suspected abuser's openness to pursuing psychiatric treatment if recommended and, if applicable, attitudes toward reunification. In general, interviewers should start out with open-ended questions, saving specific questions until the later portions of their interview.

Given the penalties associated with child abuse and that deceptive behavior is a hallmark feature of factitious disorders, abusers with FDIA are unlikely to provide an honest and straightforward account of their behaviors. Thus, abusers and nonabusers may present similarly on an interview. It is important for even expert evaluators to remain cognizant that they are at risk for being misled. Evaluators must avoid using superficial factors (such as the degree to which the suspected abuser is likeable, logical, or believable) to rule out potential abuse or neglect of a child. Research has revealed that both laypersons' and mental health professionals' ability to distinguish lies from the truth during interviews are not much better than random chance.[33,34] The weight of evidence, therefore, generally comes from the behavior analysis of the records and other collateral data.

Collateral Interviews

Interviews with people who have a history of substantial contact with a suspected abuser and/or victim, such as extended family members, school personnel, family friends, and foster placement family members, can provide helpful behavioral observations and background history. Collateral interviews can reveal behavior patterns of the suspected abusers, reveal signs of illness and wellness observed in the suspected victim or abuser, clarify inconsistencies identified within the records, provide helpful family history, and/or identify potential areas of concern that had previously gone unnoticed.

The Separation Test

The courts will often separate a child from a care provider when FDIA is suspected. This is a critical time in the evaluation of PCF because discrepancies between the child's condition before and after removal are considered relevant in some courts, as exemplified by the case described below.

In the Matter of Jessica Z is a case that was heard within the Family Court of Westchester County,

New York, in 1987. A mother was accused of repeatedly providing laxatives to her infant daughter, Jessica, resulting in chronic diarrhea, multiple surgeries, which included the placement of feeding tubes, and eventual near-fatal septic shock. Jessica's care providers became suspicious when they noticed her rapid recovery during a stay in an intensive care unit (ICU), a setting that prevented her parents from directly assisting in her care, followed by the rapid return of diarrhea once she was transferred out of the ICU. A savvy treatment provider ordered that Jessica's stool sample be analyzed and it came back positive for phenolphthaliein, a chemical compound that is commonly found in over-the-counter laxatives. Jessica was subsequently removed from her parents care and her diarrhea resolved.

The Family Court applied the concept of "res ipsa loquitur," which translated from Latin means "the thing speaks for itself," when weighing the circumstantial evidence (i.e., evidence that is not based on direct observation) referenced above. The Court ultimately ruled that the accumulated circumstantial evidence was enough to determine that Jessica's mother had most likely been surreptitiously causing her to become ill. However, not all courts rely on circumstantial evidence to the same degree, underscoring the need for considerable and persuasive evidence when providing an opinion on whether PCF has occurred.

In the case of *Jessica Z*, the separation from the parents led to invaluable information about the likelihood of ongoing abuse. Unmitigated symptoms following separation from the suspected abuser are an indicator that a child's symptoms may be legitimate. However, it is important to be mindful that children with preexisting medical conditions may only have some of their problems resolved or may only experience a change in the level of severity of symptoms after separation. In some cases, a child may have iatrogenic illnesses or conditions due to having received unnecessary treatment in the past. Such iatrogenic problems may or may not resolve following separation. Finally, there are many documented cases in which a parent has surreptitiously poisoned or coached a child during supervised visits as a means of perpetuating illness during separation.

Evaluators must be mindful of how changes in treatment around the time of separation can influence a child's symptoms. How might altering a child's psychiatric or antiseizure medication regimen around the time of separation account the observed differences in behaviors? Why did the child begin treatment in the first place? For example, if a young child is placed on antipsychotic medication because of hallucinations based solely on their mothers' report, placed in foster care once PCF is suspected, and then taken off of all antipsychotic medication, it is reasonable to think that the child may not develop any psychotic symptoms. The same child may no longer experience the side effects associated with antipsychotic medication (e.g., drowsiness, increased appetite, tremors). However, it would not make logical sense for the hallucinations to suddenly disappear *because* antipsychotic medication was discontinued. Likewise, one would not expect active seizures to abate *because* antiseizure medication is discontinued.

Clinical Evaluation of Suspected Victim

Clinical evaluations of the victim require the thoughtful creation of an evaluation and rehabilitation plan that systematically and objectively challenges claims made by the suspected abuser and/or victim. Additionally, all assessment procedures require consideration of how such tests could be undermined by the child or suspected parent. For example, clinicians might consider conducting a toxicology screen before manometry testing to ensure no gut-altering substances were provided to the child. Otherwise, clinicians might consider having an observer in the room for a pH probe test to ensure that the child only ingests the prescribed oral intake and to ensure the location of the probe is not changed. Consultation with an expert can be extremely helpful when devising such plans. Additionally, careful documentation is as important as a thorough evaluation. For example, documenting "emesis x3" does not provide critical information related to the amount or appearance of the emesis and can be interpreted to mean that someone was *informed* the child vomited, that someone *saw emesis*, or that someone actually *observed the child vomit.*

Profiling Abusers

There is a sizeable amount of literature characterizing the personality and behavior profiles of the typical parent with FDIA.[20] For example, some female caregivers with FDIA have described their identities closely tied to their children's illnesses (e.g., running support groups, maintaining a blog about the experience of caring for a sick child, volunteering at nonprofits related to their children's diagnosis), show above-average interest and/or expertise in medicine, have an uncanny ability to predict changes in illness severity, and are not relieved by normal test findings. Despite the fact that many parents with FDIA appear to display behaviors consistent with the above profile, such impressions should not be used as primary evidence that PCF has occurred. A reason for this is that many of the profile behaviors match with those of genuinely concerned parents who are not abusing their child. Furthermore, not all persons with FDIA fit the typical profile, and its use has not been shown to be sensitive or sufficiently specific when screening for potential abusers.[20]

CASE MANAGEMENT, TREATMENT, AND RECOMMENDATIONS

Merely confronting the abuser with FDIA about his/her behavior is not likely to put an end to the dangerous and deceptive behaviors.[35] In fact, confronting or casting suspicion on a suspected abuser has been known to cause some abusers to intensify their level of illness falsification to dispel skepticism. Parents with FDIA have been known to limit their children's normal growth and development, cause permanent physical injuries, and even accidentally cause their death. Children who survive this sort of abuse have also been noted to experience disrupted attachments and serious psychologic problems.[35,29,20]

Working as a Team

Working with abusers who meet criteria for FDIA and their victims requires a multidisciplinary team made up of foster care placement, therapists, physicians, case managers from child protective services, and attorneys. The team must work together to gather records and identify areas of concern as the evaluation progresses. Open communication among team members is essential, so that all players are aware of pertinent medical history, court orders, and how determinations on PCF and/or the diagnosis of FDIA were made. Team members must be prepared for attempts by the abuser to recruit supporters and to turn team members against each other. They will benefit by informing other team members when they become confused or develop doubts about the child abuse accusations so that the data can be reviewed in light of updated information, if needed.

Placement

Foster home placement is generally the most appropriate and safest option for suspected victims of a caregiver with FDIA. It is typically important the child stay with someone who is not connected with the family (e.g., friend or relative) and who might be complicit, either knowingly or unknowingly, of a parent's efforts to create illness in the child. For example, there have been cases in which a suspected abuser has recommended a family friend who was also turned out to be an abuser and/or who allowed the abuser to have access to the child. Even family members who vow to protect the child can be worn down over time by an incessant abuser who wishes to have contact with the child. Placement caregivers should not be in charge of monitoring visits, may wish not to have any contact with the abuser, and must remain vigilant against unauthorized communication between the child and abuser.

Supervised Visitation

There must be strict guidelines in place to ensure that abuse and subtle coercion do not occur during supervised visitation.[20] General guidelines for supervised visitation included the following:

1. All visits should occur at a neutral location and be monitored closely by a professional who is well acquainted with the case, understands the court orders, and is equipped to intervene if court orders or visitation guidelines are breached.
2. Parents should not be allowed to discuss health-related issues, including diet or the court case with their children.
3. Parents must not provide their child food, candy, drinks, gum, lotions, bath products, or medicine during the visit.
4. Parents should not speak ill of or attempt to compromise the child's trust in the treatment team, foster family, or other service providers.
5. All conversations with the child must be easily overheard by the monitor and all written communication must be read and cleared before being shared with the child.
6. Physical contact must be developmentally and socially appropriate.
7. All gifts should be socially and developmentally appropriate, with only one gift allowed per visit. In some counties, all gifts must be discussed in advance and approved in advance by the team.

In many cases, the child will have been removed from a suspected abuser's care before there is opportunity for an evaluator to complete the record review, summary, and behavior analysis. In addition to reviewing records pertaining to the child's ongoing medical care and analyzing the suspected abusers' behaviors during those clinical encounters, it is important to also review records and analyze behaviors that occur during supervised visitation. Monitoring for behavior problems and understanding attachment patterns can be helpful in directing therapy during supervised visitation.[39] For example, does an uninjured child who is fully capable of walking begin to limp during supervised visits? Or, does a child who was reported to have multiple severe food allergies that were subsequently proven unfounded repeatedly report having an upset stomach whenever eating in front of his/her abuser? Accounts from supervised visitation can also provide indicators of how bonded a parent is to his/her child and the degree of insight into the damaging effects of the abusive behavior. However, there is evidence that many individuals with FDIA are capable of presenting well while under close observation; thus these data are not sufficient to dismiss concerns about condition falsification.

Medical Care for Child

If the child is reunified with the abuser, the abuser(s) should be required to engage in a medical monitoring plan designed to rapidly identify the recurrence of medical setting behaviors associated with PCF. All care must be directed through a single pediatrician and his/her predetermined backup provider to avoid doctor shopping and confusion about the treatment plan. The pediatrician and backup pediatrician should be aware of the child's medical history, possess a summary of the evaluation identifying FDIA, and have access to professionals for consultation who have experience with FDIA. Because much of the FDIA-associated abuse and neglect occurs outside the medical setting, such a monitoring plan is not sufficient to ensure child safety.

School

Child victims of FDIA may be far behind in their school work as a result of repeated doctor visits, hospitalizations, withdrawal from school, and/or the cognitive effects of unnecessary treatments (e.g., antipsychotic medications; opiates, benzodiazepines, antiseizure medications). The school should be aware of the concerns related to PCF and report when the child misses class or other school activities because of reports of illness, injury, or impairment. The pediatrician or mental health clinician can educate the school regarding the child's medical and/or psychiatric status. Cognitive and educational testing can identify child's current abilities and academic needs. Child victims may benefit greatly from an individualized education program as they begin catching up in their academic work. However, care must be taken to balance the need for normalcy and reduced accommodation with providing helpful supports.

Psychotherapy for Abuser, Spouse, and Child Victim

As with other forms of child abuse and neglect, individuals who are able to be honest about the abuse and/or neglect they have perpetrated are more likely to benefit from psychotherapy. The spouses of abusers should also receive treatment as they have either colluded with the abusing parents or were unable to protect their children. Treatment approaches vary in their theoretical orientation and should be tailored to meet the parent's individual needs, with evidence-based treatment approaches used whenever possible to treat comorbidities. Couples therapy may be beneficial for parents who remain together after the abuse is discovered. Indicators for successful treatment of FDIA include the following:

1. The abuser admits to abuse and describes specifics of how he/she abused the child.
2. The abuser is able to experience an appropriate emotional response to the harm caused to the child and his/her deceptive behaviors.
3. The parent has developed strategies to identify and manage his/her needs in a manner that does not involve abusing the child.
4. The parent has demonstrated the above skills under close supervision over an extended period.

The child victim of a parent with FDIA may experience intense anger, posttraumatic stress disorder, low self-esteem, and/or enmeshment with the abuser; may readily take on the sick role; may have poor attachments; and/or may even deny that the abuse ever occurred. Older children and adolescents, those capable of abstract thought, may benefit from a therapy that objectively reviews the records or the facts of the case to reveal tendencies toward denial or misperceptions about what happened. Afterward, the child may be better able to identify how his/her experiences relate to the concerns about condition falsification.[36,20] Younger children may benefit from storytelling and play therapy as a means of understanding and coming to terms with being abused in a less traumatizing manner.

Reunification

In 1987, Dr David Jones[37] identified predictors for poor outcomes with reunification efforts for a variety of abuse types. The predictors of poor outcome include abusers who persistently deny that the abuse occurred, have a personal history of being a victim of childhood abuse, refuse to participate in recommended treatment, have a substance use disorder, have a severe personality disorder, are intellectually disabled, and/or are psychotic. Jones writes that the most significant predictor of failed attempts for reunification is a perpetrator who lacks empathy for the child or is unable to put the child's needs first. Jones adds that caregivers with FDIA who have induced illness (nonaccidental poisoning or suffocation) tend to have the poorest prognosis and the greatest likelihood of eventually killing their children.

If little or no progress is made with therapy and other efforts toward reunification within 6 months to a year, successful treatment of the abuser is less likely. In such cases, the court may wish to expedite proceedings to terminate parental rights.[20] However, in cases where progress is being made, reunification services should continue to be provided, and movements toward reunification should proceed slowly with close monitoring. Before reunification is attempted, reassessment by an expert who is not part of the treatment team is highly recommended. Follow-up should continue for years after a child is reunified with the previously abusing caregiver to make sure the child is safe and to monitor the parent's mental health status.[38] Clinical experience suggests that risk for relapse increases with subsequent births and increased stress.

CONCLUSION

Those with a diagnosis of FDIA engage in a complex set of behaviors that can unintentionally have deadly consequences for victims. It is important that clinicians who have a reasonable suspicion for PCF report it to the appropriate agencies, as abuse and neglect associated with this diagnosis often goes undetected. A thorough record review and behavior analysis, a psychiatric interview, and a team approach, as described earlier, are recommended to properly identify and address the issues associated with FDIA. Because of the skill of some individuals to present as normal caregivers, FDIA cannot be ruled out solely based on normal psychologic testing or psychiatric interview. National guidelines are available to assist interested professionals.[40]

DISCLOSURE STATEMENT

Disclosure of any relationship with a commercial company that has a direct financial interest in subject matter or materials discussed in article or with a company making a competing product.

REFERENCES

1. *Diagnostic and Statistical Manual of Mental Disorders.* 5th ed. Washington DC: American Psychiatric Association; 2013.
2. Meadow R. Munchausen syndrome by proxy the hinterland of child abuse. *Lancet.* 1977;310(8033):343–345. https://doi.org/10.1016/s0140-6736(77)91497-0.
3. Google Trends data, accessed 5/14/17.
4. Ayoub C, Alexander R. For APSAC munchausen by proxy task force, definitional issues in munchausen by proxy. *APSAC Advis.* 1998;11:7–10.

5. Roesler TA, Jenny C. *Medical Child Abuse.* American Academy of Pediatrics; 2008.

6. Flaherty EG, Macmillan HL. Caregiver-fabricated illness in a child: a manifestation of child maltreatment. *Pediatrics.* 2013;132(3):590–597. https://doi.org/10.1542/peds.2013-2045.

7. McClure RJ, Davis PM, Meadow SR, Sibert JR. Epidemiology of Munchausen syndrome by proxy, non-accidental poisoning, and non-accidental suffocation. *Arc Dis Child.* 1996;75(1):57–61. https://doi.org/10.1136/adc.75.1.57.

8. Ferrara P, Vitelli O, Bottaro G, et al. Factitious disorders and Münchausen syndrome. *J Child Health Care.* 2013;17(4):366–374. https://doi.org/10.1177/1367493512462262.

9. Feldman MD, Brown RM. Munchausen by Proxy in an international context. *Child Abuse Neglect.* 2002;26(5):509–524. https://doi.org/10.1016/s0145-2134(02)00327-7.

10. Sheridan MS. The deceit continues: an updated literature review of Munchausen syndrome by proxy. *Child Abuse Neglect.* 2003;27(4):431–451. https://doi.org/10.1016/s0145-2134(03)00030-9.

11. Levin AV, Sheridan MS, eds. *Munchausen Syndrome by Proxy: Issues in Diagnosis and Treatment.* Jossey-Bass; 1995.

12. Carlson RJ. Factitious psychiatric disorders: diagnostic and etiologic considerations. *Psychiatr Med.* 1984;2(4):383.

13. Sanders M. Symptom coaching: factitious disorder by proxy with older children. *Clin Psychol Rev.* 1995:15.

14. Bools C, Neale B, Meadow R. Munchausen syndrome by proxy: a study of psychopathology. *Child Abuse Negl.* 1994;18(9):773–788.

15. Elmer KB, George RM, Peterson K. Therapeutic update: use of risperidone for the treatment of monosymptomatic hypochondriacal psychosis. *J Am Acad Dermatol.* 2000;43(4):683–686.

16. Meehan WJ, Badreshia S, Mackley CL. Successful treatment of delusions of parasitosis with olanzapine. *Arch Dermatol.* 2006;142(3):352–355.

17. Trabert W. 100 years of delusional parasitosis. *Psychopathology.* 1995;28(5):238–246.

18. Green M, Solnit AJ. Reactions to the threatened loss of a child: a vulnerable child syndrome. *Pediatrics.* 1964;34(1):58–66.

19. Ayoub CC. Emotional impact of Munchausen by proxy on the child victims: a five-year follow-up study. In H. Schreier (Chair), Munchausen by proxy: psychiatric presentations, treatment findings, what to do when a new child is born. In: *Symposium meeting of the American Academy of Child & Adolescent Psychiatry, Chicago.* October 1999.

20. Sanders MJ, Bursch B. Forensic assessment of illness falsification, Munchausen by proxy, and factitious disorder, NOS. *Child Maltreat.* 2002;7(2):112–124.

21. Bass C, Jones D. Psychopathology of perpetrators of fabricated or induced illness in children: case series. *Br J Psychiatry.* 2011;199(2):113–118.

22. Johnson JG, Patricia C, Brown J, Smailes EM, Bernstein DP. Childhood maltreatment increases risk for personality disorders during early adulthood. *Arch Gen Psychiatry.* 1999;56(7):600–606.

23. Ehlers W, Plassmann R. Diagnosis of narcissistic self-esteem regulation in patients with factitious illness (Munchausen syndrome). *Psychother Psychosom.* 1994;62(1–2):69–77.

24. Gordon DK, Sansone RA. A relationship between factitious disorder and borderline personality disorder. *Innov Clin Neurosci.* 2013;10(11–12):11.

25. Everson MD, Sandoval JM. Forensic child sexual abuse evaluations: assessing subjectivity and bias in professional judgments. *Child Abuse Neglect.* 2011;35(4):287–298.

26. Bursch B. Munchausen by proxy and factitious disorder imposed on another. *Psychiatr Times.* 2014;31(8):16–27.

27. Meadow R. Suffocation, recurrent apnea, and sudden infant death. *J Pediatr.* 1990;117(3):351–357.

28. Kahn A, Groswasser J, Rebuffat E, et al. Sleep and cardiorespiratory characteristics of infant victims of sudden death: a prospective case-control study. *Sleep.* 1992;15(4):287–292.

29. Samuels MP, Southall DP. Child abuse and apparent life-threatening events. *Pediatrics.* 1995;96:167–168.

30. Truman TL, Ayoub CC. Considering suffocatory abuse and Munchausen by proxy in the evaluation of children experiencing apparent life-threatening events and sudden infant death syndrome. *Child Maltreat.* 2002;7(2):138–148.

31. Hyman PE, Bursch B, Beck D, DiLorenzo C, Zeltzer LK. Discriminating Munchausen syndrome by proxy from chronic digestive disease in toddlers. *Child Maltreat.* 2002;7(2):132–137.

32. Mash C, Frazier T, Nowacki A, Worley S, Goldfarb J. Development of a risk-stratification tool for medical child abuse in failure to thrive. *Pediatrics.* 2011;128(6):e1467–e1473. https://doi.org/10.1542/peds.2011-1080.

33. Rosenhan DL. On being sane in insane places. *Science.* 1973;179(4070):250–258.

34. ten Brinke L, Stimson D, Carney DR. Some evidence for unconscious lie detection. *Psychol Sci.* 2014;25(5):1098–1105.

35. Bools CN, Neale BA, Meadow SR. Follow-up of victims of fabricated illness (Munchausen syndrome by proxy). *Arch Dis Child.* 1993;69(6):625–630.

36. Bursch B. Individual psychotherapy with child victims. In: Schreier H, ed. *Munchausen by Proxy: psychiatric presentations, treatment findings: what to do when a new child is born. Symposium Meeting of the American Academy of Child and Adolescent Psychiatry.* 1999.

37. Jones DP. The untreatable family. *Child Abuse Negl.* 1987;11(3):409–420.

38. Berg B, Jones D. Outcome of psychiatric intervention in factitious illness by proxy (Munchausen's syndrome by proxy). *Arch Dis Child.* 1999;81(6):465–472.

39. Haight WL, Kagle JD, Black JE. Understanding and supporting parent-child relationships during foster care visits: Attachment theory and research. *Social work.* 2003;48(2):195–207.

40. APSAC Taskforce (2017). APSAC Practice Guidelines: Munchausen by proxy: Clinical and Case Management Guidance. https://www.apsac.org/guidelines-form

CHAPTER 10

Pediatric Sleep Disorders

TEMITAYO O. OYEGBILE, MD, PHD

INTRODUCTION

Sleep is one of the most important activities that growing children engage in. By age 3 years, children will have spent more time sleeping than any other activity and will have spent more than half of their lives asleep. As they get older, they continue to require a substantial amount of sleep into their adolescent years. This significant sleep requirement is vital for cognitive, physical, and psychologic development across childhood. Given the high level of sleep requirement in this age range, the impact of insufficient sleep and/or poor-quality sleep can be considerable. This insufficient or poor-quality sleep can manifest as attention deficit disorders with short easily disrupted attention spans, emotional lability/mood changes, psychiatric illness, hyperactivity, behavioral/conduct disorders, and poor academic performance. Up to 25% of the pediatric population experiences a form of sleep disturbance, regardless of the disorder type.[1]

There are major developmental changes in sleep architecture, sleep patterns, and sleep behavior throughout childhood.[2] As children mature, they slowly attain adult-type sleep patterns, including less daytime sleep/naps and shorter sleep duration. Rapid eye movement (REM) sleep decreases from 50% of total sleep time to the normal adult pattern of 25% of sleep time and slow-wave sleep, which is highest in early childhood, drops off dramatically after puberty, and continues to decline thereafter throughout the life span.[3]

This chapter endeavors to discuss normal sleep patterns in children at different age ranges and then discusses sleep pathology, specifically focusing on common pediatric sleep disorders. We will then discuss the interconnection between psychiatric disorders and sleep disorders. Finally we will have a short discussion on specific psychiatric disorders and their effects on sleep.

NORMAL SLEEP DEVELOPMENT

It is important to recognize that sleep is an active process, which involves cycling of physiologic diverse stages throughout the night, and the specific stages are dependent on the particular stages in development.

Newborns (0–2 Months)

Newborns generally sleep approximately 16–20 h per day.[4] The newborns sleep cycle is much shorter than the adult sleep cycle such that newborns sleep in 1- to 4-h periods followed by wake periods of 1–2 h. This sleep pattern does not follow any nocturnal or diurnal patterns, which explains why newborns awaken frequently throughout the night. At this time the circadian sleep-wake rhythms are not yet developed and do not emerge until around 2–4 months of age; therefore, environmental cues play no significant role in sleep onset or maintenance at this developmental stage. Newborn awakenings are dependent on hunger and satiety such that formula-fed newborns tend to wake up less frequently than breast-fed newborns. On average, formula-fed newborns awaken every 3–5 h, whereas breast-fed newborns awaken every 2–3 h. This is likely due to the higher caloric density of formula compared with breast milk. As such, formula-fed newborns feel fuller longer than breast-fed newborns.

Unlike older children and adults, newborns enter into REM sleep immediately on falling asleep. They exhibit mainly REM sleep (active sleep) and non-REM sleep (quiet sleep) only on electroencephalogram (EEG). Sleep architecture patterns, such as deep sleep/slow-wave sleep, do not develop until later in development. During active REM sleep, newborns may exhibit grimaces, smiles, sucking, twitching, and jerking. Parents may sometimes interpret this as a disrupted or abnormal sleep pattern or may interpret it as not sleeping; however, this is a normal and expected sleep pattern.

At this developmental age, most sleep concerns are generally parental perceptions of problematic sleep patterns, which are actually a discrepancy between developmentally appropriate sleep behaviors and parental expectations of "normal" sleep. Other sleep concerns in newborns at this developmental age may include excessive fussiness and difficultly consoling due to medical issues such as colic, formula intolerance due to food allergies, metabolic disorders, seizures, and gastroesophageal reflux disorders.

Infants (2–12 Months)

Infants generally sleep approximately 9–12 h at night and 2–5 h in total during the day (1–4 naps).[4] There can be a significant individual variability in sleep amount during this developmental stage. At 2–3 months of age, infants sleep in 3- to 4-h periods, whereas by 4–6 months, infants lengthen their sleep periods to 6–8 h uninterrupted. Therefore by 6 months of age, some infants may be able to sleep 8 h through the night. During this developmental stage, active/REM sleep declines in total duration and quiet/non-REM sleep begins to separate into three distinct stages of non-REM sleep, specifically stages N1, N2, and N3 (also known as slow-wave sleep). During this period, infants are expected to reach multiple developmental milestones, including physical, cognitive, and social milestones. They are also expected to reach to specific sleep development milestones—sleep consolidation and sleep regulation. Sleep consolidation involves the ability to sleep for a continuous period generally concentrated during the night. In other words, the children should begin "sleeping through the night." By 9 months of age, roughly 70%–80% of infants will have achieved this sleep development milestone.[2] Sleep regulation involves the ability of the infant to "self-soothe" as they fall asleep at the beginning of the night and in the middle of the night if they awaken. In other words, infants at this age should master the ability to fall asleep and returned to sleep independently after normal night arousal/awakenings.

It is important to note that other developmental milestones, which are being acquired during this period, may temporarily disrupt sleep, but these disruptions should not persist. For instance, as the infant learns to roll over and crawl (gross motor developmental milestones), they may spend some of their sleep/nap time enjoying their emerging independence. Furthermore, cognitive developmental milestones, including development of object permanence can lead to separation anxiety and eventually develop into bedtime resistance, sleep onset/settling difficulties, and problematic nighttime awakenings. Up to 25%–50% of infants at this developmental stage experience transient and/or chronic sleep problems.[2] Risk factors for these sleep problems persisting and becoming chronic include "difficult" temperament, maternal depression, family stress, and medical conditions being experienced by the infant. Clear bedtime routines and use of transitional objects such as pacifiers and blankets can reduce these separation concerns. Other sleep disorders noted at this developmental age include sleep-onset association disorder and rhythmic movement disorders (discussed in the following).

Toddlers (12 Months–3 Years)

Toddlers generally sleep about 12–13 h in a 24-h period.[4] Napping remains an important factor in daily sleep at this developmental stage. Morning naps tend to drop off usually around age 18 months; however, the afternoon naps remain usually lasting about 1.5–3.5 h. Developmentally, toddlers are progressing quite drastically. At this age, they have significantly increased mobility so that they can climb out of their crib at night. As such, transitioning from the crib to the bed may be critical at this age. At this stage, toddlers are increasing their language and cognitive skills dramatically daily, and this may interfere with nighttime bedtime routines when they endeavor to oppose the usual bedtime routines. Fortunately at this age, children are beginning to understand consequences, as well as cause and effect, and thus behavioral interventions can be beneficial at this stage. On the other hand, toddlers begin to develop imagination and fantasy, which can lead to bedtime fears, as well as the development of autonomy and independence that can all result in increased bedtime resistance. Separation anxiety can also adversely affect sleep. Therefore, transitional objects can remain very important to reduce anxiety. At this time, parents frequently resort to cosleeping to reduce the bedtime resistance. Unfortunately this may sometimes lead to regression in sleep behavior and sleep-onset association insomnia.

Sleep problems at this stage occur in 25%–30% of toddlers with bedtime resistance and nighttime awakenings accounting for most of the problems.[2] At this developmental stage, behavioral insomnias of childhood such as sleep-onset association disorder and limit-setting sleep disorder are common.[5] In addition, rhythmic movement disorders such as head banging, body rolling, and body rocking can be prevalent.

Preschoolers (3–5 Years)

Preschoolers generally require 11–12 h of sleep in a 24-h period.[4] Napping time persists in about 92% of children at age 3 years and drops to 27% by age 5 years. The duration and frequency of napping after age 5 years gradually peters off until napping is given up completely. By this age, sleep architecture during nighttime sleep will begin to follow a more adult pattern but still have a high proportion of both slow-wave sleep and REM sleep. Given the rapid cognitive, physical, and social development at this age, children are able to express their needs more clearly, which may lead to worsening in limit-setting problems and bedtime resistance. Therefore, it is important to maintain a set bedtime routine with consistent sleep and wake times and is imperative to normalize sleep-wake patterns. Continued development of imagination and fantasy can worsen fears and anxiety around bedtime.

Preschoolers experience sleep disorders in about 15%–30% of the population.[2] This is a critical time to address sleep problems and sleep disorders, as habits are developing at this age and sleep difficulty may become chronic. Common sleep disorders among preschoolers include nighttime fears, nightmares, behavioral insomnias, including sleep-onset association disorder and limit-setting sleep disorder, obstructive sleep apnea (OSA)/sleep-disordered breathing, and partial arousal parasomnias, which include sleepwalking and sleep terrors[5] (see the following).

School-Aged Children (6–12 Years)

School-aged children require about 10–11 h per 24-h period.[4] By this age, their sleep architecture is almost identical to the distribution of sleep stages in adults. Naps are infrequent by this age, as school-aged children normally have a very high physiologic level of alertness. Therefore daytime sleepiness at this age is highly suggestive of sleep deprivation/disruption due to a sleep disorder. At this age, children are beginning to develop more autonomy and responsibility for their self-care. As a result, it is important to continue to instill healthy sleep habits at this developmental stage. Children are more likely to begin to use caffeine by way of sodas and other caffeinated drinks, and this can lead to a regular sleep-wake cycles. Furthermore, extracurricular activities, peer relationships, and media/electronics become increasingly important and begin to compete for sleep time. Nighttime fears may begin to escalate at this age, as children become more cognitively aware of real dangers such as fires, burglary, and death. The increased pressure to perform well academically can also impair normal sleep. Interestingly, based on teacher and parental surveys, children who are classified as "poor sleepers" tend to exhibit more behavioral and mood problems overall.

Sleep problems may be considered fairly rare at this age group, and common sleep disorders include nightmares, anxiety-related sleep-onset delay, partial arousal parasomnias, OSA, sleep-disordered breathing, behaviorally induced insufficient sleep syndrome, and poor sleep hygiene.[5]

Adolescents (12–18 Years)

Adolescents generally require about 9–9.25 h of sleep nightly; however, studies show that adolescents generally get only 7 h of sleep in a 24-h period.[6] This sleep deprivation may exacerbate the emotional difficulties frequently experienced at this age. Furthermore, slow-wave sleep decreases by around 40% between ages 10 and 20 years. During this developmental stage, adolescents are undergoing significant biologic changes during sleep. For instance, during puberty, there is a significant increase in secretion of hormones, including growth hormone, and these hormonal changes are dependent on circadian rhythms. In addition, adolescents undergo a physiologic circadian phase delay of at least 2 h such that they begin to develop later sleep-onset times and later wake times.[7] Unfortunately, extensive academic, extracurricular, social, and occupational demands can require adolescents not only to sleep late but also to awake early, which tends to be in opposition to their naturally delayed circadian rhythm. This can lead to significant chronic insufficient sleep and poor sleep hygiene. Because of increased autonomy and decreased adult supervision, adolescents tend to engage in "weekend oversleep" to make up for the significant sleep debt they accumulate during the week. As such, they develop an increasing discrepancy between weekday and weekend bedtime and wake time schedules. In addition, adolescents have a physiologic predisposition to develop decreased daytime alertness in mid- to late puberty. Overall, these factors lead to increased daytime sleepiness, poor nighttime sleep, which ultimately leads to impaired mood, creativity, attention, impulse control, memory, and academic performance.[7]

There is roughly a 20% prevalence of sleep problems in this age group, with those experiencing chronic medical and/or psychiatric disorders at the highest risk.[6] Common sleep disorders at this stage include behaviorally induced insufficient sleep syndrome, inadequate sleep hygiene, insomnia, delayed sleep phase syndrome (DSPS), restless leg syndrome (RLS), and narcolepsy.

PEDIATRIC SLEEP DISORDERS

It is important to note that younger children with sleep disorders respond differently to chronic sleep disruption compared with older children and adolescents. A sleepy toddler or preschooler exhibits paradoxic hyperactivity, irritability, and impulsivity, whereas sleepy older children exhibit signs and symptoms similar to that of adults with chronic sleep disruption such as low energy and drowsiness. Regardless, there are nonspecific signs and symptoms, which children of all ages manifest with chronic inadequate sleep:

- mood changes
- negative sense of well-being
- excessive daytime sleepiness manifesting as drowsiness or unscheduled naps

- fatigue
- somatic complaints
- cognitive impairment
- poor school performance

This can lead to increased stress, abnormal sensation/reaction to pain, poor eating habits, among other adverse reactions. To be clear, no sleep disorder is confined to the pediatric age range; however, some sleep disorders occur primarily in childhood and may manifest differently in a nonpediatric population.

Clinical Evaluation

Accurate diagnoses and treatment of pediatric sleep disorders are dependent on a comprehensive clinical evaluation. This includes assessing both waking and sleeping behaviors. An initial assessment should include

- a detailed sleep history
- medical history
- family history of sleep disorders
- social history
- psychologic/psychiatric assessment
- developmental screening
- physical examination

Age of onset, the associated circumstances, degree of debilitation, persistence/worsening, triggers, and ameliorating factors should be included in this assessment. In addition, usual sleep/wake habits, napping habits, bedtime/nighttime awakenings, and symptoms of daytime sleepiness and/or irritability should be documented. Duration of sleep periods, frequency, timing, sleep changes during weekends and vacations, stressors, and school performance should also be assessed. Sleep diaries and sleep habit questionnaires may also be beneficial. It is also important to assess symptoms of snoring, overnight gasping for air, episodes of stopped breathing, sleepwalking, sleep talking, and bed-wetting.

Common Pediatric Sleep Disorders During the First 3 Years of Life

Behavioral insomnia of childhood

Behavioral insomnia of childhood is defined as difficulty falling asleep, staying asleep, or both, which is a consequence of poor limit setting or inappropriate sleep-onset associations.[3]

Limit-setting behavioral insomnia. This disorder is characterized by parents or caregivers who are unwilling or unable to institute appropriate sleep routines and enforce bedtime limits. Inability to set limits during bedtime routines can result in sleep deterioration. The child will constantly find reasons to lengthen the duration of the bedtime routine by making unnecessary excuses such as requests for a glass of water, more stories, use of the bathroom, and food. Parents will describe a child with noncompliant behavior who verbally protests parental requests, has bedtime resistance, repeatedly demands parental attention after bedtime, has delayed sleep onset usually over 30 min, has frequent nighttime awakenings, and has poor daytime function due to insufficient sleep. This disorder is common in preschool and early school-aged children. Prevalence is up to 30% of preschoolers and about 15% of school-aged children. Without intervention, it can become a chronic problem.

Diagnosis and treatment. Through extensive history taking, the diagnosis can easily be made. Medical history and physical examination are usually benign except for possible oppositional defiant disorder or attention-deficit hyperactivity disorder (ADHD). For children with limit-setting behavioral insomnia, it will be incumbent on the parents to learn to be firm with their limit setting by establishing a regular bedtime and ensuring the bedtime routines have a clear endpoint. Maintaining good sleep hygiene practices and daytime sleep habits such as avoiding naps is beneficial. Reinforcing good behavior with positive behavioral modification using stickers or star charts or other prizes may rapidly elicit the awaited response.[4]

Sleep-onset association behavioral insomnia. In this disorder, the child learns to fall asleep only with specific associations, usually parents, and has an inability to self-soothe during nighttime awakenings without that specific association. This disorder is primarily stressful for the parents, and nighttime awakenings can be quite bothersome and disruptive to parental sleep. The disorder tends to be a reflection of the established patterns of interactions between the parent and child around the time of bedtime. The child becomes accustomed to parental intervention to enable them to fall asleep. As such the child becomes reliant on the parent to make the sleep transition successfully regardless of the time of the night. Using a commonly described analogy from leaders in the field, most adults fall asleep with a pillow and if they awaken in the middle of the night and find the pillow is gone, they will wake up and look for it. When the pillow is found, they can easily fall back to sleep. Based on this analogy, in the child's eyes, the presence of the parent while falling asleep is equivalent to the pillow. Consequently, a child with sleep-onset association behavioral insomnia will wake up and look around for his or her "pillow" and will be unable to fall back to sleep until the pillow/parent is located. This can cause distress, leading to a full awakening and agonizing crying by the child until the parent appears. Once the parent returns to the room, the child is easily able to fall back to sleep. Sleep-onset association behavioral insomnia is primarily seen in infants and young children. Up to 50% of 6- to 12-month-olds, 30% of 1-year-olds, and 20% of toddlers exhibit symptoms of this disorder.[5]

Diagnosis and treatment. Diagnosis is usually made through careful history taking. Medical history and physical examination are usually benign. There are multiple options for intervention that can be employed here. These include (1) *extinction*, which involves letting the child "cry it out" until they learn to self-soothe; (2) *gradual extinction*, which involves progressively ignoring the child for longer and longer periods until the child learns to self-soothe; and (3) *fading of adult intervention*, in which the parent positions themselves further and further away from the child at bedtime until eventually they are no longer in the room.[3] Engaging in regular bedtime routines, avoiding prolonged daytime naps, and an introduction of other transitional objects such as blankets, dolls, and stuffed animals are important. Furthermore, a discontinuation of nighttime feedings is important to reduce the chances of a "learned hunger" nighttime habit. Children with sleep-onset association behavioral insomnia usually rapidly respond to simple gradual behavioral interventions, which helps the child to develop new sleep association habits that do not include the parent.

Common Pediatric Disorders in Children Ages 3–8 Years

Obstructive sleep apnea syndrome in childhood

OSA in childhood is a disorder in which children/adolescents experience decreased upper airway patency (upper airway obstruction) and/or an inability to maintain patency of the upper airway (decreased upper airway diameter and muscle tone) while asleep.[5] This obstruction and loss of tone can lead to a decrease in airflow and reduction in oxyhemoglobin saturation, along with hypercarbia. In children, this disorder is most frequently associated with large tonsils and adenoids. Childhood OSA syndrome manifests differently from that of adults. Children with OSA can have clinically significant sleep-disordered breathing with only brief obstructive events and without significant changes in blood oxygen hemoglobin levels. These children will have frequent brief awakenings specifically just to reopen the airway, and this results in fragmented and unrefreshing sleep. This disorder can lead to significant

nighttime and daytime symptoms. Nighttime symptoms include loud continuous snoring, paradoxic chest to abdomen motion, and abnormal sleeping positions such as sleeping with the neck hyperextended, nocturnal sweating, witnessed apnea, witnessed difficulty breathing during sleep, gasping for air, restless sleep, or occasionally patients have no witnessed nighttime symptoms at all.[5] Daytime symptoms include nasal congestion/obstruction, mouth breathing, failure to thrive, hyponasal speech, behavioral problems, and excessive daytime sleepiness (though less frequent). The results of this disturbance both during the night and daytime lead to difficulties in focus, attention, aggression and irritability, enuresis, partial arousal parasomnias, difficulty awakening the patient in the morning, emotional lability, and other signs of chronic insufficient sleep.[8]

The prevalence rate of OSA is about 3% of preschool-age children and the peak age of occurrences between 2 and 6 years, which is usually a period when adenotonsillar hypertrophy and lymphoid hyperplasia are common.[9] There is a second peak of OSA in adolescence due to other risk factors such as obesity.[1] The presentation in adolescence is similar to that of adults. There may be a male preponderance in younger children. In addition, a family history of OSA and/or disruptive snoring is frequently elicited. Certain special populations are more likely to experience this disorder such as trisomy 21, Prader-Willi syndrome, certain neuromuscular disorders, and children with obesity.[14]

Diagnosis and treatment. To correctly diagnose OSA in childhood, a good clinical history is required to elicit information on daily sleep habits, breathing concerns while sleeping, daytime symptoms, school performance, and previous airway surgery. Specifically, it is imperative to assess the nature and quality of snoring, parental observations of witnessed apnea, retractions, and inspiratory struggles. There is frequently a family history of OSA and/or loud snoring. The physical examination may reveal an overweight or obese child, or alternatively a child with failure to thrive, midface hypoplasia, retro- or micrognathia, chronic nasal congestion with swollen turbinates, deviated septum, and oftentimes tonsillar and adenoid hypertrophy is observed. Diagnosis is confirmed by a polysomnogram, which will provide an accurate description of the type of apnea (obstructive vs. central vs. mixed), the prevalence of the breathing problems during REM sleep or supine sleep, the degree of oxygen desaturation, the degree of hypercarbia, any concerning cardiac arrhythmias, and evidence of sleep fragmentation.[9] Treatment would include surgical evaluation for potential tonsillectomy and adenoidectomy and pharmacologic therapy—specifically use of medication such as steroid sprays to reduce inflammation and swelling, which will eventually lead to a reduction in airway obstruction and increase airway patency.[8] Weight management is also strongly recommended if the child is obese or overweight. If symptoms do not improve with the above options, mechanical therapies such as continuous positive airway pressure may be considered.[9]

Partial arousal parasomnias

One of the most frequent sleep-related problems observed at this developmental stage is partial arousal events.[4] These are partial arousals from deep non-REM sleep and may occur more frequently during the transition between slow-wave deep sleep and REM sleep. This disorder is seen most frequently in preschool and school-age children and tends to resolve by the adolescent years. Partial arousals can manifest as sleepwalking (calm or agitated), confusional arousals, or sleep terrors.[10] These disorders are all similar to each other, as they all represent a sudden partial awakening from deep sleep and all tend to occur 1–2 h after sleep onset.[10] During these episodes, there is automated behavior, relative nonreactivity to external stimuli, a high threshold to arouse, amnesia for the events, disorientation when awakened, confusion, and an inability to recall any associated dreams. Another key feature of these events is that they resolve just as suddenly as they begin because these children rapidly fall back into deep sleep. These disorders do differ by the specific behavioral manifestation and the developmental stage. Sleep terrors frequently develop around age 18 months.[4] Sleepwalking tends to present in preschoolers and school-age children. Up to 40% of children sleepwalk at least on one occasion, with 3%–4% having more frequent episodes.[5] Confusional arousals tend to occur at any stage during childhood. Overall, these partial arousal events tend to diminish after the onset of puberty and frequently completely resolve before adulthood.

These events tend to occur as a result of multiple factors, including age, overtiredness, inherited factors, and anxiety. The chances of experiencing partial arousals depend on the amount and intensity of a child's slow-wave sleep, which is known to be associated with developmental stage. Slow-wave sleep is the highest and most intense between ages 3 and 5 years.[2] This is also around the time when daytime naps are reducing. Consequently, the change in sleep schedules, potential bad sleeping habits, stress, and overtiredness can increase the likelihood of partial arousal events. In addition, a strong family history of partial arousal parasomnias can also play a key role in determining whether this disorder will develop.

Confusional arousals. Confusional arousals are thought to be very frequent in children under age 5 years; the arousal usually presents as a movement or moaning, which progresses to crying and occasionally calling out.[10] Wild irrational thrashing can sometimes be seen in older children. The child is frequently sweating with eyes open or closed. Patient will have a look of confusion, agitation, and distress. Coddling or speaking softly frequently does not provide reassurance and may actually lead to increased distress in the child. Attempts to wake up the patient, turn on the lights, or yell also tend to be unsuccessful. The episode will last anywhere from 1 to 2 min up to 40 min; however, the average duration is 5–15 min.[10]

Sleep terrors. Sleep terrors are considered a variation of confusional arousals.[10] These events also occur suddenly with the child abruptly bolting upright from sleep and letting out a bloodcurdling scream. The child will seem aroused and appear fully awake with a racing heartbeat, dilated pupils, and extremely agitated behavior.[12] They appear to be in fear. During that period, they appear awake; however, they are confused and do not recognize parents or family members and are often inconsolable. Occasionally they will run out of bed as if attempting to avoid unseen danger. These events usually last minutes and can be quite worrisome and terrifying to parents. There is complete amnesia of the event the next morning.

Sleepwalking disorder. There are two types of sleepwalking disorders—calm sleepwalking disorder and agitated sleepwalking disorder.[10] In calm sleepwalking disorder, the child quietly stands up from bed while asleep and calmly walks around, usually quiet and unnoticed. The child's movements are poorly coordinated and not purposeful. There is a paucity of speech; however, the child may answer to his or her name but generally remains incoherent. The child may engage in inappropriate behavior such as urinating in the closet or next to the toilet. Young children frequently are able to quietly be escorted back to bed. The event frequently lasts only a few minutes. Older children frequently awaken during the sleepwalking and are embarrassed to find themselves in an unanticipated location or circumstance. Regardless, they are easily able to return back to bed and to sleep. In agitated sleepwalking disorder, the child suddenly becomes upset and agitated while walking around during sleep. The presence of speech is greater; however, speech tends to be garbled and unintelligible. The event may last anywhere between 1 and 30 min and eventually resolves with the child awakening and returning to bed. Overall agitated sleepwalking tends to occur more frequently in older children.

Treatment. Overall these partial arousal parasomnias will resolve without intervention over time. In the meantime, behavioral interventions play a huge role in reducing the frequency and intensity of these events.[10,12] Increasing total sleep time and adhering to a strict sleep-wake cycle while removing potential sources of sleep disruption can significantly assist in providing a relaxing emotionally safe state for the child as he or she falls asleep. In cases where the partial arousal events are more concerning, such as sleepwalking and getting into danger, safety precautions such as alarms that trigger when the child leaves his/her bed may be essential. In addition, medications such as benzodiazepines may be considered if behavioral interventions are not sufficient.

Rhythmic movement disorders
Rhythmic movement disorders are defined as repetitive and stereotyped movements that occur primarily during sleep-wake transitions, especially at bedtime.[11] These disorders include body rocking, head banging, and body rolling. These disorders are generally considered benign and commonly occur in typically developing children. If these kinds of movements occur during the daytime, unrelated to sleep transitions, or occur in children with developmental delays, further evaluation by a neurologist may be warranted. Rhythmic movement disorders are not only benign but also the evidence of injury is rare. It is estimated that two-thirds of infants have engaged in a type of rhythmic behavior, and 3%–15% of children have self-soothed through head banging.[11] The onset is usually before 1 year of age. By age 18 months, 50% of children will have discontinued these behaviors, and by age 4 years, only 8% of children will have persistent evidence of these disorders.[12] Males tend to engage in these behaviors more frequently than females with a male to female ratio of 4:1.[11] Parents frequently present to clinic as they are very concerned and it is important to spend time reassuring the family that this is normal, common, benign, and self-limited. Bringing attention to these behaviors in front of the child can sometimes reinforce the behaviors and therefore intentionally disregarding the behaviors while the child is present is recommended to avoid developing bad habits. Occasionally, there can be an underlying sleep disorder such as sleep-disordered breathing that needs to be treated to reduce these

behaviors. Pharmacologic agents, such as benzodiazepines, hydroxyzine, and try cyclic antidepressants, are rarely necessary.

Restless legs syndrome
RLS is a disorder that is dependent on a circadian pattern.[13] Patients experience abnormal sensations deep in the legs, which subsequently lead to an irresistible urge to move. The symptoms are worst at rest and are lessened with voluntary movement. Patients primarily experience these sensations in the evening, and the sensations can be quite vexing but generally not painful. Because of this intense urge to move, patients experience difficulty initiating sleep and maintaining sleep. This can lead to excessive daytime sleepiness and poor daytime function. On polysomnogram, periodic limb movements are frequently noted. These limb movements during sleep can be quite disruptive and may cause frequent arousals, which can further contribute to the inadequate and insufficient sleep.

This disorder may manifest because of an underlying vitamin/mineral deficiency. Specifically, a deficiency in iron, vitamin B_{12}, and/or folate may cause the symptoms. Children presenting with RLS frequently have a strong family history of the disorder.[13]

Diagnosis and treatment. RLS is primarily diagnosed clinically through an extensive history and physical examination. This disorder is frequently initially misdiagnosed as growing pains or hyperactivity as patients cannot sit quietly for long periods in the evening. The fatigue and drowsiness, which can develop because of insufficient sleep and stress, can worsen the symptoms of RLS. Treatment includes reducing stress, improving sleep hygiene, and managing behaviors using therapies such as massage and relaxation. Alternatively, if behavioral management is not sufficient, medications such as clonidine, gabapentin, and dopamine agonists may be of help.[12]

Common Pediatric Disorders in Children in Preteens and Young Adolescents
Insufficient sleep
Insufficient sleep is the most common cause of sleepiness in adolescents.[6] It is defined as obtaining an insufficient number of hours in bed and can lead to chronic sleep deprivation. Daytime sleepiness, stress, and other related symptoms can lead to prolonged daytime naps and "catch-up" weekend sleep, which can promote abnormal circadian rhythms, resulting in an erratic sleep-wake schedule. These erratic sleep patterns result in fragmented overnight sleep, inability to fall asleep early especially on school nights; this subsequently results in a repeated cycle of poor inadequate sleep.

Consequences of this disorder include falling asleep in class, oversleep in the morning, fatigue, irritability, mood lability, and other symptoms of chronic sleep restriction.[7]

Treatment. The best treatment for insufficient sleep is to make behavioral changes to ensure adequate sleep. It is important to get the family involved in understanding and acknowledging the consequences of insufficient sleep and its relationship to poor daytime function. Strategies to improve sleep including a behavioral contract agreed to by the family specifying specific number of hours in bed and targeting poor sleep habits would be beneficial.[1] In addition, rewards for successes versus negative consequences for failures will help to increase the chances of success of the contract.

Circadian rhythm disorders—delayed sleep phase syndrome

DSPS is the most common circadian rhythm disorder in adolescents.[1] It usually develops during early puberty and manifests as a tendency to stay up late and sleep in late. The circadian system in adolescents can be highly susceptible and when entrained into a specific phase position, it can be very difficult to shift to an earlier time. This can result in a long delay in falling asleep and a strenuous effort to awaken early in the morning. Children and adolescents frequently take long afternoon naps to make up for this loss of sleep time. Unfortunately, these long afternoon naps encourage continuation of an unhealthy cycle, as DSPS patients lose their drive to sleep during normal bedtime hours after taking a long late afternoon nap. These long afternoon naps lead to a lack of sleepiness until late at night, and this leads to restricted sleep when the patient is required to awaken early in the morning. This subsequently leads to daytime fatigue/sleepiness and thus another long afternoon nap to catch up on sleep. This unhealthy cycle is not without consequences. At this age range, there are many new inexperienced drivers who are required to operate vehicles early in the morning to get to school, during a period that falls within their natural sleep cycle.[7,12] Studies have shown that motor vehicle accidents are most frequent during early morning commutes, especially by young inexperienced drivers. Patients also frequently have trouble organizing themselves such that they frequently miss early morning appointments and have difficulty making it to school on time.

Diagnosis and treatment. The diagnosis of DSPS is determined by a comprehensive assessment of a pa-

tient's activities.[2] A detailed sleep diary would reveal a pattern that may be less evident from just history taking. Treatment involves both eliminating the sleep debt and restoring a normal bedtime, sleep-onset time, and rise time. The child/adolescent and family have to be willing and motivated to make significant behavioral changes, including prioritizing sleep hygiene, as well as providing help for stress management and priority setting. If behavioral management is not sufficient, chronotherapy may be considered.[12] This involves resetting the biologic clock and involves intense management of the sleep schedule to result in a gradual realignment to the desired sleep schedule and then maintenance of this new realignment. Maintenance of the realigned sleep schedule can be very challenging. Daytime naps must be avoided, and adequate sleep hygiene must be followed closely to successfully maintain a normal sleep schedule. Occasionally, melatonin may be beneficial to assist with the realignment.

Pediatric narcolepsy

Narcolepsy frequently develops early childhood and fully matures by mid-adolescence or young adulthood. Narcolepsy is the second most prevalent cause of hypersomnolence in adolescents. Narcolepsy is characterized by a tetrad of symptoms, including (1) excessive daytime sleepiness sometimes with irresistible sleep attacks; (2) cataplexy, which is characterized by a sudden loss of muscle tone often preceded by strong emotions.[5] Patients may describe symptoms such as facial weakness or knees buckling with sudden change of emotions such as hearing a joke or sudden surprise or anger; (3) hypnagogic or hypnopompic hallucinations, which are perceptual distortions that occur as the patient is awakening or falling asleep; and (4) sleep paralysis at sleep onset, which is a sensation of being awake but not being able to move.[5] Adolescents usually do not manifest all four of these symptoms; however, excessive daytime sleepiness tends to be the most prominent symptom. These patients will have an adequate night's sleep of 8–9 h in bed and will be able to fall back to sleep within hours of awakening. Narcolepsy patients exhibit REM sleep during daytime naps on the EEG, which is abnormal and is a defining pathognomonic sign of narcolepsy. Narcolepsy patients often have emotional and behavioral disturbances as prominent features of the disorder. This can lead to incorrect diagnosis of a psychiatric disorder before the narcolepsy has been recognized.

Diagnosis and treatment. Narcolepsy is currently diagnosed by assessing the clinical findings, as well as characteristic features on an overnight polysomnogram and subsequent MSLT (multiple sleep latency test). Adolescents with this disorder are vulnerable to adolescent social pressures and tend to require more counseling and support for psychosocial concerns. Patients with narcolepsy perform best when they are allowed to take naps throughout the day, even while at school. Furthermore, important academic courses should be scheduled during periods of greatest alertness. Stimulant medications work best to alleviate excessive daytime sleepiness in children and adolescents with this disorder. Furthermore, tricyclic antidepressant medications and monoamine oxidase inhibitors (MAOIs) are recommended to manage cataplexy, sleep paralysis, and hypnopompic or hypnagogic hallucinations.[5]

Insomnia

Childhood-onset insomnia or idiopathic insomnia often develops in adolescence and is very different from the behavioral insomnias of childhood discussed earlier.[4] Studies have shown that adolescents with childhood-onset insomnia have an inability to completely shut down the arousal mechanisms in the brain while asleep. As a result, there is an imbalance between arousal and sleep systems and leads to a constant hyperarousal state and persistent hyposomnolence. Adolescents with insomnia often complain of impaired vigilance and attention, poor concentration, low energy, bad mood, and increased fatigue; however, they rarely complain of daytime sleepiness. Occasionally, some patients may develop hyperactivity. Insomnia patients frequently have a family history of poor sleep/insomnia.

Treatment. Children and adolescents with insomnia benefit most from close monitoring of sleep and bedtime routines, improving sleep hygiene, and normalizing of sleep schedules.[5] In addition, it is important to avoid alcohol and use of other drugs, as these may significantly impair sleep. Furthermore, relaxation therapy, massage, yoga, biofeedback, and psychotherapy are beneficial for children and adolescents with this disorder.

Sleep bruxism

Sleep bruxism is characterized by stereotyped movements of the mouth while asleep, resulting in grinding or clenching of the teeth.[5] It is frequently related to stress and emotional tension. Bruxism usually appears between ages 10 and 20 years. Parents will describe loud grinding noises while patient is asleep, and the patient exhibits a clenched jaw while asleep.

Patients may complain of jaw tenderness, waking up with a headache, or temporomandibular joint problems. Furthermore, inspection of the teeth may show excessive wear.

Treatment. Treatment includes reducing stress and anxiety, nocturnal alarms, and/or interocclusal appliances.

PEDIATRIC PSYCHIATRIC DISORDERS AND SLEEP

Sleep difficulty is common in psychiatric disorders. There is a strong, complex, and bidirectional interconnection between psychiatric disorders and sleep.[15] Specifically, disruption in sleep can be a major heralding sign for many psychiatric disorders. For instance, insomnia is a defining symptom of psychiatric disorders, such as depression, generalized anxiety, mania, and panic disorder. On the other hand, sleep disorders are frequently associated with psychiatric symptoms and a longer duration of certain sleep disorders is correlated with increased lifetime risk of experiencing psychiatric illness. It is also well known that sleep deprivation can improve or exacerbate many psychiatric disorders. Furthermore, many psychiatric disorders and sleep disorders are treated with the same pharmacologic agents. For instance, stimulant medications, which are frequently used for narcolepsy and hypersomnia disorders, are also used for treatment of attention deficit disorders and occasionally depressive disorders. Antidepressant medications are frequently used to treat insomnia, as well as cataplexy and sleep paralysis, which are symptoms experienced by patients with narcolepsy. Also, mood-stabilizing medications, frequently used in patients with bipolar disorder, are regularly used to induce sleep in sleep-deprived patients. To add to this very complex relationship, for patients who experience a psychiatric and sleep disorder simultaneously, the sleep disorder may impede the treatment of the psychiatric disorder and vice versa. It is thus imperative that both psychiatric and sleep disorders be treated simultaneously to successfully improve the patient's overall condition.

Sleep Disturbance in Attention Deficit Hyperactivity Disorder

Children with ADHD frequently have sleep problems.[16] The most frequent sleep difficulty in patients with ADHD is sleep-onset delay and restless sleep. The reasons for this sleep difficulty remain unclear; however, it is well-documented that the regions within the central nervous system that regulate sleep and attention/arousal are closely linked. Therefore, the sleep difficulty may be intrinsic to ADHD. However, it also may be related to comorbid psychiatric disorders, such as depression and/or oppositional defiant disorder. Alternatively, the sleep disturbance may be secondary to concomitant stimulant medications. It is important to note that at least 25% of children with ADHD have a primary sleep disorder such as OSA, RLS, or narcolepsy, which may account for a portion of their behavioral concerns.[16] Therefore, patients who have sleep disturbance and ADHD should be evaluated by a sleep physician to rule out other frequently associated sleep disorders that may cause hyperactivity and inattentiveness. If the patient has sleep disturbance because of the stimulant medications, strict regulation of the timing of day that the medication is administered (i.e., taking medication immediately on awakening with avoidance of late afternoon doses) may be beneficial. Otherwise, the child may fare better with a nonstimulant agent.

Sleep Disturbance in Autism

Children with autism have a very high frequency of sleep problems. The most frequent sleep difficulty in patients with autism includes severe sleep-onset and sleep-maintenance insomnia. It is estimated that up to 70% of children with pervasive developmental delay and autism experience significant sleep problems.[14] The sleep problems are likely intrinsic abnormalities in sleep regulation and circadian rhythms associated with the disorder. Furthermore, medications used to treat associated symptoms, cognitive delays, sensory deficits, and increased parental stress may play a role in exacerbating the sleep problems. Children with autism often are unable to tolerate a polysomnogram because of sensory integration concerns. Therefore, the evaluation of sleep disturbance in children with autism may have to be based primarily on medical history and physical examination, especially if there are significant cognitive delays. Studies have shown that parents may over-report sleep concerns in autistic children likely due to increased levels of parental stress; therefore, behavioral interventions for sleep problems in autistic children are the mainstay of treatment. It is highly recommended so that both parents and children with autism can develop healthy sleep habits, and this increases the parents' sense of competence, control, and ability to cope. It is important to recommend targeted behavioral interventions that focus on the specific needs of the child such as a weighted blanket for autistic children with significant sensory concerns, strictly enforced

daytime and bedtime routines/schedules for autistic children with significant obsessive-compulsive disorder concerns, chronotherapy for autistic children with circadian dysregulation, and applied behavior analysis therapy, including visual supports, sticker charts, and established bedtime routines for autistic children with significant emotional lability, and/or a combination of targeted behavioral interventions.[14] Occasionally, pharmacologic agents such as melatonin may be included in the treatment regimen to help ease the transition to sleep.

It is important to note that children with autism are frequently treated with psychotropic medications, which can lead to excessive weight gain and eventually result in OSA. In this situation, evaluation for symptoms of OSA and empiric treatment may be the best option to improve sleep problems.

Sleep Disturbance in Generalized Anxiety Disorder

The most frequent sleep difficulty in patients with generalized anxiety disorder (GAD) is sleep-onset insomnia.[17] Over 50% of children with GAD experience sleeping difficulty, both falling asleep and staying asleep. These patients describe difficulties relaxing around the time of bedtime, shutting off their minds, and an inability to stop worrying as they fall asleep. There is limited evidence available providing guidance on how to manage insomnia in children with GAD. Behavioral treatments such as cognitive behavioral therapy for sleep can be very effective. Pharmacologic agents such as benzodiazepines, trazodone, and tricyclic antidepressants that treat the GAD may also be beneficial to secondarily target insomnia.[12]

Sleep Disturbance in Posttraumatic Sleep Disorder

Children with posttraumatic stress symptoms (PTSD) invariably experience significant sleep difficulties, and disrupted sleep is a hallmark of PTSD.[12] Some studies have suggested that sleep disturbance may be an integral component in the development of the disorder. There is no evidence that preexisting insomnia/sleep disturbance plays a role in the development of PTSD; however, sleep disturbance occurring soon after the traumatic event may play a role in how the brain consolidates emotional/anxiety-provoking memories in the temporal lobe where memories are typically housed. A vast number of studies have been conducted on PTSD and there have been vastly differing conclusions; however, one fairly consistent finding is that individuals with PTSD who undergo a polysomnogram frequently experience disrupted sleep with significant amounts of time spent awake in bed. Furthermore, individuals with PTSD have an alteration in their REM sleep such that their REM density is much higher than average. The reasons for this finding remain unclear; however, high REM density is a frequent finding in other psychiatric disorders such as depression. It is important to note that the polysomnogram frequently does not mirror a patient's self-report of sleep disturbance, as the patients frequently describe more sleep problems overnight than those are captured on the polysomnogram. Treatments for PTSD-related sleep disturbance have a wide range of outcomes, and the few studies that have been devoted to the treatment of PTSD-related sleep disturbance have found multiple different conclusions, as there is a high frequency of comorbid conditions and heterogeneity of the symptoms associated with the disorder.[17] Currently, sertraline and fluoxetine have been shown to be fairly efficacious, as well as lamotrigine, which is an anticonvulsant. These medications may calm anxiety and stabilize mood so as to allow an individual to more easily induce sleep onset. In general, medications that are FDA-approved hypnotic agents for primary insomnia have been frequently utilized for PTSD-related sleep disturbance, such as benzodiazepines and sedating antidepressants. Children and adolescents with PTSD may also benefit from an α-1-adrenergic antagonist for the treatment of nightmares, which can improve sleep by reducing sleep fragmentation.[17]

Sleep Disturbance in Panic Disorder

Individuals with panic disorder report disturbances in sleep, which differ from that of individuals with GAD.[15] Those with panic disorder report frequent sleep/nocturnal panic attacks, which may occur multiple times a night, causing recurrent difficulty maintaining sleep. Nocturnal panic attacks tend to arise from non-REM sleep similar to sleep terrors and are independent from nightmares, which generally occur during REM sleep. The child will suddenly awaken out of non-REM sleep and then have a panic attack, which is much like the awake panic with the associated fear and somatic symptoms. Over time, children may develop a fear of going to bed, which can lead to insufficient sleep over time and this may exacerbate both daytime and sleep anxiety. Relaxation therapy may be beneficial to reduce fears before bedtime. Polysomnogram findings indicate that individuals with panic disorder have poor sleep efficiency (i.e., spend more time in bed, awake instead of asleep), likely due to prolonged latency to sleep onset.

Similar to PTSD, there tends to be discordance between polysomnogram findings and the patient's sleep complaints.[15] Of note, REM sleep physiology does not appear to be affected by panic disorder. The key to treating sleep disturbance associated with panic disorder is to focus on treating the panic disorder itself. When treatment of the panic symptoms improves, sleep onset and sleep maintenance will improve as well. Cognitive behavioral therapy can also be beneficial to improve sleep in children with panic disorder.

Sleep Disturbance and Mood Disorders
Major depression

Sleep complaints and fatigue are some of the hallmarks of major depression.[15] These sleep concerns include insomnia, hypersomnia, or a combination of both; however, insomnia is the most common sleep complaint in depression. During a depressive episode, children tend to experience a decrease in total sleep time over a 24-h period and nonrestorative sleep, along with daytime fatigue and sedation. The sleep disturbance may actually precede the mood episode. During a major depressive episode, the polysomnogram shows abnormal REM sleep, sleep continuity, and slow-wave sleep disturbances. REM sleep, which usually occurs about 90 min after falling asleep, occurs significantly sooner after sleep onset in children with depression, indicating a reduction in REM latency. In addition, there is an increase in REM density, an increase in overall ratio of REM sleep to total sleep, and a longer duration of the first REM period. In addition, depressed children show increased latency to sleep onset, frequent overnight awakenings, and decreased slow-wave sleep. Interestingly, insomnia tends to be one of the earliest symptoms to improve on starting depression treatment and this is mirrored by the improvement in the polysomnogram. Specifically, slow-wave sleep and total sleep time improve the most. It is important to note that MAOIs, tricyclic antidepressants, and electroconvulsive therapy are potent suppressors of REM sleep.[17]

Bipolar disorder

Manic episodes are typically characterized by a fairly abrupt decreased need for sleep and decreased total sleep time in a 24-h period.[17] There appears to be a bidirectional relationship between mania and insomnia such that insomnia may cause mania, while mania further exacerbates insomnia. Because of this, treatments for mania include early and aggressive treatment of sleep disturbance. During a manic episode, the polysomnogram shows finding similar to that of major depression, with the one potential exception being the significantly truncated total sleep time. Of note, mood stabilizers such as lithium increase slowing sleep, delay REM sleep onset, and suppress total REM sleep.

SUMMARY

In summary, this chapter has aimed to review normal pediatric sleep patterns and the changes that occur through all major developmental stages of childhood, reviewed the major pediatric sleep disorders, and finally addressed the interconnection between psychiatric disorders and sleep in some detail. It is evident that this area requires further research to fully understand the connection between pediatric psychiatric disorders and sleep disturbances. In the future, treatments for sleep disturbance in typically developing children and children with psychiatric illnesses will be better tailored to fit the individual's specific needs.

For further reading

- Clinical Sleep Disorders by Carney, Berry, and Geyer
- Principles and Practice of Pediatric Sleep Medicine by Sheldon, Ferber, and Kryger
- Principles and Practice of Sleep Medicine by Kryger, Roth, and Dement

REFERENCES

1. Carskadon MA. The second decade. In: Guilleminault C, ed. *Sleeping and Waking Disorders: Indications and Techniques.* Menlo Park, CA: Addison Wedley; 1982.
2. Mindell JA, Carskadon MA, Owens JA. Developmental features of sleep. *Child Adolesc Psychiatr Clin N Am.* 1999;8(4):695–725.
3. Kuhn BR, Weidinger D. Interventions for infant and toddler sleep disturbance: a review. *Child Fam Behav Ther.* 2000;22(2):33–50.
4. Sheldon S, Spire JP, Levy HB. *Pediatric Sleep Medicine.* Philadelphia: W.B. Saunders; 1992.
5. Sheldon S, Kryger M, Ferber R, Gozal D. *Principles and Practice of Pediatric Sleep Medicine.* Philadelphia: W.B. Saunders; 2014.
6. Carskadon MA, Harvey K, Duke P, et al. Pubertal changes in daytime sleepiness. *Sleep.* 1980;2(4):453–460.
7. Carskadon MA, Dement WC. Sleepiness in the normal adolescent. In: Guilleminault C, ed. *Sleep and its Disorders in Children.* New York: Raven Press; 1987:53–66.
8. Torretta S, Rosazza C, Pace ME, Iofrida E, Marchisio P. Impact of adenotonsillectomy on pediatric quality of life: review of the literature. *Ital J Pediatr.* 2017;43:107.
9. Marcus CL. Sleep-disordered breathing in children. *Am J Respir Crit Care Med.* 2001;164:16–30.
10. Mindell JA, Owens JA. *A Clinical Guide to Pediatric Sleep: Diagnosis and Management of Sleep Problems.* Philadelphia, PA: Lippincott Williams & Wilkins; 2003:88–96. Chapter 10: Sleepwalking and sleep terrors.
11. Mindell JA, Owens JA. *A Clinical Guide to Pediatric Sleep: Diagnosis and Management of Sleep Problems.* Philadelphia, PA: Lippincott Williams & Wilkins; 2003:97–101. Chapter 11: Headbanging and bodyrocking.
12. Owens JA, Witmans M. Sleep problems. *Curr Probl Pediatr Adolesc Health Care.* 2004;34:154–179.
13. Mahowald MW. Restless leg syndrome and periodic limb movements of sleep. *Curr Treat Opt Neurol.* 2003;5:251–260.
14. Johnson C. Sleep problems in children with mental retardation and autism. *Child Adolesc Psychiatr Clin N Am.* 1996;5:673–681.
15. Avidan AY, Zee PC. *Handbook of Sleep Medicine.* Philadelphia, PA: Lippincott Williams & Wilkins; 2006:165–184. Chapter 7: Sleep disorders in children.
16. Chervin RD, Archbold KH, Dillon JE, et al. Inattention, hyperactivity and symptoms of sleep-disordered breathing. *Pediatrics.* 2002;109:449–456.
17. Carney PR, Berry RB, Geyer JD. *Clinical Sleep Disorders.* Philadelphia, PA: Lippincott Williams & Wilkins; 2005:136–146. Chapter 11: Pediatric and Adolescent Presentations.

CHAPTER 11

Concussion in Children and Adolescents

NASSIM ZECAVATI, MD, MPH

INTRODUCTION

Of the millions of male and female youth who participate in sports yearly within the United States, approximately 2 million children and adolescents sustain concussions, accounting for over 160,000 emergency room visits and hospitalizations annually.[1,2] There is increasing evidence of the adverse effects of a single concussion on cognition and postconcussive symptoms, including poor attention, headaches, and fatigue.[3–6] After a single concussion, a subsequent concussion is more likely and multiple concussions are often sustained in a short period.[6] Given the morbidity associated with concussion, prompt diagnosis and treatment are crucial to promoting a complete recovery and preventing cumulative and long-term brain injury. This chapter provides an overview of the etiology of concussion and recommendations for screening, diagnosis, and treatment.

DEFINITION/SYMPTOM CRITERIA

The Quality Standards Subcommittee of the American Academy of Neurology defines concussion as a trauma-induced alteration that may or may not involve loss of consciousness.[7] Concussions are considered a mild traumatic brain injury (TBI) and can occur with contact to the head or with acceleration/deceleration forces. In the 2016 Berlin Consensus Statement on Concussion in Sport, an expert panel defined concussion as follows: "Sport related concussion (SRC) is a traumatic brain injury induced by biomechanical forces. Several common features that may be utilized in clinically defining the nature of a concussive head injury include:

- SRC may be caused either by a direct blow to the head, face, neck or elsewhere on the body with an impulsive force transmitted to the head.
- SRC typically results in the rapid onset of short-lived impairment of neurological function that resolves spontaneously. However, in some cases, signs and symptoms evolve over a number of minutes to hours.

- SRC may result in neuropathological changes, but the acute clinical signs and symptoms largely reflect a functional disturbance rather than a structural injury and, as such, no abnormality is seen on standard structural neuroimaging studies.
- SRC results in a range of clinical signs and symptoms that may or may not involve loss of consciousness. Resolution of the clinical and cognitive features typically follows a sequential course. However, in some cases symptoms may be prolonged.

The clinical signs and symptoms cannot be explained by drug, alcohol, or medication use, other injuries (such as cervical injuries, peripheral vestibular dysfunction, etc.) or other comorbidities (e.g., psychological factors or coexisting medical conditions).[8]"

The *Diagnostic and Statistical Manual of Mental Disorders, Fifth Edition*, characterizes concussion as a neurocognitive disorder, which is placed on a spectrum with more severe conditions. Diagnosis is based on a clinical presentation of a mild or major neurocognitive disorder. The distinction between these conditions is not based on the initial severity of TBI but instead on the severity of posttraumatic cognitive impairments and their effects on everyday function.[9] Although the exact terminology and definition of concussion may vary among experts, the general consensus is that even relatively mild head injury without the loss of consciousness is sufficient to warrant the diagnosis of concussion.

PREVALENCE/EPIDEMIOLOGY

Approximately, one-half of all patients with concussion or mild TBI are between the ages of 15 and 34 years.[10] Patients vulnerable to injury include children less than 5 years of age and those with lower socioeconomic status, lower cognitive function, and a history of prior hospital admissions.[10] Since 2000, there has been a significant increase in the diagnosis of concussion in the outpatient and emergency department settings in children and adolescents with 4 in 1000 children aged 8–13 years sustaining an SRC.[11] This may be due in part to increased awareness of concussion by patients, coaches/athletic directors, and healthcare providers.

Although boys playing collision sports (football, rugby, ice hockey, lacrosse) have historically had the highest incidence of concussion, girls playing soccer, lacrosse, and field hockey have also emerged as high-risk groups. When considering the role of gender in concussion, data suggest that adolescents with concussion exhibit gender differences with respect to risk factors, recovery, and symptomatology. Females are more likely to present with a concussion, experience more discomfort from a concussion, and seek treatment for postconcussive headaches.[12] On the other hand, males are more likely to sustain a concussion from a contact sport and experience loss of consciousness, confusion, and amnesia with a concussion more frequently than females.[12]

At the front line of concussion care is the primary care physician who routinely provides care for pediatric patients who have sustained a concussion during sports or other recreational activities. In one observational study of over 1000 high school students with SRC, approximately 60% of patients were managed by a primary care physician, whereas about 10% were managed by a specialist such as a pediatric neurologist or sports medicine physician.[13]

ETIOLOGY/PATHOPHYSIOLOGY

The pathophysiology of concussion is complex with neuropathology showing variable findings. Although axonal injury can occur at the time of a severe TBI, milder forms of axonal damage may occur in concussion. Studies indicate impaired axonal transport, leading to axonal swelling, Wallerian degeneration, and transection.[14] Excitatory neurotransmitters such as acetylcholine, glutamate, and aspartate are released potentiating injury.[15] Neuroimaging studies have shown that patients with concussion have more extensive areas of abnormality as measured by functional MRI, suggesting a structural and/or physiologic derangement in concussion.[16]

SCREENING/DIAGNOSIS

In the outpatient setting, the diagnosis of concussion is made after a detailed history is elicited, which documents trauma, either from a direct blow to the head or from a blow to another part of the body with rapid

rotation of the head.[8] Soon after the injury, the signs and symptoms of concussion begin to surface, representing an acute change from the patient's baseline. According to the CDC[17] concussion signs may include the following:

- Can't recall events *prior to* or *after* a hit or fall.
- Appears dazed or stunned.
- Forgets an instruction, is confused about an assignment or position, or is unsure of the game, score, or opponent.
- Moves clumsily.
- Answers questions slowly.
- Loses consciousness *(even briefly)*.
- Shows mood, behavior, or personality changes.

The following concussion symptoms may be reported:

- Headache or "pressure" in head.
- Nausea or vomiting.
- Balance problems or dizziness, or double or blurry vision.
- Bothered by light or noise.
- Feeling sluggish, hazy, foggy, or groggy.
- Confusion, or concentration or memory problems.
- Just not "feeling right," or "feeling down."

Most athletes are not immediately aware that they have sustained a concussion and may return to play and to school before symptoms are recognized. A common misconception is that concussion must be associated with loss of consciousness. In fact, most SRCs are not associated with loss of consciousness.[4] After a suspected concussion, an athlete should be evaluated by a healthcare provider with concussion training, preferably on site at the time of injury.

Several free standardized concussion assessment tools are available to healthcare providers. A validated tool is the Sport Concussion Assessment Tool 5 (SCAT5), which was revised by an expert panel as part of the Fifth International Consensus Conference on Concussion in Sport held in Berlin in 2016.[18] This tool is specifically designed to aid physicians and licensed healthcare individuals in assessing concussion in the acute and outpatient setting in athletes age 13 years and older. A child version of the SCAT5 is available for athletes 12 years and younger. This tool aids providers in recognizing a suspected concussion, enabling prompt removal from play. The SCAT5 recommends periodically reassessing the athlete to monitor for deterioration as concussion signs and symptoms evolve over time. This tool includes an on field and off field/office assessment consisting of a series of steps. At the sideline, the first step is to quickly screen for the presence of any red flags that may necessitate urgent medical care. Red flags include neck pain, double vision, weakness, severe or increasing headache, seizure, loss of consciousness greater than 1 min, deteriorating conscious state, vomiting, or restlessness and agitation. The presence of any of these red flags indicates a need for immediate transfer to the closest emergency department. High-impact injuries in which there is concern for intracranial hemorrhage or skull fracture (palpable skull deformity, drainage of cerebrospinal fluid from the nose) also warrant urgent transfer/medical evaluation. Once the initial assessment has ruled out the red flags above, the second step in the SCAT5 is to observe physical signs such as imbalance, motor incoordination, disorientation, and facial injury. This is followed by a brief memory assessment and examination consisting of the Glasgow Coma Scale (GCS) and cervical spine assessment. Although the SCAT5 should not be used by itself to make or exclude a diagnosis of concussion, it is a valuable tool that healthcare providers can use to assist in making a clinical diagnosis of concussion. For patients seen in the office following the acute injury, a 22-item symptom scale is administered, in addition to a cognitive and neurologic screen, including a balance examination. Although standardized tools such as the SCAT5 should not be used as a stand-alone method to measure recovery or make decisions regarding return to play, they are valuable in objectively measuring the signs and symptoms of concussion and can facilitate a clinical diagnosis of concussion. Additional historical information that is important to identify in children and adolescents with suspected concussion includes how the injury was obtained, including location and force of impact, the timing of symptoms, and whether there is a history of head injury or concussion. Patients with developmental delay and with neurologic deficits at baseline may be at increased risk for concussion due to slow reaction time and impaired visual motor skills. In addition to the SCAT5, all patients should receive a thorough neurologic examination, including mental status examination, cranial nerve function, sensory and motor function, and most importantly gait and balance.

Baseline Testing

At the current time, baseline assessment of neurocognitive function is the norm before participation in intramural contact and collision sports in middle school and high school; however, this remains controversial with differing recommendations from key opinion leaders. The benefit of baseline neuropsychologic testing is that it allows providers to distinguish a concussion from baseline processing delays as may

be present in a learning disability or attention deficit hyperactivity disorder (ADHD). A commonly used neuropsychologic test is the Immediate Post-concussion Assessment and Cognitive Assessment (ImPACT). ImPACT is a computer-based test that assesses an individual's cognitive function and cumulatively documents current concussion symptoms measured by the Post-Concussion Symptoms Scale. The test is administered via a Web-enabled desktop computer and with the assistance of a clinical nurse who has undergone test administration training. The neurocognitive assessment consists of a demographic questionnaire, concussion symptom inventory, and a neurocognitive performance test. The data obtained from the neurocognitive component examine variables such as reaction time, processing speed, verbal memory, visual memory, and total symptom score. A patient's baseline performance on this neuropsychologic test is compared with a postinjury assessment to monitor for acute changes.

DIFFERENTIAL DIAGNOSES

The differential diagnosis for concussion is broad, as the signs and symptoms of concussion are not unique and may be present in a number of conditions. The most serious injury that overlaps with concussion is intracranial hemorrhage such as subdural or epidural hematoma. Often, these conditions are associated with focal neurologic deficits, altered mental status, and worsening symptoms. Other conditions that may present similar to concussion include dehydration, heat stroke, hypoglycemia, syncope, and primary headache disorders such as migraine headache. An important consideration in the diagnosis and treatment of concussion is the presence of a comorbid psychiatric disorder such as ADHD, depression, and/or anxiety. There is a growing body of evidence that suggests concussion affects mood, affect and sleep all of which significantly influence a patient's recovery following concussion. Even more complex is the relationship between gender and sleep following a concussion. Data suggest that females are at increased risk of developing significant sleep disturbance after a single concussion, whereas males may not report sleep disturbance until cumulative concussions have been sustained.[19] Recent data have also shown that among concussed children and adolescents, females who were more likely to require medical treatment for a postconcussive mood disorder had higher levels of sleep disturbance compared with males.[19] Thus, a subset of female athletes with concussion are at increased risk for comorbid sleep conditions, highlighting the need for close follow-up in these patients and coordinated care between various subspecialists, including physical medicine, neurology, and psychiatry.

WORKUP/CLINICAL FINDINGS

Neuroimaging in pediatric and adolescent patients following concussion often takes place in the emergency department setting. Most patients undergo head CT, given availability and sensitivity to intracranial hemorrhage. Because most patients with concussion have normal head imaging, it is important to consider head imaging in high-risk patients such as those with a GCS of <15, suspected skull fracture, recurrent vomiting, prolonged amnesia, seizure, or focal neurologic sign.[20] For patients with normal head CT but with impaired GCS and seizure, inpatient observation is suggested. The vast majority of patients with concussion, however, will have a normal head CT and experience typical postconcussion symptoms, permitting observation in the outpatient setting.

Physical Examination

The physical examination in children and adolescents with concussion is often normal. Depending on the nature of the injury, there may be a concomitant neck injury and thus the cervical spine, in particular, should be assessed and cleared. The cervical spine can be cleared clinically if there is no midline cervical spine tenderness, no focal neurologic deficit, normal alertness, no intoxication, and no painful, distracting injury in a patient who is able to move his/her head in flexion/extension and rotate 45 degrees to both sides without pain. If there is uncertainty, the cervical spine can be cleared by X-ray or CT. In addition to a general physical examination, the patient should undergo a comprehensive neurologic examination, including mental status, cranial nerves, motor, sensory, cerebellar, and gait. As discussed earlier, a standardized assessment tool such as the SCAT5 is a useful tool and can be administered serially to assess for change.

TREATMENT

Most children and adolescents diagnosed with concussion can be safely monitored in the outpatient setting unless red flags are present such as GCS of <15, suspected skull fracture, recurrent vomiting, prolonged amnesia, seizure, or focal neurologic sign. Pediatric patients must have a reliable caretaker at home who is able to observe changes in signs and symptoms. With conservative management that includes both physical and cognitive rest, many patients return to baseline within a few days. Standard concussion treatment entails resting until all symptoms fully resolve followed by a graded program of exertion before medical clearance and return to play. A subset of patients with concussion, however, will develop postconcussion syndrome. Postconcussion syndrome, which includes headache, dizziness, neuropsychiatric changes, and cognitive impairment.[21] There is a wide range (30%–80%) in the reported incidence of postconcussion syndrome with differing theories on the pathogenesis of postconcussion syndrome, which include structural, biochemical, and possibly psychogenic origins. In clinical practice, an almost identical injury can result in vastly different outcomes with some patients making a complete recovery in a short period and others having persistent and protracted postconcussion syndrome. It is possible that patients with postconcussion syndrome have comorbid psychiatric conditions that are either unmasked or exacerbated by concussion. Studies have shown that poor coping skills, limited social support, and negative perceptions are more common in patients with postconcussion syndrome compared with patients who do not develop persistent symptoms following a concussion.[22] Treatment of postconcussion syndrome is multifaceted. Physical therapy with graded increase in aerobic activity/exertion is recommended. Headaches can be treated with prophylactic medications such as amitriptyline. If depression and anxiety are prominent features, a selective serotonin reuptake inhibitor can be helpful. Avoiding analgesic overuse is important. Narcotics and benzodiazepines should be strictly avoided given the potential for abuse and dependency. The author's experience is that appropriate academic accommodations for young athletes are extremely effective in facilitating recovery. This includes a flexible school day with extended test-taking time and extended time to turn in school work. Communication and collaboration with school teachers, nurses, and guidance counselors is key in supporting a student's recovery following concussion.

The diagnosis and treatment of concussion and postconcussion syndrome continues to evolve, as data in this young field grow and best practices are developed. For healthcare providers, keeping abreast of the latest recommendations for screening, diagnosing, and treating concussion will be essential given the significant public health concern that concussion poses.

REFERENCES

1. Bryan MA, Rowhani-Rahbar A, Comstock RD, Rivara F. Sports- and recreation-related concussions in US youth. *Pediatrics*. June 20, 2016. pii: e20154635.
2. CDC. Nonfatal traumatic brain injuries from sports and recreation activities – United States, 2001-2005. *Morb Mortal Wkly Rep*. 2007;56:733–737.
3. Covassin T, Elbin R, Kontos A, Larson E. Investigating baseline neurocognitive performance between male and female athletes with a history of multiple concussion. *J Neurol Neurosurg Psychiatry*. 2010;81:597–601.
4. Collins MW, Grindel SH, Lovell MR, et al. Relationship between concussion and neuropsychological performance in college football players. *JAMA*. 1999;282(10):964–970.
5. Guskiewicz KM, McCrea M, Marshall SW, et al. Cumulative effects associated with recurrent concussion in collegiate football players. The NCAA concussion study. *JAMA*. 2003;290:2549–2555.
6. Collins MW, Lovell M, Iverson G, Cantu R, Maroon J, Field M. Cumulative effects of concussion in high school athletes. *Neurosurgery*. 2002;51:1175–1179.
7. The Quality Standards Subcommittee of the American Academy of Neurology.
8. *Consensus Statement on Concussion in Sport—the 5th International Conference on Concussion in Sport Held in Berlin*. October 2016.
9. Wortzel HS, Arciniegas DB. The DSM-5 approach to the evaluation of traumatic brain injury and its neuropsychiatric sequelae. *NeuroRehabilitation*. 2014;34(4):613–623. https://doi.org/10.3233/NRE-141086.
10. Kraus JF, McArthur DL. Epidemiologic aspects of brain injury. *Neurol Clin*. 1996;14(2):435.
11. Bakhos LL, Lockhart GR, Myers R, et al. Emergency department visits for concussion in young child athletes. *Pediatrics*. 2010;126(3):e550–e556.
12. Tanveer S, Zecavati N, Delasobera EB, Oyegbile TO. Gender differences in concussion and postinjury cognitive findings in an older and younger pediatric population. *Pediatr Neurol*. 2017;70:44–49.
13. Meehan 3rd WP, d'Hemecourt P, Collins CL, et al. Assessment and management of sport-related concussions in United States high schools. *Am J Sports Med*. 2011;39(11):2304.
14. Povlishock JT, Katz DI. Update of neuropathology and neurological recovery after traumatic brain injury. *J Head Trauma Rehabil*. 2005;20(1):76.
15. Hayes RL, Dixon CE. Neurochemical changes in mild head injury. *Semin Neurol*. 1994;14(1):25.
16. McAllister TW, Sparling MB, Flashman LA, et al. Neuroimaging findings in mild traumatic brain injury. *J Clin Exp Neuropsychol*. 2001;23(6):775.
17. Centers for Disease Control and Prevention. Concussion Signs and Symptoms. Available at: https://www.cdc.gov/headsup/basics/concussion_symptoms.html.
18. Echemendia RJ, Meeuwisse W, McCrory P, et al. The sport concussion assessment tool 5th edition (SCAT5). *Br J Sports Med*. 2017.
19. Oyegbile TO, Delasobera BE, Zecavati N. Gender differences in sleep symptoms and concussion. *Sleep Med*. 2017. [pending publication].
20. Stiell IG, Clement CM, Rowe BH, et al. Comparison of the Canadian CT head rule and the New Orleans criteria in patients with minor head injury. *JAMA*. 2005;294(12):1511.
21. Bazarian JJ, Wong T, Harris M, et al. Epidemiology and predictors of post-concussive syndrome after minor head injury in an emergency population. *Brain Inj*. 1999;13(3):173.
22. McCauley SR, Boake C, Levin HS, et al. Postconcussional disorder following mild to moderate traumatic brain injury: anxiety, depression, and social support as risk factors and comorbidities. *J Clin Exp Neuropsychol*. 2001;23(6):792.

CHAPTER 12

Pediatric Delirium

JESSICA CRAWFORD, MD • MICHELLE GOLDSMITH, MD, MA • JOSHUA WORTZEL, MSC • RICHARD SHAW, MD

INTRODUCTION

In everyday parlance, delirium is a familiar term. For example, one might say someone is delirious with grief, or someone else might be described as deliriously happy. Although these forms of delirium may look different (i.e., one is somnolent and sad and the other is frenetically gleeful), these behaviors share a common definition that is encapsulated using the term delirium (i.e., an incoherence of thought and speech accompanied by behavioral dysregulation). As this chapter will discuss, the medical definition of delirium is not far from this colloquial one in terms of its phenotypic variability.

Pediatric delirium is a medical emergency that requires immediate management; however, in the hospital and outpatient settings, it often goes underdiagnosed.[1] Mortality rates in untreated delirium range from 12.5% to 29% in affected children.[2] There is ongoing effort to codify the clinical presentation of pediatric delirium with age-appropriate assessment tools to allow for more timely diagnosis and treatment.[3] Adult and pediatric delirium types share many similarities; however, pediatric practitioners should be familiar with the significant differences.[4,5]

The goal of this chapter is to provide an overview of medical delirium, as it relates to the pediatric population. It is intended for physicians and healthcare providers in primary care and hospital settings. Topics addressed include definition and symptom criteria, epidemiology, pathophysiology, assessment and screening, diagnostic dilemmas, treatment, sequelae, prevention, and integrative care. The incidence of delirium has been shown to be decreased by improving multidisciplinary education and collaboration,[6] which is an additional aspiration of this chapter.

DEFINITION/SYMPTOM CRITERIA

Delirium is a neuropsychiatric condition involving acute behavioral and mental status changes associated with underlying medical illness.[7] The symptoms that meet the *Diagnostic and Statistical Manual, Fifth Edition*

(*DSM-5*)[8] diagnostic criteria (see Table 12.1) are applicable to both adults and children.[9] As in adults, pediatric delirium may present with three motoric subtypes: hyperactive, hypoactive, and mixed delirium (see Table 12.2).[10] Of note, there is a new fourth "informal" category identified in adults called a nonmotoric subtype; however, this has not been described in children. The frequency of these subtypes is well studied in adult populations[11,12]; however, a gap in the literature exists for pediatric patients.

To date, the most comprehensive data regarding pediatric delirium are from a descriptive study of patients seen by a single pediatric intensive care unit (PICU) psychiatric consult service over a 4-year period at the University Hospital of Maastricht in the Netherlands.[13] These data are presented below; however, further studies are needed to strengthen these preliminary findings.

Hyperactive delirium is characterized by an elevated level of psychomotor activity and mood liability.[7] Symptoms include confusion, psychosis, disorientation, agitation, hypervigilance, hyperalertness, fast or loud speech, combativeness, and behavioral problems, such as pulling out catheters and lines.[7] Patients with hyperactive delirium are often quite disruptive and quickly come to the attention of caregivers. Hyperactive delirium is reported to have a prevalence rate of 35% by Schieveld and colleagues in the above study.

Hypoactive delirium, in contrast, is notable for reduced levels of psychomotor activity, ranging from sluggishness and apathy to lethargy, confusion, and stupor.[7,14] These patients are more sedate and less disruptive, and consequently their delirium is more likely to be overlooked by care providers or misdiagnosed as depression. The aforementioned study identified 22.5% of patients in the cohort with this subtype.[13]

Mixed delirium describes patients with features of both hyper- and hypoactive delirium or those who fluctuate between the two states.[15,16] These patients can also present with relatively normal psychomotor activity and solely express disruption of attention and awareness.[7] Mixed delirium can also masquerade

TABLE 12.1	
DSM-5 Definition of Delirium	
A	Disturbance in attention (i.e., reduced ability to direct focus, sustain, and shift attention) and awareness (reduced orientation to the environment).
B	The disturbance develops over a short period (usually hours to a few days), represents an acute change from baseline attention and awareness, and tends to fluctuate in severity during the course of a day.
C	An additional disturbance in cognition (e.g., memory deficit, disorientation, language, visuospatial ability, or perception).
D	The disturbances in Criteria A and C are not better explained by a preexisting, established, or evolving neurocognitive disorder and do not occur in the context of a severely reduced level of arousal, such as coma.
E	There is evidence from the history, physical examination, or laboratory findings that the disturbance is a direct physiologic consequence of another medical condition, substance intoxication or withdrawal (i.e., due to a drug of abuse or a medication), exposure to a toxin, or is due to multiple etiologies.

From *Neurocognitive Disorders*. 5th ed. Washington, DC: American Psychiatric Association; 2013. *Diagnostic and statistical manual of mental disorders*, with permission.

TABLE 12.2	
Motoric Subtypes of Delirium	
Hyperactive	Proof of at least two of the following behaviors over the prior 24 hours that deviate from baseline: • Increased movement/motor activity • Less coordinated/controllable activity • Restlessness • Wandering (if the patient is mobile)
Hypoactive	Proof of at least two of the following behaviors over the prior 24 hours that deviate from baseline: • Reduced amount or speed of activity • Reduced awareness of surrounding • Reduced amount or speed of speech • Reduced alertness
Mixed motor	Proof of hyperactive and hypoactive features over the prior 24 hours that deviate from baseline

Adapted from Meagher D, Moran M, Raju B, et al. A new data-based motor subtype schema for delirium. *J Neuropsychiatry Clin Neurosci*. 2008;20(2):185–193, with permission.

TABLE 12.3		
Risk Factors for Developing Delirium		
Predisposing Factors	**Precipitating Factors**	**Environmental Factors**
Age	Electrolyte	Immobility
Genetic	imbalance	Light/noise
predisposition	Hypoxia	Reduced social
Neurologic	Acidosis	interaction
disease	Hypoalbuminemia	Pain
Psychiatric	Fever	Use of IV lines
illness	Hypotension	Physical
Visual	Sepsis	restraints
impairment	Infection	
Hearing	Polypharmacy	
impairment	Oversedation	
Surgery	Medication	
	withdrawal	
	Sleep deprivation	

From Wolfe J, Hinds P, Sourkes P. *Textbook of Interdisciplinary Pediatric Palliative Care E-Book: Expert Consult Premium Edition*. Philadelphia: Elsevier Health Sciences; 2011, with permission.

as generalized systemic symptoms, possibly presenting with pain, anxiety, and nausea, which occasionally makes it more difficult for medical professionals to recognize. The majority of cases (42.5%) in the Schieveld study were classified with this subtype.[13]

A 2008 study comparing the phenomenology of pediatric delirium with that of adult delirium found delirium in children to have faster onset and more severe perceptual disturbances, mood lability, and agitation. Less severe cognitive deficits, sleep-wake cycle disturbance, and variability of symptoms over time were noted in pediatric patients when compared with adults.[5]

PREVALENCE/EPIDEMIOLOGY

The epidemiology and risk factors associated with pediatric delirium remain difficult to determine because of a lack of universal hospital screening and recognition.[2,17,18] (See Table 12.3 for general risk factors for developing delirium.) However, several studies in the recent years elucidate this area. In a prospective, 10-week,

observational study, all children in Cornell University's PICU were assessed for delirium over the course of their hospitalization.[19] Silver and colleagues showed that the prevalence of delirium was 21% among this cohort of patients (newborns to 21-year-olds). The greatest risk factors for developing delirium included the presence of developmental delay (odds ratio [OR] = 3.45 [1.54, 7.76]), the need for mechanical ventilation (OR = 3.86 [1.81, 8.24]), and age 2–5 years (OR = 8.80 [1.82, 42.53] compared with adolescents >13 years of age).[19]

In a similarly designed study looking at delirium in Columbia University's pediatric cardiothoracic intensive care unit (ICU), the prevalence of delirium (49%) was significantly higher.[20] Patel and colleagues corroborated that developmental delay was a risk factor for delirium in their patients (OR = 3.38 [1.18–9.66]). Better nutrition (OR = 0.19 [0.04–0.84] with albumin >3 mg/dL) and older age (compared with 0–2 years, 2–5 years had OR = 0.30 [0.12–0.72], 5–13 years with OR = 0.30 [0.10–0.87], and >13 years with OR = 0.06 [0.02–0.22]) were protective factors. The risk factors identified in these two studies parallel risk factors identified in adults, which include preexisting cognitive impairment, medications with high anticholinergic effects, sleep deprivation, hypoxia, metabolic abnormalities/poor nutrition, and a history of alcohol or drug abuse.[21]

As expected with patients studied in more acutely ill settings (i.e., PICU and cardiothoracic ICU), these two studies report a prevalence of pediatric delirium that is much higher than earlier reports (see Chapter 28: Delirium by Wolfe and colleagues,[22] for an in-depth comparison of these earlier studies). The largest of these earlier single-center, retrospective studies reported a 9% prevalence of delirium in a sample of 1027 pediatric patients referred for psychiatric consultation.[9] Another study in a pediatric sample of 877 critical care patients reported an even lower prevalence of 4.6%.[13] These older, more conservative estimates are likely more representative of delirium frequencies among generally hospitalized children. That said, these newer studies use more sensitive screening techniques that likely identify patients who would have previously gone undiagnosed. The true prevalence of delirium among hospitalized children probably falls between these estimates. A later section in this chapter discusses some of the new advances made in screening for improved sensitivity in diagnosis of pediatric delirium.[3]

PATHOPHYSIOLOGY/ETIOLOGY

Delirium is a behavioral manifestation of global encephalopathy and cognitive slowing caused by multiple dysregulated neural pathways and physiologic processes (see Table 12.4 for some of the most common etiologies).[23] No single mechanism of delirium

TABLE 12.4
Common Etiologies of Delirium

Infectious	• Bacterial: sepsis, urinary tract infection, peritonitis, neurosyphilis, cellulitis • Viral: Lyme disease, herpes zoster, HIV • Either: pneumonia, meningitis, endocarditis
Metabolic	• Electrolyte imbalance: Hypo/hypernatremia, hypo/hypercalcemia, hypo/hypermagnesemia • Metabolic derangement: Hypo/hyperglycemia, hypercapnia, hypoxemia • Systemic organ dysfunction: Hypo/hyperthermia, hepatic failure, thyroid failure, renal failure
Neurologic	• Stroke • Intracranial tumor • Intracranial bleed: epidural hematoma, subdural hematoma, intracerebral hemorrhage, subarachnoid hemorrhage • Nonconvulsive epilepsy
Iatrogenic	• Prescription medications: opioids, sedative hypnotics, polypharmacy • Nonprescription medications: antihistamines • Drugs of abuse: ethanol, heroin, hallucinogens • Withdrawal: ethanol, benzodiazepines

Adapted from Rockwood K. Causes of delirium. *Psychiatry*. 2008;7(1):39–41; Francis J, Young B, Aminoff MJ, Schmader KE, Wilterdink JL. Diagnosis of delirium and confusional states. *UpToDate*. 2014, with permission.

has yet been identified, although numerous theories have been put forward. Neurotransmitter deficiency/dysregulation, neuroinflammation, and oxidative stress are among the most substantiated mechanisms pertinent to children.[24] Most cases of delirium likely arise from a mix of some or all of these factors. For those seeking a more detailed discussion of these topics, see Maldonado.[24]

Neurotransmitter Deficiency/Dysregulation

Delirium is conceptualized as a by-product of aberrations in a number of different neurotransmitters, many of which are the downstream consequences of acetylcholine (ACh) and dopamine (DA) dysregulation. In animal models, a deficiency in cholinergic function relative to other neurotransmitters has been shown to alter arousal, attention, and memory.[25] Samples of plasma and cerebrospinal fluid (CSF) taken directly from delirious patients show low levels of ACh,[26] and resolving delirium correlates with decreased serum anticholinergic activity.[27] Inversely, DA levels are increased in delirium, as measured by increased homovanillic acid (a DA metabolite) in the CSF of delirious patients.[28] Dopaminergic antagonists are often effective in treating delirium, further suggesting this axis is critical to the pathogenesis of delirium.[29] Glutamine, gamma-aminobutyric acid (GABA), and serotonin have also been implicated in the pathogenesis of delirium, perhaps as upstream or downstream consequences of ACh and DA dysregulation.[21] For example, GABAergic agents such as benzodiazepines and barbiturates are shown to exacerbate delirium, probably at least in part by interrupting central cholinergic muscarinic transmission in the basal forebrain and hippocampus,[30] and excess DA is known to potentiate the neurotoxic excitatory effects of glutamate that contribute to delirium.[31]

Neuroinflammation

Peripheral inflammation is theorized to play a large role in the pathogenesis of delirium. Infection, surgery, and trauma induce brain parenchymal cells to release proinflammatory cytokines that increase blood-brain barrier permeability, which allows inflammatory cytokines and chemokines to enter the central nervous system.[32] These cytokines, which include interleukin (IL)-1, IL-2, interferon, and tumor necrosis factor, activate microglia to deleteriously modulate astrocyte and neuronal activity.[33] By a separate mechanism, these cytokines also set in motion a cascade of neurodegenerative metabolites: they activate indoleamine-2,3-dioxygenase, which decreases tryptophan levels and subsequently 5-hydroxytryptamine and melatonin production, which ultimately leads to increased kynurenine and other neurotoxic metabolites in the brain.[34] These cytokines also exacerbate neurotransmitter dysregulation by inhibiting ACh-dependent neuronal pathways, which, as discussed above, precipitates agitation, perceptual disturbances, seizures, and delirium.[35,36]

Oxidative Stress

Oxidative metabolism is required in many biologic processes to convert toxic chemicals into benign ones, such that when insufficient oxygen is available, these toxins (i.e., oxygen-free radicals, arachidonic acid metabolites, and cytokines) accumulate within tissues and cause potential damage.[37] This process, oxidative stress, can occur in a multitude of conditions, ranging from trauma, severe illness, frank hypoxia,

to infection.[24] The brain is particularly susceptible to oxygen-free radical damage, which chemically alters lipids in the myelin sheaths.[38] Impaired oxidative metabolism has been shown to be a predisposing factor for delirium[39]; this is supported by epidemiologic findings indicating that patients requiring ventilation are at a greater risk for developing delirium.[19] It seems likely that the residual cognitive deficits reported in many recovered delirious patients are at least in part due to this irreversible, oxidative stress–induced brain damage.[40,41]

ASSESSMENT

Screening

With the prevalence of delirium varying widely based on clinical environment and severity of underlying medical illness, screening for delirium has been proposed as evaluating for an additional vital sign with every shift change or more often in the ICU setting. Based on a change in mental status or from findings based on routine screening, a consult to assess for delirium may arise. Psychiatrists typically field these consults and also screen for depression and anxiety, which may occur comorbidly or be mistaken for hypoactive and hyperactive delirium, respectively. All assessments for delirium include a review of the medical record, laboratory work, imaging, and outside records interview with the patient, parents, primary care givers, and clinical staff. Nursing and parent reports provide valuable information about levels of consciousness and sleep disturbance. Additionally, parents offer a point of comparison about their child's affect, disposition, behavior, and functioning. Frequently, examining clinicians hear parents say "my child is not acting like my child" or "this is not my child."

More recently a wider array of screening tools for delirium in pediatric patients is now available. These tools stem from research in many clinical specialties, including psychiatry, nursing, intensive care, pulmonology, palliative care, and anesthesiology. Table 12.5 contrasts the most widely used pediatric delirium assessment measures. Of note, the Delirium Rating Scale-Revised-98 (DRS-R-98) is a validated instrument for diagnosis and serial assessment in pediatric patients.[42] More recently in 2011 and then in 2016, the Vanderbilt Delirium and Cognitive Impairment Study Group has validated the Pediatric Confusion Assessment Method (p-CAM) and Preschool Confusion Assessment Measure (ps-CAM) (2016) for use in children down to age 5 years and age 6 months, respectively.[43]

TABLE 12.5
Scales Used in the Assessment of Pediatric Delirium

Scale	Objective and Intended Use	Development	Areas Assessed and Items Rated	Validity and Strengths	Questions and Possible Limitations
Pediatric Anesthesia Emergence Delirium Scale (PAEDS)[120]	Assessment of emergence delirium postsedation.	Sikich and Lerman[120] 5 of 27 proposed items were validated for the measurement of delirium emerging from anesthesia	Assesses: • Disturbance of consciousness • Change in cognition Items rated: • Eye contact with the caregiver • Purposeful actions • Awareness of surroundings • Restlessness • Inconsolability	Deemed valid and reliable in children in its intended clinical context Used with children 2 years and older	Based on the subjective rating by clinician. Lacks validation against DSM-IV criteria for diagnosis of delirium. Most easily identifies hyperactive delirium and may fail to detect cases of hypoactive or mixed delirium.
Pediatric Confusion Assessment Measure (p-CAM)[121]	Diagnosis and screening of delirium in PICU patients intubated or not. Ratings may be completed by clinicians without psychiatric specialty training.	Vanderbilt Delirium and Cognitive Impairment Study Group Adaptation of the adult CAM-ICU[122,123] The Richmond Agitation Sedation Scale (RASS)[124] is used in conjunction with the p-CAM	Assesses: • Level of consciousness via the RASS • Content of consciousness Items rated • Acute alteration or fluctuation from baseline mental status • Inattention (cardinal feature) • Altered level of consciousness	For children 5 years and older or with developmental delay Adapted from the CAM-ICU to be age appropriate Validations studies completed in 2011	Suitable for use in nonsedated patients. Low scores on the RASS may lead to failure to recognize cases of hypoactive delirium. Clinicians will need to use the RASS in conjunction with developmentally appropriate visual aids that are downloadable.
Preschool Confusion Assessment Measure (ps-CAM)[125]	Diagnosis and screening of delirium in PICU patients intubated or not. Ratings may be completed by clinicians without psychiatric specialty training.	Vanderbilt Delirium and Cognitive Impairment Study Group Adaption of the p-CAM[121]	Assesses: • Level of consciousness via the RASS • Content of consciousness Items rated: • Acute alteration or fluctuation from baseline mental status • Inattention (cardinal feature) • Altered level of consciousness Disorganized systems/thinking	For children 6 months to 5 years, or with developmental delay Adapted from the p-CAM to be age appropriate Validation studies completed in 2016	Suitable for use in nonsedated patients. Low scores on the RASS may lead to failure to recognize cases of hypoactive delirium. Clinicians will need to use the RASS in conjunction with developmentally appropriate visual aids that are downloadable and/or a hand-held mirror.

Continued

TABLE 12.5
Scales Used in the Assessment of Pediatric Delirium—cont'd

Cornell Assessment for Pediatric Delirium (CAPD)[3]	A developmentally focused nurse administered bedside validated screen for delirium.	Traube et al.[3] An adaptation of the PAEDS 111 PICU patients Ages 0–21 over 10 weeks Overall prevalence of delirium was 20.6% in study population	Assesses: • Orientation • Arousal • Cognition Items rated: • Eye contact • Purposefulness of movements • Awareness of surroundings • If consolable • Communicates needs • Psychomotor activity • Latency of response to interactions	Validated for children Additional developmental anchor points provided in 2015 guide screeners and improve reliability[126]	More easily detects all subtypes of delirium than the PAEDS. Question based, differentiating it from other scales. Highly developmentally focused and useful for children younger than 2 years of age. Does not account for degree of sedation.
Delirium Rating Scale-Revised-98 (DRS-R-98)[49]	Initial assessments of delirium and sequential ratings over time to track clinical progress and response to treatment.	Trzepacz et al.[127] and Turkel et al.[42]	Assesses: • DSM criteria for delirium Items rated: • Two items to assess onset and temporality • Eight items to assess symptoms	Deemed valid and reliable in children Used widely with adults and available in multiple languages Used for diagnosis and ongoing assessment of illness course	Turkel et al.[128] report that hallucinations and delusions occur less frequently in children than in adults and may not be required symptoms in the diagnosis of pediatric delirium. Total scores did not predict mortality or length of hospital stay in pediatric patients in contrast to studies of adult patients.
Pediatric Risk of Mortality (PRISM II)[129] Pediatric Index of Mortality (PIM)[130]	Originally designed to predict mortality in critically ill patients.	Schieveld et al.[131] Four-year prospective study in an ICU setting following 877 consecutive admissions	Assesses: • Medical stability • Severity of illness Items rated: • Vital signs • Acid/base status • Ventilation status • Pupillary dilatation (spelling) • Coagulation • Electrolytes	Ability of scale to predict pediatric delirium: PRISM • sensitivity 76% • specificity 62% PIM • sensitivity 82% • specificity 62%	Low number of children with delirium in the study (40/877; 4.6%). Low positive predictive value. High negative predictive value. Useful in predicting the likely nonoccurrence of delirium.

The Montreal Cognitive Assessment (MoCA) and the Mini-Mental State Examination (MMSE), both of which evaluate cognitive abilities adjusted for education levels, are used to distinguish delirium from other neurocognitive disorders in adult patients aged 18 years and older. These assessments have been studied and validated for adults; however, versions modified for pediatric patients have not been as extensively examined for validity and reliability. One study suggests that the MMSE scores reach a plateau at a mental age of approximately 10 years and is a suitable instrument for screening higher mental function in children at the age of 4 years and above in the outpatient setting.[44]

Electroencephalogram Findings

The electroencephalogram (EEG) demonstrates diffuse slowing in patients with metabolic encephalopathy or delirium. Focal slowing usually reflects an underlying localized structural brain abnormality. The EEG may lack specificity for etiology, but there are some patterns that are linked to metabolic abnormalities, such as triphasic waves in hepatic encephalopathy. When the assessment, mental status examination, and collateral information are consistent with delirium, the EEG does not usually provide additional useful diagnostic information. However, if the mental status remains altered despite a persistently negative medical workup, the EEG could reveal nonconvulsive status epilepticus, which may be occurring at higher rates than originally suspected.[45] The highest yield for an EEG in patients with an altered mental status without a clear cause is a normal finding (as seen with psychiatric disorders) and therefore rules out ictal encephalopathies and other possible organic causes of a confusional state.[46]

Developmental Concerns

Delirium in children can be difficult to differentiate from other neuropsychiatric conditions. From a developmental perspective, children are apt at baseline to exhibit mood, personality, or behavioral changes because of hospitalization. Variations from baseline readily develop in the pediatric (and adult) population because of the absence of a familiar environment, typical and predictable routine, and familiar relationships. An overstimulating and restrictive setting then replaces this former stability, with little or no consistent schedule (i.e., meals, school, play, naps, and sleep), and an influx of new faces from staff and providers who often, though unintentionally, disrupt the parent-child bond for treatment purposes. Depending on a child's age, he/she may lack psychologic insight or expressive abilities to accurately communicate what

is being experienced, and internal mental states may manifest behaviorally, such as through regression or acting out. Therefore, during hospitalization, awareness of a child's baseline functioning and coping skills is essential in diagnosing and differentiating delirium from other disorders.

DIAGNOSTIC DILEMMAS
Delirium Versus Catatonia

Physicians who treat critically ill patients are often faced with the difficulty of distinguishing delirium from other states that include altered mental status. We pay close attention to the diagnostic challenge between delirium and catatonia, which can occur together, as the treatment for each syndrome may worsen the other. Table 12.6 adapted with permission from Saddawi-Konefka et al. provides an additional comparison between delirium and other altered neurocognitive states.[47]

The *DSM-5* attempts to differentiate between the conditions of delirium and catatonia offering 5 diagnostic criteria for delirium (listed in Table 12.1) and 12 symptoms characteristic of catatonia, 3 of which must cooccur to make a catatonia diagnosis.[7] Nevertheless, these two diagnoses can still share many similar clinical features,[48] and they may even develop concurrently.[49] For example, in one study of 205 delirium patients, over 39% of the cohort exhibited two or more catatonic features, the most common being excitement (73%), immobility/stupor (21%), mutism (16%), and negativism (10%).[50] Delirium and catatonia also have similar motoric subtypes that further complicate diagnosis (i.e., hyperactive, hypoactive, and mixed types for delirium, and excited and retarded/stuporous poles for catatonia).[51]

While the diagnostic criteria for delirium and catatonia may be challenging, the distinction between them is crucial, as the treatment of one can exacerbate the other (i.e., neuroleptics, the mainstay of delirium treatment,[29] can potentiate catatonia and result in neuroleptic malignant syndrome [NMS],[52] whereas benzodiazepines, the treatment of choice for catatonia,[53] may worsen symptoms of delirium[54]). There is currently no fail-safe method for distinguishing between the two diagnoses a priori, but close observation for pathognomonic psychomotor findings of catatonia can be helpful. Catatonia typically lacks a pattern of ebb and flow to the level of consciousness; however, a waxing and waning quality to the characteristic psychomotor features of catatonia has been observed.[47]

TABLE 12.6
Differential Diagnosis of Altered Mental Status

Differential	Syndrome Description	Key Distinguishing Features
Delirium	An acute confused state with waxing and waning orientation and arousal.	Psychomotor features of catatonia will be absent. The waxing and waning in delirium describes arousal/orientation, whereas in catatonia it refers to the motoric dysregulation.
Catatonia	A state of altered sensorium coupled with characteristic psychomotor dysregulation possibly negativistic and/or agitated in presentation.	Key psychomotor abnormalities, such as posturing, stereotypies, waxy flexibility (catalepsy), verbigeration, and echolalia/praxia. The Bush-Francis Catatonia Rating Scale remains the favored psychometric instrument.[1,2]
Neuroleptic malignant syndrome (NMS)	A form of malignant catatonia characterized by fever, "lead-pipe" rigidity, and autonomic instability that results from administration of a dopamine antagonist.	This is a form of malignant catatonia and may be indistinguishable. With NMS, there will be a culprit drug with temporal association to onset. NMS is also more often associated with elevation of creatinine kinase (to greater than four times the upper limit of normal). Initial treatment of both is identical.
Serotonin syndrome	A condition characterized by confusion, autonomic dysregulation (fever, hypertension, tachycardia), and motoric signs (myoclonus, hyperreflexia, tremor) due to drugs that lead to excess serotonin.	While serotonin syndrome has cognitive and autonomic features that may appear similar to those of catatonia, the motoric features should not include rigidity, waxy flexibility, etc.
Complex partial seizures	A form of seizure that affects arousal and can include automatisms, staring, and verbigeration.	Seizures can be difficult to distinguish from catatonia and can often be the cause of a superimposed catatonia. Electroencephalogram is useful. Both are acutely treated with IV benzodiazepines. Note that catatonia will not respond to phenytoin.
Metabolic disturbance	An imbalance that may present with a wide spectrum of potential varied features (e.g., multifocal clonus with hyperammonemia, lethargy with hyponatremia).	Differentiation is based on suspicion of potential metabolic imbalance and assessment of laboratories (i.e., basic electrolytes, magnesium, calcium, blood urea nitrogen, creatinine, liver panel, and ammonia).
Central nervous system (CNS) infection	A collection of infections that may present differently depending on the infection and location.	CNS infections typically lack speech latency, waxy flexibility, and other motor signs present with catatonia. Imaging, lumbar puncture, and serologies are also helpful.
Cerebrovascular events	Ischemic neurologic events with acute changes and often focal neurologic symptoms.	Differentiation is based on neurologic examination with focal features (not present in catatonia) and imaging.
CNS neoplasm	Many forms that can result in acute, subacute, or chronic changes because of direct invasion or mass effect.	Differentiation is based on neurologic examination with focal features (not present in catatonia) and imaging.
Autoimmune encephalopathy	A syndrome resulting from various etiologies (e.g., paraneoplastic) that has variable presentation, usually including severe altered mental status.	The psychomotor features of catatonia are typically not seen in isolated autoimmune encephalopathy.
Neurodegenerative disorders	A collection of disorders caused by neuron death, including, among others, dementia, Parkinson disease, and Huntington disease.	Onset is typically subacute to chronic. The motoric features of Parkinson disease are distinct in that they include cogwheeling and tremor, whereas catatonia does not.

TABLE 12.6
Differential Diagnosis of Altered Mental Status—cont'd

Differential	Syndrome Description	Key Distinguishing Features
Paratonia	Increased motor tone that may be seen with neurodegenerative disorders, encephalopathy, secondary to medications, or idiopathic in nature, as with advanced age.	Motor symptoms will be limited to increased tone. There should be no speech latency, waxy flexibility, gegenhalten, etc.
Critical illness myopathy/ neuropathy	Syndromes of widespread motor weakness.	These will present with muscle flaccidity, while catatonia will present with increased tone.
Pharmacologic sedation	Hypoarousal due to medical sedation.	Psychomotor features of catatonia will be absent.
Vegetative state	A wakeful unconscious state due to traumatic brain injury, neurodegenerative conditions, or congenital features, such as negativism and waxy abnormalities.	Catatonic patients will typically have some interaction with their environment (e.g., negativism) and display psychomotor flexibility.

Adapted from Saddawi-Konefka D, Berg SM, Nejad SH, Bittner EA. Catatonia in the ICU: an important and underdiagnosed cause of altered mental status. A case series and review of the literature. *Crit Care Med*. 2014;42(3):e234–e241, with permission.

In a delirious patient with observed catatonic psychomotor features, antipsychotics should be avoided, and an initial trial of benzodiazepines should be attempted.[51] The risk of inducing NMS outweighs the risk of exacerbating delirium, and a well-designed and closely observed trial of intravenous lorazepam can rapidly provide a response to catatonia. This intervention alone does not make the diagnosis because, as mentioned, these entities can occur concomitantly. If a robust trial of benzodiazepines proves ineffective in mitigating hallmark catatonic motoric dysregulation, there should be concern for worsening underlying delirium, and electroconvulsive shock therapy (ECT) may provide a safer alternative treatment.[51,55] Nevertheless, ECT is not without the risk of exacerbating delirium,[56] and further research is needed to provide an evidence-based approach to diagnosing and treating patients with concurrent features of catatonia and delirium.

Delirium Versus Psychiatric Illness

Hypoactive delirium, with characteristic symptoms such as decreased activity and speech, withdrawal, and apathy, may mimic depression and as a result may be confused with symptoms of depression[4]; however, hypoactive delirium can be distinguished from depression by the waxing and waning symptoms and altered levels of consciousness, both of which are not observed in depression. Alternatively, hyperactive delirium, with symptoms such as hypervigilance, hyperalertness, fast or loud speech, and agitation, may often be erroneously interpreted as anxiety, which can manifest in extreme symptoms in hospitalized children. However, patients suffering from anxiety or related disorders can be soothed and consoled by parents, whereas children with delirium generally cannot. In addition, in severe cases where pharmacologic intervention is indicated, patients typically respond with some degree of immediate anxiety symptom relief with benzodiazepines. By contrast, benzodiazepines are likely to worsen and exacerbate delirium symptoms, and there is, at best, minimal correlation between psychotherapeutic interventions and symptom improvement in delirium. Rating scales support the mental status examination and may need to be administered repeatedly, given the waxing and waning quality of delirium.

TREATMENT
Nonpharmacologic Management

Treatment of delirium is widely acknowledged to fall into three primary domains: identification and treatment of underlying causes, nonpharmacologic interventions (which may represent both preventive and treatment measures), and pharmacologic interventions aimed at reducing the clinical impact of delirium and its associated morbidity and mortality.[2] See Table 12.7 for examples of nonpharmacologic management of delirium. Regulation of sleep and early mobilization are the two nonpharmacologic interventions that have some recent evidence for their efficacy in the adult population. A 2014 study by Patel et al.[57] found that a light and noise reduction program in the ICU reduced sleep deprivation and delirium, decreasing the incidence and duration of delirium (55/167 [33%] before versus 24/171 [14%] after, $P < .001$; 3.4 [1.4] days before versus 1.2 [0.9] days after, $P = .021$), while increased sleep efficiency was associated with a lower OR of developing delirium (OR 0.90, 95% CI 0.84–0.97). In another study by Schweickert et al.,[58] daily interruption of sedation for physical and occupational therapy in mechanically ventilated patients was associated with improved functional outcomes at hospital discharge and shorter duration of delirium (median 2.0 days, interquartile range 0.0–6.0 vs. 4.0 days in intervention group vs. 2.0–8.0 in the group receiving standard of care; $P = .02$). Other environmental measures include removing immobilizing lines and devices (IV lines, physical restraints) as early as possible to facilitate stimulation and minimize isolation.[59] Depending on the developmental age of the child, the most powerful environmental stimulation and reorienting measures may be a favorite toy or stuffed animal or a parent at bedside to provide comfort and reassurance.

Pharmacologic Management

Pharmacologic management of delirium typically includes both removal medications that can cause or exacerbate delirium and, if necessary, the use of certain medications to target the clinical symptoms and behavioral sequelae that pose a danger to the patient and can interfere with treatment. The removal or minimization of medications as one intervention in the treatment of delirium is a common clinical practice in pediatric patients similar to that in adults; however, the clinical outcomes have not been studied extensively in the pediatric population. Nonetheless, it is intuitive that medications that may, even in healthy individuals, cause some cognitive blunting or sedation may also contribute to delirium. Particularly, consistent with the hypothesis of delirium as a disruption in ACh transmission, anticholinergic medications are minimized or removed. Notably, many medications not typically considered "anticholinergic" do indeed have anticholinergic effects; examples include furosemide, ranitidine, and clindamycin.[59] Other medications that can cause or exacerbate delirium typically include benzodiazepines and other sedative hypnotics, opiates, steroids, antihistamines, and some antibiotics. When caring for a child in the inpatient and outpatient setting with altered mental status, it is important to review patient's medication list for medications that could contribute to delirium. The use of over-the-counter medications such as diphenhydramine (Benadryl) is a common course of altered mental status in children. In a recent prospective, longitudinal study of all children admitted to the PICU over 1 year, which included 1547 patients assessed for delirium twice daily, a multivariate analysis showed that administration of benzodiazepines and anticholinergics were independent predictors of delirium with $P < .001$ and $P = .006$, respectively.[60] In one study, every 5-mg dose increase of midazolam-equivalent benzodiazepines

TABLE 12.7 Nonpharmacologic Management of Delirium in Pediatric Patients	
Intervention Type	**Specific Interventions**
Sensory and environmental modification	Favorite or soothing music Gentle touch and massage Minimize immobilizing lines, catheters, and restraints Minimize noise Calming and clear speech Lighting in accordance with circadian rhythm Familiar objects to patient in the room

Caregiver measures	Proper body alignment
	  Assist with passive range of motion
	  Avoid immobility
	Time and place reorientation
	  Boards to communicate by pointing to pictures or words
	  Clocks
	  Photos
	  Daily schedules to promote sleep-wake cycle
	Sleep protocols
	Play favorite movies and/or shows
	Parental/significant other presence/participation in care
	Scheduled medicine to minimize interruption of patient's routine

From Wolfe J, Hinds P, Sourkes B. *Textbook of Interdisciplinary Pediatric Palliative Care E-Book: Expert Consult Premium Edition.* Elsevier Health Sciences; 2011, with permission.

in an otherwise alert patient was associated with 4% higher odds of that patient developing delirium the subsequent day.[54,61]

Benzodiazepine Withdrawal–Induced Delirium

Although it is necessary to minimize and discontinue the use of benzodiazepines as soon as possible, it is also necessary to be cautious when weaning them, as doing as decreasing the dose too quickly may contribute to delirium.[62] Slow benzodiazepine tapers are considered the best preventative measure for benzodiazepine withdrawal–induced delirium, and there are established guidelines for how this should be done in pediatric patients.[63] In a study of PICU patients in Montreal Children's Hospital, adverse withdrawal reactions from benzodiazepines were prevented by conducting daily weans that were determined by each child's duration of use. For children receiving continuous infusions for 1–3 days, doses were weaned by 20% daily. Likewise, children with infusions for 4–7 days received 13%–20% daily weans; 8–14 days received 8%–13%; 15–21 days received 8%; and more than 21 days received 2%–4%.[63] The authors note that these weans may have been conservative, as many of the patients were being concurrently weaned from opioids, which is often the case in sedated patients. Typically, when benzodiazepines are used for many days for sedation in the ICU, tapers that are specific to the patient's clinical status will be designed, considering the total dose and duration of use. For a patient at high risk for withdrawal, a possible initial wean could be a 10% reduction in total daily dose per day, with the daily percentage reduction adjusted depending on response.[63] There is some evidence to suggest that anticonvulsive agents such as carbamazepine may be useful in the setting of a more rapid benzodiazepine taper to minimize the risk of developing delirium. However, much of this work was conducted decades ago,[64] suggesting that this is an area in need of further study.[65]

Treatment of Behavioral Symptoms With Medications

In addition to a thorough evaluation of the patient's medication list to remove or minimize medications that could cause delirium, there is a practice of medication provision aimed at treatment of symptoms of delirium. Even in adults, the pharmacologic treatment of delirium is somewhat controversial, as the evidence base showing robust and replicated improvements in morbidity and/or mortality attributable to pharmacologic treatment of delirium is lacking. For example, a double-blind, placebo-controlled trial randomizing 101 mechanically ventilated patients to receive haloperidol, ziprasidone, or placebo for up to 14 days found no significant difference in the number of days alive or without delirium or coma between the groups.[66]

However, from a practical standpoint, many of the behavioral problems that arise from the disorientation and impaired attention found in delirium necessitate intervention. These behaviors include attempting to get out of bed, pulling out IVs and oxygen tubing, refusing necessary interventions such as blood draws or wound care, and interfering with bandages and wound healing. These behaviors also tend to disturb other patients in close proximity and can pose a threat or danger to staff attempting to provide care. In addition, patients experiencing delirium appear to be suffering psychological distress, which is also a source of stress to the patient's family members.

Antipsychotics, in particular haloperidol, tend to be the most frequently used medications in the treatment of hyperactive delirium. Haloperidol has some advantages, which include the availability of an IV formulation and possible efficacy in treating the proposed underlying increase in dopamine neurotransmission that may be present in hyperactive delirium. However, there is little concrete evidence in the literature or research studies that illuminates whether this is an accurate proposed mechanism of efficacy.[67] Although some past trials support the use of haloperidol for treatment or prophylaxis of delirium, overall the evidence is inconclusive or contradictory.[68] Although antipsychotic medications are clinically shown to be effective in reducing agitation and perhaps consequently decreasing psychologic sequelae, whether medication treatment lessens its duration or associated morbidity and mortality is not yet determined. The Society of Critical Care Medicine's 2013 Clinical Practice Guidelines for Pain, Agitation and Delirium concluded that there was no good evidence supporting the use of haloperidol to treat delirium in the ICU, and the use of atypical antipsychotics had only low-quality evidence.[69] Nevertheless, antipsychotics continue to be prescribed for delirium based on practitioners' preference, theoretical benefit, and treatment of symptoms, including positive symptoms of psychosis.[70]

A recent metaanalysis of randomized controlled trials of antipsychotics in adult patients with delirium found that treatment with antipsychotic medications was superior to placebo/usual care controls and that second-generation antipsychotics (e.g., risperidone, olanzapine) are more beneficial regarding efficacy and safety outcomes compared with haloperidol.[71] The binding profile of second-generation antipsychotics, with action affecting availability of not only dopa-mine but also serotonin and other neurotransmitters, may play a role in balancing disruptions in multiple neurotransmitter systems in delirium and its subtypes. Modern practices incorporate a greater use of second-generation antipsychotics when there is ability to take medications by mouth, in part because of their favor-able short-term side effect profile, including fewer extrapyramidal side effects and less cardiac toxicity.[72,73]

In children, as in adults, antipsychotics are often first-line agents used to manage symptoms of delirium, although antipsychotic medications do not have FDA approval for treatment of delirium in either population and there is limited research in children overall. Stud-ies examining the pharmacologic treatment of delirium in pediatric populations suggest that these atypical anti-psychotics are safe and effective in infants, as well as in children and adolescents.[74,75] For example, in a study published in 2012 by Turkel et al.,[76] a retrospective chart review of 75 patients aged 1–18 years treated with an atypical antipsychotic (olanzapine, risperidone, or que-tiapine) and monitored with two DRS-R-98 ratings during their hospitalization at initiation and cessation of antipsy-chotic medication demonstrated decreases in DRS-R-98 scores, and adverse effects were only noted in one patient (a mild dystonia that improved with dose reduction).

Table 12.8 provides suggested dosing for haloperi-dol IV and risperidone and olanzapine orally or PO in the pediatric population. When using these medica-tions, ECGs should be monitored because of the risk of

---

TABLE 12.8
Pharmacologic Management Guidelines for Pediatric Delirium

1–6 years or 10–30 kg	
Agitated or NPO (nothing by mouth)	Haloperidol (0.01–0.02 mg/kg, max 0.6 mg) IV q1h × 3 days PRN (as needed) agitation or psychotic symptoms
1–3 years or 10–20 kg: Do not exceed 1 mg/24 h	
>3–6 years or 20–30 kg: Do not exceed 2 mg/24 h	
Not agitated and PO	Risperidone (0.0125–0.025 mg/kg; max 0.5 mg) PO q6h × 3 days PRN agitation or psychotic symptoms
1–3 years or 10–20 kg: Do not exceed 1 mg/24 h	
>3–6 years or 20–30 kg: Do not exceed 2 mg/24 h	
>6–10 years or 30–40 kg	
Agitated or NPO	Haloperidol (0.3–0.8 mg/dose) IV q1h ×3 days PRN agitation or psychotic symptoms
Do not exceed 4 mg/24 h	
Not agitated and PO	Risperidone (0.375–1 mg/dose) PO q6h × 3 days PRN agitation or psychotic symptoms
Do not exceed 3 mg/24 h	
Delirium with insomnia (patients 7–10 years)	Olanzapine 1.25 mg or 2.5 mg PO at bedtime × 3 days
>10 years or >40 kg	
Agitated or NPO	Haloperidol (0.4–1.0 mg/dose) IV q1h × 3 days PRN agitation or psychotic symptoms
Do not exceed 7 mg/24 h	
Not agitated and PO	Risperidone (0.5–1 mg/dose) PO q6h × 3 days PRN agitation or psychotic symptoms
Do not exceed 4 mg/24 h	
Delirium with insomnia	Olanzapine 2.5 or 5 mg PO at bedtime × 3 days

From *Pharmacologic Treatment of Delirium*. The Cardiovascular Intensive Care Unit (CVICU); 2017 Available at: https://intranet.lpch.org/pdf/de partments/cvicu/guidebook/pharmacologicTreatmentOfDelirium.pdf.

QTc prolongation, particularly with the IV formulation of haloperidol, which may place the patient at risk for torsades de point. A QTc interval greater than 450 ms or greater than 25% over baseline may warrant a cardiology consultation and reduction or discontinuation of the antipsychotic medication.[77]

Because of the risk of cardiac effects, tolerability, or other clinical issues or contraindications, antipsychotics are often deferred even when treatment for delirium is indicated. In these cases, beyond preventative measures and sleep aids, other medications have been tried in the adult population. For example, valproic acid has been used in patients with delirium. The rationale for the use of this agent includes its modulatory effects on neurotransmitter systems, inflammation, and oxidative stress implicated in the pathophysiology of delirium.[78] In adolescents, ketamine, an *N*-methyl-D-aspartate receptor antagonist and effective dissociative agent, has been used as a calming and sedating agent in cases of agitated delirium in the pediatric emergency room.[79]

Pharmacologic Strategies to Reduce the Incidence of Delirium

To decrease the risk of delirium in ventilated patients by reducing reliance on medications that can cause or worsen delirium, including benzodiazepines, opioids, and propofol, α-2-agonists have been proposed as safer alternatives and have been gaining favor as sedatives in this population. Recent reviews on α-2-agonists, dexmedetomidine[80] and clonidine,[81] have found them, overall, to be efficacious and safe despite potential adverse effects on blood pressure and heart rate in this critically ill population.

α-2-Agonists have also been proposed and studied in the prevention and treatment of pediatric emergence delirium (ED). ED is a postoperative phenomenon characterized by a disturbance in awareness and attention to the environment and manifests as disorientation, hyperactive behavior, and hypersensitivity. It is more common in the pediatric population than in the adult,[82] with incidence of ED in children found to be 11.5%.[83] A 2014 review found dexmedetomidine to be promising in preventing and treating ED.[84] Avoiding use of potent inhalation anesthetics and instead administering total intravenous anesthesia can help prevent ED.[84]

Supporting the regular sleep-wake cycle through use of exogenous melatonin and ramelteon, a synthetic melatonin receptor agonist, shows promise in preventing and decreasing duration of delirium.[74,85] A 2016 metaanalysis of randomized controlled trials of exogenous melatonin for delirium prevention found that it reduced the incidence of delirium in patients on medical wards.[86] Studies in children have found that melatonin given preoperatively may decrease ED.[87]

Integrative Management

An integrated approach to managing delirium is now being studied in adult critical care.[88] Adult ICU clinical care guidelines by the Society of Critical Care Medicine suggest a multifaceted approach to preventing, assessing, and treating delirium, involving managing pain, awakening and breathing trials, early mobility, and family engagement, known as the "ABCDEF bundle"[89] (see Table 12.9).

TABLE 12.9
Integrative Approach to Managing Delirium: "ABCDEF Bundle"

A	Assess, prevent, and manage pain • Self-report of pain level • Validated pain assessment tools • Use of analgesics less likely to contribute to delirium
B	Both spontaneous awakening trials and spontaneous breathing trials • Target sedation level for individual patients • Use of sedation scales • Trials of discontinuing sedatives to lighten sedation • Timely removal of mechanical ventilation
C	Choice of analgesia and sedation • Patient comfort as primary goal • Use of safest pain medications and sedatives • Avoid oversedation and promote extubation
D	Delirium: assess, prevent, and manage • Identify and reduce risk factors (see Table 12.3) • Daily assessment using validated tools (see Table 12.5) • Environmental measures (see Table 12.7) • Pharmacologic measures for behavioral management (see Table 12.8)
E	Early mobility and exercise • Goal activity level based on RASS score • Early mobility performed by part of interdisciplinary team • From passive range of motion to ambulation
F	Family engagement and empowerment • Good communication with family • Family as part of the care team

RASS, Richmond Agitation Sedation Scale.
Adapted from Vanderbilt University Medical Center. *Delirium Prevention and Safety: Starting with the ABCDEF's.* http://www.icudelirium.org/medicalprofessionals.html, with permission; 2013.

When developing a treatment plan for pediatric patients with delirium, evaluation of the risks versus benefits of proposed interventions is indicated. If mental status changes are mild and there is no acute concern for safety, environmental measures and supportive nonpharmacologic care might be all that is necessary.

SEQUELAE

With more survivors of critical illness associated with advances in medicine, there is a growing interest in outcomes post-ICU, including in the cognitive and psychologic domains. The adult literature on delirium discusses the range of outcomes from full recovery to death with many variable degrees of cognitive and functional deficits in between.[90]

Cognitive Outcomes

The association between delirium and long-term cognitive impairment is well established, but it is not clear whether delirium itself is causal in cognitive impairment or an epiphenomenon.[91] Well-designed studies have shown that patients with delirium have not returned to baseline cognitive function at 6 months[92] and that longer duration of delirium is associated with higher rates of cognitive impairment 1 year after discharge, after adjusting for numerous cofounding variables.[93,94] Studies using self-report questionnaires of ICU survivors who suffered from delirium reported that they made more social blunders and they had significantly more long-term cognitive problems compared with ICU survivors who had not been delirious.[95]

In the pediatric literature, a lack of a validated tool for assessing pediatric delirium until recently has limited the understanding of the effects of delirium in this population, as outcome studies of pediatric survivors of critical illness could not examine delirium as an independent risk factor.[96] There are some data on the short-term effects of critical illness and forms of nontraumatic brain injury other than delirium, including meningoencephalitis. A 2013 study of 88 children admitted to intensive care with meningoencephalitis, septic illness, or other critical illnesses assessed 3–6 months after discharge were found to have significant underperformance on neuropsychologic measures ($P < .02$), including intellectual function, memory, and attention compared to healthy controls; furthermore, teachers rated these children to be worse academic performers and have more difficulties with school work ($P < .01$), and below average on tasks of executive function[97], which persisted one year after discharge.[98]

Psychiatric Outcomes

Psychologic distress is common after delirium, including symptoms of posttraumatic stress, anxiety, and depression, leading to increased interest in rates of psychiatric disorders and how to treat them in survivors of critical illness.[99] A 2016 review examining the literature on the relationship between critical care and development of posttraumatic stress disorder (PTSD) found delirium during admission and delusional and traumatic memory (in-ICU frightening and/or psychotic experiences) to be the two risk factors for PTSD, along with younger age, female gender, previous psychiatric history, and the use of mechanical restraint.[100] Sedation with benzodiazepines, an independent risk factor for delirium, is associated with increased risk of post-ICU PTSD.[101]

Many studies indicate an association between delirium episodes and subsequent symptoms of anxiety and depression.[102] A recent review found an association with depression after delirium but was inconclusive with regard to anxiety and PTSD.[103] It is also important to consider how the patient's psychologic distress in the hospital might relate to functional outcomes. For example, a 2013 study found that in-hospital acute stress symptoms were independently associated with greater impairment in cognitive functioning assessed at 12 months after discharge ($P = .03$).[104]

There have been a few studies on children's mental health after discharge from critical care that generally parallel the adult literature of ICU survivorship in terms of psychiatric vulnerability. A 2010 review of studies on pediatric critical illness survivors found that significant PTSD symptoms ranged from 10% to 28%.[105] In a 2008 study, children's delusional memories, including disturbing hallucinations, were associated with duration of use of opiates/benzodiazepines and risk of posttraumatic stress, among children interviewed 3 months after discharge from the PICU.[106] A 2015 study found that children admitted to PICU were at increased risk (between 20% and 80%) of developing a psychiatric disorder, posttraumatic stress symptoms, and sleep disturbance when compared with healthy controls.[107]

As usual when discussing children's well-being, the mental health of parents is crucial, and attention to the family system and parental health is necessary in understanding and treating pediatric delirium. Indeed, the severity of PTSD symptoms in children survivors of critical illness has been associated with parental psychopathology.[108] The child's trauma related to the experiences of frightening procedures, severe pain, and environmental and other factors is summarily experienced by their parents. A 2004 study comparing psychiatric outcomes in children and parents following PICU admission with those following general pediatric ward admission showed much higher rates of PTSD symptoms 6–12 months after discharge (21% compared with 0% of children and 27% compared with 7% of parents, respectively).[109] Studies have shown evidence of persistent posttraumatic stress in families many months following discharge from PICU,[110] with one study pointing to as high as 84% of parents having subclinical symptoms of PTSD persisting 1 year after their child was discharged from PICU.[111]

Treatment of long-term behavioral health problems associated with critical illness and delirium is a growing area of investigation. Models for addressing post-ICU PTSD symptoms in adults have included strategies of avoiding the overuse of sedation, improving identification of symptoms, providing psychologic support, introducing coping and mindfulness strategies, and encouraging mental healthcare post-ICU.[112] Post-PICU interventions designed for parents and children have had features of providing psychoeducation, offering intervention to high-risk families, providing parent support after discharge, and targeting PTSD symptoms.[113]

Decreasing the burden of delirium and its sequelae ideally involves psychologic support for the child and family from in-hospital stay to well beyond discharge. Even when children recover from significant posttraumatic stress and cognitive symptoms, it is difficult to estimate how ramifications of delirium and critical illness may affect their life trajectories. Challenges abound, including impacts on self-esteem and self-image and interrupted social and academic development. It behooves child health providers to recognize this toll and to facilitate adaptation and promote resilience in these children and their families.

CLOSING

Delirium not only affects individuals and families but also has a large impact on society. Prolonged hospital stays, complicated inpatient care, specialized aftercare, and poor functional and cognitive recovery related to delirium contribute to high healthcare costs.[90,114–116] A study conducted at New York Presbyterian Hospital on pediatric delirium inpatient costs found that delirium was associated with 85% increase in PICU costs ($P<.0001$) after controlling for other variables, including the severity of illness and PICU length of stay.[117] In the adult population, the national economic burden of delirium has been estimated to range from 38 to 152 billion dollars per year,[118] exceeding the national healthcare costs associated with diabetes mellitus, which is estimated to be 91.8 billion dollars annually.[119]

The broad reach of delirium warrants creation of better clinical interventions designed to enhance its prevention, management, and treatment. Pediatric care providers facing problems related to delirium can be attuned to delirium's challenges and aim to improve quality of life of affected children and families.

REFERENCES

1. Smith HA, Fuchs DC, Pandharipande PP, Barr FE, Ely EW. Delirium: an emerging frontier in the management of critically ill children. *Crit Care Clin.* 2009;25(3):593–614.
2. Hatherill S, Flisher AJ. Delirium in children and adolescents: a systematic review of the literature. *J Psychosom Res.* 2010;68(4):337–344.
3. Traube C, Silver G, Kearney J, et al. Cornell Assessment of Pediatric Delirium: a valid, rapid, observational tool for screening delirium in the PICU. *Crit Care Med.* 2014;42(3):656–663.
4. Turkel SB, Trzepacz PT, Tavaré CJ. Comparing symptoms of delirium in adults and children. *Psychosomatics.* 2006;47(4):320–324.
5. Leentjens AF, Schieveld JN, Leonard M, Lousberg R, Verhey FR, Meagher DJ. A comparison of the phenomenology of pediatric, adult, and geriatric delirium. *J Psychosom Res.* 2008;64(2):219–223.
6. Pretto M, Spirig R, Milisen K, DeGeest S, Regazzoni P, Hasemann W. Effects of an interdisciplinary nurse-led Delirium Prevention and Management Program (DPMP) on nursing workload: a pilot study. *Int J Nurs Stud.* 2009;46(6):804–812.
7. Neurocognitive Disorders. *Diagnostic and statistical manual of mental disorders.* 5th ed. Washington, DC: American Psychiatric Association; 2013.
8. Association AP. *Diagnostic and Statistical Manual of Mental Disorders: DSM-5.* Washington, D.C: American Psychiatric Association; 2013.
9. Turkel SB, Tavaré CJ. Delirium in children and adolescents. *J Neuropsychiatry Clin Neurosci.* 2003;15(4):431–435.
10. Meagher D, Moran M, Raju B, et al. A new data-based motor subtype schema for delirium. *J Neuropsychiatry Clin Neurosci.* 2008;20(2):185–193.
11. Meagher DJ, Leonard M, Donnelly S, Conroy M, Adamis D, Trzepacz PT. A longitudinal study of motor subtypes in delirium: frequency and stability during episodes. *J Psychosom Res.* 2012;72(3):236–241.
12. Velthuijsen EL, Zwakhalen SM, Mulder WJ, Verhey FR, Kempen GI. Detection and management of hyperactive and hypoactive delirium in older patients during hospitalization: a retrospective cohort study evaluating daily practice. *Int J Geriatr Psychiatry.* 2017. https://doi.org/10.1002/gps.4690.
13. Schieveld JN, Leroy PL, van Os J, Nicolai J, Vos GD, Leentjens AF. Pediatric delirium in critical illness: phenomenology, clinical correlates and treatment response in 40 cases in the pediatric intensive care unit. *Intensive Care Med.* 2007;33(6):1033–1040.

14. Boettger S, Breitbart W. Phenomenology of the subtypes of delirium: phenomenological differences between hyperactive and hypoactive delirium. *Palliat Support Care.* 2011; 9(02):129–135.

15. Gupta A, Saravay S, Trzepacz P, Chirayu P. 11. Delirium motoric subtypes. *Psychosomatics.* 2005;46(2):158.

16. Gupta N, de Jonghe J, Schieveld J, Leonard M, Meagher D. Delirium phenomenology: what can we learn from the symptoms of delirium? *J Psychosom Res.* 2008;65(3):215–222.

17. Silver G, Traube C, Kearney J, et al. Detecting pediatric delirium: development of a rapid observational assessment tool. *Intensive Care Med.* 2012;38(6):1025–1031.

18. Silver GH, Kearney JA, Kutko MC, Bartell AS. Infant delirium in pediatric critical care settings. *Am J Psychiatry.* 2010;167(10):1172–1177.

19. Silver G, Traube C, Gerber LM, et al. Pediatric delirium and associated risk factors: a single-center prospective observational study. *Pediatr Crit Care Med.* 2015;16(4):303.

20. Patel AK, Biagas KV, Clarke EC, et al. Delirium in children after cardiac bypass surgery. *Pediatr Crit Care Med.* 2017;18(2):165–171.

21. Maldonado JR. Pathoetiological model of delirium: a comprehensive understanding of the neurobiology of delirium and an evidence-based approach to prevention and treatment. *Crit Care Clin.* 2008;24(4):789–856.

22. Wolfe J, Hinds P, Sourkes B. *Textbook of Interdisciplinary Pediatric Palliative Care: Expert Consult Premium Edition.* Elsevier Health Sciences; 2011.

23. Rockwood K. Causes of delirium. *Psychiatry.* 2008;7(1): 39–41.

24. Maldonado JR. Neuropathogenesis of delirium: review of current etiologic theories and common pathways. *Am J Geriatr Psychiatry.* 2013;21(12):1190–1222.

25. Ruivo LMT-G, Baker KL, Conway MW, et al. Coordinated acetylcholine release in prefrontal cortex and hippocampus is associated with arousal and reward on distinct timescales. *Cell Rep.* 2017;18(4):905–917.

26. Plaschke K, Thomas C, Engelhardt R, et al. Significant correlation between plasma and CSF anticholinergic activity in presurgical patients. *Neurosci Lett.* 2007;417(1):16–20.

27. Flacker JM, Cummings V, Mach JR, Bettin K, Kiely DK, Wei J. The association of serum anticholinergic activity with delirium in elderly medical patients. *Am J Geriatr Psychiatry.* 1999;6(1):31–41.

28. Ramirez-Bermudez J, Ruiz-Chow A, Perez-Neri I, et al. Cerebrospinal fluid homovanillic acid is correlated to psychotic features in neurological patients with delirium. *Gen Hosp Psychiatry.* 2008;30(4):337–343.

29. Flurie RW, Gonzales JP, Tata AL, Millstein LS, Gulati M. Hospital delirium treatment: continuation of antipsychotic therapy from the intensive care unit to discharge. *Am J Health Syst Pharm.* 2015;72(23 suppl 3):S133–S139.

30. Pain L, Jeltsch H, Lehmann O, Lazarus C, Laalou F, Cassel J. Central cholinergic depletion induced by 192 IgG-Saporin alleviates the sedative effects of propofol in rats. *Br J Anaesth.* 2000;85(6):869–873.

31. Trzepacz P. Is there a final common neural pathway in delirium? Focus on acetylcholine and dopamine. Paper presented at: Seminars in clinical neuropsychiatry; 2000.

32. Rudolph JL, Ramlawi B, Kuchel GA, et al. Chemokines are associated with delirium after cardiac surgery. *J Gerontol A Biol Sci Med Sci.* 2008;63(2):184–189.

33. Cerejeira J, Firmino H, Vaz-Serra A, Mukaetova-Ladinska EB. The neuroinflammatory hypothesis of delirium. *Acta Neuropathol.* 2010;119(6):737–754.

34. Stone T, Behan W, Jones P, Darlington L, Smith R. The role of kynurenines in the production of neuronal death, and the neuroprotective effect of purines. *J Alzheimer's Dis.* 2001;3(4):355–366.

35. Becher B, Bechmann I, Greter M. Antigen presentation in autoimmunity and CNS inflammation: how T lymphocytes recognize the brain. *J Mol Med.* 2006;84(7):532–543.

36. Dimitrijevic OB, Stamatovic SM, Keep RF, Andjelkovic AV. Effects of the chemokine CCL2 on blood–brain barrier permeability during ischemia–reperfusion injury. *J Cereb Blood Flow Metab.* 2006;26(6):797–810.

37. Karlidag R, Unal S, Sezer OH, et al. The role of oxidative stress in postoperative delirium. *Gen Hosp Psychiatry.* 2006;28(5):418–423.

38. Uttara B, Singh AV, Zamboni P, Mahajan R. Oxidative stress and neurodegenerative diseases: a review of upstream and downstream antioxidant therapeutic options. *Curr Neuropharmacol.* 2009;7(1):65–74.

39. Seaman JS, Schillerstrom J, Carroll D, Brown TM. Impaired oxidative metabolism precipitates delirium: a study of 101 ICU patients. *Psychosomatics.* 2006;47(1):56–61.

40. Jackson JC, Gordon SM, Hart RP, Hopkins RO, Ely EW. The association between delirium and cognitive decline: a review of the empirical literature. *Neuropsychol Rev.* 2004;14(2):87–98.

41. Berr C, Balansard B, Arnaud J, Roussel AM, Alpérovitch A. Cognitive decline is associated with systemic oxidative stress: the EVA study. *J Am Geriatr Soc.* 2000;48(10): 1285–1291.

42. Turkel SB, Braslow K, Tavare CJ, Trzepacz PT. The delirium rating scale in children and adolescents. *Psychosomatics.* 2003;44(2):126–129.

43. Center VUM. *Pediatric Delirium*; 2013. http://www.icudelirium.org/pediatric.html.

44. Besson PS, Labbe EE. Use of the modified mini-mental state examination with children. *J Child Neurol.* 1997;12(7):455–460.

45. Sutter R, Stevens RD, Kaplan PW. Continuous electroencephalographic monitoring in critically ill patients: indications, limitations, and strategies. *Crit Care Med.* 2013;41(4):1124–1132.

46. Kaplan PW. The EEG in metabolic encephalopathy and coma. *J Clin Neurophysiol.* 2004;21(5):307–318.

47. Saddawi-Konefka D, Berg SM, Nejad SH, Bittner EA. Catatonia in the ICU: an important and underdiagnosed cause of altered mental status. A case series and review of the literature. *Crit Care Med.* 2014;42(3): e234–e241.

48. Penland HR, Weder N, Tampi RR. The catatonic dilemma expanded. *Ann Gen Psychiatry.* 2006;5(1):14.

49. Francis A, Lopez-Canino A. Delirium with catatonic features: a new subtype? *Psychiatr Times.* 2009;26 (7):32.

50. Grover S, Ghosh A, Ghormode D. Do patients of delirium have catatonic features? An exploratory study. *Psychiatry Clin Neurosci.* 2014;68(8):644–651.

51. Oldham MA, Lee HB. Catatonia vis-à-vis delirium: the significance of recognizing catatonia in altered mental status. *Gen Hosp Psychiatry.* 2015;37(6):554–559.

52. Van Den Eede F, Van Hecke J, Van Dalfsen A, Van den Bossche B, Cosyns P, Sabbe BG. The use of atypical antipsychotics in the treatment of catatonia. *Eur Psychiatry.* 2005;20(5):422–429.

53. Rosebush PI, Mazurek MF. Catatonia and its treatment. *Schizophr Bull.* 2010;36(2):239–242.

54. Zaal IJ, Devlin JW, Hazelbag M, et al. Benzodiazepine-associated delirium in critically ill adults. *Intensive Care Med.* 2015;41(12):2130–2137.

55. van den Berg KS, Marijnissen RM, van Waarde JA. Electroconvulsive therapy as a powerful treatment for delirium: a case report. *J ECT.* 2016;32(1):65–66.

56. Reti IM, Krishnan A, Podlisky A, et al. Predictors of electroconvulsive therapy postictal delirium. *Psychosomatics.* 2014;55(3):272–279.

57. Patel J, Baldwin J, Bunting P, Laha S. The effect of a multicomponent multidisciplinary bundle of interventions on sleep and delirium in medical and surgical intensive care patients. *Anaesthesia.* 2014;69(6):540–549.

58. Schweickert WD, Pohlman MC, Pohlman AS, et al. Early physical and occupational therapy in mechanically ventilated, critically ill patients: a randomised controlled trial. *Lancet (London, England).* 2009;373(9678): 1874–1882.

59. Maldonado JR. Delirium in the acute care setting: characteristics, diagnosis and treatment. *Crit Care Clin.* 2008;24(4):657–722,vii.

60. Traube C, Silver G, Gerber LM, et al. Delirium and mortality in critically ill children: epidemiology and outcomes of pediatric delirium. *Crit Care Med.* 2017;45(5):891–898.

61. Wilson JE, Brummel NE, Stollings JL. Benzodiazepine-associated delirium dosing strategy or cumulative dose? *Intensive Care Med.* 2015;41(12):2245–2246.

62. Starer J, Chang G. Hyperammoneic encephalopathy, valproic acid, and benzodiazepine withdrawal: a case series. *Am J Drug Alcohol Abuse.* 2010;36(2):98–101.

63. Ducharme C, Carnevale FA, Clermont M-S, Shea S. A prospective study of adverse reactions to the weaning of opioids and benzodiazepines among critically ill children. *Intensive Crit Care Nurs.* 2005;21(3):179–186.

64. Ries RK, Roy-Byrne PP, Ward NG, Neppe V, Cullison S. Carbamazepine treatment for benzodiazepine withdrawal. *Am J Psychiatry.* 1989;146(4):536–537.

65. Zullino DF, Khazaal Y, Hattenschwiler J, Borgeat F, Besson J. Anticonvulsant drugs in the treatment of substance withdrawal. *Drugs Today.* 2004;40(7):603–620.

66. Girard TD, Pandharipande PP, Carson SS, et al. Feasibility, efficacy, and safety of antipsychotics for intensive care unit delirium: the MIND randomized, placebo-controlled trial. *Crit Care Med.* 2010;38(2):428–437.

67. Meagher DJ, McLoughlin L, Leonard M, Hannon N, Dunne C, O'Regan N. What do we really know about the treatment of delirium with antipsychotics? Ten key issues for delirium pharmacotherapy. *Am J Geriatr Psychiatry.* 2013;21(12):1223–1238.

68. Santos KC, Silva DB, Sasaki NA, Benega MA, Garten R, Paiva TM. Molecular epidemiology of influenza A(H1N1)PDM09 hemagglutinin gene circulating in Sao Paulo State, Brazil: 2016 anticipated influenza season. *Rev Inst Med Trop Sao Paulo.* 2017;59:e9.

69. Barr J, Fraser GL, Puntillo K, et al. Clinical practice guidelines for the management of pain, agitation, and delirium in adult patients in the intensive care unit. *Crit Care Med.* 2013;41(1):263–306.

70. Tomichek JE, Stollings JL, Pandharipande PP, Chandrasekhar R, Ely EW, Girard TD. Antipsychotic prescribing patterns during and after critical illness: a prospective cohort study. *Crit Care (London, England).* 2016;20(1):378.

71. Kishi T, Hirota T, Matsunaga S, Iwata N. Antipsychotic medications for the treatment of delirium: a systematic review and meta-analysis of randomised controlled trials. *J Neurol Neurosurg Psychiatry.* 2016;87(7):767–774.

72. Yoon HJ, Park KM, Choi WJ, et al. Efficacy and safety of haloperidol versus atypical antipsychotic medications in the treatment of delirium. *BMC Psychiatry.* 2013;13:240.

73. Sonnier L, Barzman D. Pharmacologic management of acutely agitated pediatric patients. *Paediatr Drugs.* 2011;13(1):1–10.

74. Turkel SB, Hanft A. The pharmacologic management of delirium in children and adolescents. *Paediatr Drugs.* 2014;16(4):267–274.

75. Turkel SB, Jacobson JR, Tavare CJ. The diagnosis and management of delirium in infancy. *J Child Adolesc Psychopharmacol.* 2013;23(5):352–356.

76. Turkel SB, Jacobson J, Munzig E, Tavare CJ. Atypical antipsychotic medications to control symptoms of delirium in children and adolescents. *J Child Adolesc Psychopharmacol.* 2012;22(2):126–130.

77. Delirium WGo. *Practice Guideline for the Treatment of Patients with Delirium;* 1999. http://psychiatryonline.org/ pb/assets/raw/sitewide/practice_guidelines/guidelines/ delirium.pdf.

78. Sher Y, Miller Cramer AC, Ament A, Lolak S, Maldonado JR. Valproic acid for treatment of hyperactive or mixed delirium: rationale and literature review. *Psychosomatics.* 2015;56(6):615–625.

79. Kowalski JM, Kopec KT, Lavelle J, Osterhoudt K. A novel agent for management of agitated delirium: a case series of ketamine utilization in the pediatric emergency department. *Pediatr Emerg Care.* 2017;33(9):58–59.

80. Tsaousi GG, Lamperti M, Bilotta F. Role of dexmedetomidine for sedation in neurocritical care patients: a qualitative systematic review and meta-analysis of current evidence. *Clin Neuropharmacol.* 2016;39(3):144–151.

81. Jing Wang G, Belley-Cote E, Burry L, et al. Clonidine for sedation in the critically ill: a systematic review and meta-analysis (protocol). *Syst Rev.* 2015;4:154.

82. Kim HJ, Kim DK, Kim HY, Kim JK, Choi SW. Risk factors of emergence agitation in adults undergoing general anesthesia for nasal surgery. *Clin Exp Otorhinolaryngol.* 2015;8(1):46–51.

83. Stamper MJ, Hawks SJ, Taicher BM, Bonta J, Brandon DH. Identifying pediatric emergence delirium by using the PAED Scale: a quality improvement project. *AORN J.* 2014;99(4):480–494.

84. Dahmani S, Delivet H, Hilly J. Emergence delirium in children: an update. *Curr Opin Anaesthesiol.* 2014;27(3):309–315.

85. Luther R, McLeod A. The effect of chronotherapy on delirium in critical care - a systematic review. *Nurs Crit Care.* 2017. https://doi.org/10.1111/nicc.12300.

86. Chen S, Shi L, Liang F, et al. Exogenous melatonin for delirium prevention: a meta-analysis of randomized controlled trials. *Mol Neurobiol.* 2016;53(6):4046–4053.

87. Kain ZN, MacLaren JE, Herrmann L, et al. Preoperative melatonin and its effects on induction and emergence in children undergoing anesthesia and surgery. *Anesthesiology.* 2009;111(1):44–49.

88. Carrothers KM, Barr J, Spurlock B, Ridgely MS, Damberg CL, Ely EW. Contextual issues influencing implementation and outcomes associated with an integrated approach to managing pain, agitation, and delirium in adult ICUs. *Crit Care Med.* 2013;41(9 suppl 1):S128–S135.

89. Center VUM. *ICU Delirum for Medical Professionals*; 2013. http://www.icudelirium.org/medicalprofessionals.html.

90. Maldonado JR. Acute brain failure: pathophysiology, diagnosis, management, and sequelae of delirium. *Crit Care Clin.* 2017;33(3):461–519.

91. Girard TD, Dittus RS, Ely EW. Critical illness brain injury. *Annu Rev Med.* 2016;67:497–513.

92. Saczynski JS, Marcantonio ER, Quach L, et al. Cognitive trajectories after postoperative delirium. *N Engl J Med.* 2012;367(1):30–39.

93. Girard TD, Jackson JC, Pandharipande PP, et al. Delirium as a predictor of long-term cognitive impairment in survivors of critical illness. *Crit Care Med.* 2010;38(7):1513–1520.

94. Pandharipande PP, Girard TD, Jackson JC, et al. Long-term cognitive impairment after critical illness. *N Engl J Med.* 2013;369(14):1306–1316.

95. van den Boogaard M, Schoonhoven L, Evers AW, van der Hoeven JG, van Achterberg T, Pickkers P. Delirium in critically ill patients: impact on long-term health-related quality of life and cognitive functioning. *Crit Care Med.* 2012;40(1):112–118.

96. Schieveld JN, van Tuijl S, Pikhard T. On nontraumatic brain injury in pediatric critical illness, neuropsychologic short-term outcome, delirium, and resilience. *Crit Care Med.* 2013;41(4):1160–1161.

97. Als LC, Nadel S, Cooper M, Pierce CM, Sahakian BJ, Garralda ME. Neuropsychologic function three to six months following admission to the PICU with meningoencephalitis, sepsis, and other disorders: a prospective study of school-aged children. *Crit Care Med.* 2013;41(4):1094–1103.

98. Als LC, Tennant A, Nadel S, Cooper M, Pierce CM, Garralda ME. Persistence of neuropsychological deficits following pediatric critical illness. *Crit Care Med.* 2015;43(8):e312–e315.

99. Davydow DS. Posttraumatic stress disorder in critical illness survivors: too many questions remain. *Crit Care Med.* 2015;43(5):1151–1152.

100. Morrissey M, Collier E. Literature review of post-traumatic stress disorder in the critical care population. *J Clin Nurs.* 2016;25(11–12):1501–1514.

101. Davydow DS, Gifford JM, Desai SV, Needham DM, Bienvenu OJ. Posttraumatic stress disorder in general intensive care unit survivors: a systematic review. *Gen Hosp Psychiatry.* 2008;30(5):421–434.

102. Davydow DS. Symptoms of depression and anxiety after delirium. *Psychosomatics.* 2009;50(4):309–316.

103. Langan C, Sarode DP, Russ TC, Shenkin SD, Carson A, Maclullich AM. Psychiatric symptomatology after delirium: a systematic review. *Psychogeriatrics.* 2017;17(5):327–335.

104. Davydow DS, Zatzick D, Hough CL, Katon WJ. In-hospital acute stress symptoms are associated with impairment in cognition 1 year after intensive care unit admission. *Ann Am Thorac Soc.* 2013;10(5):450–457.

105. Davydow DS, Richardson LP, Zatzick DF, Katon WJ. Psychiatric morbidity in pediatric critical illness survivors: a comprehensive review of the literature. *Arch Pediatr Adolesc Med.* 2010;164(4):377–385.

106. Colville G, Kerry S, Pierce C. Children's factual and delusional memories of intensive care. *Am J Respir Crit Care Med.* 2008;177(9):976–982.

107. Als LC, Picouto MD, Hau SM, et al. Mental and physical well-being following admission to pediatric intensive care. *Pediatr Crit Care Med.* 2015;16(5):e141–e149.

108. Davydow DS. The burden of adverse mental health outcomes in critical illness survivors. *Crit Care (London, England).* 2010;14(1):125.

109. Rees G, Gledhill J, Garralda ME, Nadel S. Psychiatric outcome following paediatric intensive care unit (PICU) admission: a cohort study. *Intensive Care Med.* 2004;30(8):1607–1614.

110. Colville G, Pierce C. Patterns of post-traumatic stress symptoms in families after paediatric intensive care. *Intensive Care Med.* 2012;38(9):1523–1531.

111. Nelson LP, Gold JI. Posttraumatic stress disorder in children and their parents following admission to the pediatric intensive care unit: a review. *Pediatr Crit Care Med.* 2012;13(3):338–347.

112. Long AC, Kross EK, Davydow DS, Curtis JR. Posttraumatic stress disorder among survivors of critical illness: creation of a conceptual model addressing identification, prevention, and management. *Intensive Care Med.* 2014;40(6):820–829.

113. Baker SC, Gledhill JA. Systematic review of interventions to reduce psychiatric morbidity in parents and children after PICU admissions. *Pediatr Crit Care Med.* 2017;18(4):343–348.

114. Ely EW, Gautam S, Margolin R, et al. The impact of delirium in the intensive care unit on hospital length of stay. *Intensive Care Med.* 2001;27(12):1892–1900.

115. Witlox J, Eurelings LS, de Jonghe JF, Kalisvaart KJ, Eikelenboom P, van Gool WA. Delirium in elderly patients and the risk of postdischarge mortality, institutionalization, and dementia: a meta-analysis. *JAMA.* 2010;304(4):443–451.

116. Leslie DL, Inouye SK. The importance of delirium: economic and societal costs. *J Am Geriatr Soc.* 2011;59(suppl 2):S241–S243.

117. Traube C, Mauer EA, Gerber LM, et al. Cost associated with pediatric delirium in the ICU. *Crit Care Med.* 2016;44(12):e1175–e1179.

118. Leslie DL, Marcantonio ER, Zhang Y, Leo-Summers L, Inouye SK. One-year health care costs associated with delirium in the elderly population. *Arch Intern Med.* 2008;168(1):27–32.

119. Hogan P, Dall T, Nikolov P. Economic costs of diabetes in the US in 2002. *Diabetes Care.* 2003;26(3):917–932.

120. Sikich N, Lerman J. Development and psychometric evaluation of the pediatric anesthesia emergence delirium scale. *Anesthesiology.* 2004;100(5):1138–1145.

121. Smith HA, Boyd J, Fuchs DC, et al. Diagnosing delirium in critically ill children: validity and reliability of the pediatric Confusion Assessment Method for the Intensive Care Unit. *Crit Care Med.* 2011;39(1):150–157.

122. Inouye SK, van Dyck CH, Alessi CA, Balkin S, Siegal AP, Horwitz RI. Clarifying confusion: the confusion assessment method. A new method for detection of delirium. *Ann Intern Med.* 1990;113(12):941–948.

123. Ely EW, Margolin R, Francis J, et al. Evaluation of delirium in critically ill patients: validation of the Confusion Assessment Method for the Intensive Care Unit (CAM-ICU). *Crit Care Med.* 2001;29(7):1370–1379.

124. Sessler CN, Gosnell MS, Grap MJ, et al. The Richmond Agitation-Sedation Scale: validity and reliability in adult intensive care unit patients. *Am J Respir Crit Care Med.* 2002;166(10):1338–1344.

125. Smith HA, Gangopadhyay M, Goben CM, et al. The preschool confusion assessment method for the ICU: valid and reliable delirium monitoring for critically ill infants and children. *Crit Care Med.* 2016;44(3):592–600.

126. Silver G, Kearney J, Traube C, Hertzig M. Delirium screening anchored in child development: the Cornell assessment for pediatric delirium. *Palliat Support Care.* 2015;13(4):1005–1011.

127. Trzepacz PT, Mittal D, Torres R, Kanary K, Norton J, Jimerson N. Validation of the Delirium Rating Scale-revised-98: comparison with the delirium rating scale and the cognitive test for delirium. *J Neuropsychiatry Clin Neurosci.* 2001;13(2):229–242.

128. Turkel SB, Trzepacz PT, Tavare CJ. Comparing symptoms of delirium in adults and children. *Psychosomatics.* 2006;47(4):320–324.

129. Pollack MM, Ruttimann UE, Getson PR. Pediatric risk of mortality (PRISM) score. *Crit Care Med.* 1988;16(11):1110–1116.

130. Shann F, Pearson G, Slater A, Wilkinson K. Paediatric index of mortality (PIM): a mortality prediction model for children in intensive care. *Intensive Care Med.* 1997;23(2):201–207.

131. Schieveld JN, Lousberg R, Berghmans E, et al. Pediatric illness severity measures predict delirium in a pediatric intensive care unit. *Crit Care Med.* 2008;36(6):1933–1936.

CHAPTER 13

Pediatric Catatonia

MEGHAN STARNER, MD • MAXINE AMES, MD • ALEXANDER J. GORDON, BA • MARY LYNN DELL, MD • ELORA HILMAS, PHARM D • JOSEPHINE ELIA, MD

INTRODUCTION

Catatonia is a syndrome with characteristic features, involving motor, speech, behavioral, and autonomic dysregulation. It is associated with neurodevelopmental, medical, neurologic, and neuropsychiatric disorders, as well as medication toxicity[1] or withdrawal.[2] Catatonia has similar characteristics and causes in children as in adults, but its recognition has lagged.[3] It is frequently not recognized in the medical[4] and psychiatric pediatric settings.[5]

BACKGROUND

In 1874, Karl Kahlbaum used the term "catatonia" to describe patients in a psychiatric ward with motor, speech, affective, and behavioral abnormalities.[6] Subsequently, catatonia was used to define a subgroup of patients with schizophrenia.[7] As catatonia was beginning to be recognized outside of the spectrum of psychiatric hospitals, Alan Gelenberg advised physicians, in a report in the Lancet in 1976, to consider catatonia in medical disorders.[8] Further reports in the literature of catatonia in a variety of medical conditions, including infections, metabolic disorders, autoimmune disorders, and others,[9,10] led to the revisions in the *Diagnostic and Statistical Manual of Mental Disorders, Fourth Edition* (*DSM-IV*), recognizing catatonia not only within the context of schizophrenia and mood disorders but also with general medical conditions.[11] *DSM-5* further differentiated catatonia from an independent condition to a specifier for neuropsychiatric and medical conditions.[12,13]

PREVALENCE

In adults, catatonia has been reported in 7%–15% of patients in psychiatric hospitals[14] and in approximately 35% of patients with schizophrenia.[15,16] In an outpatient psychiatric population, 5.5% of adolescents were reported to have catatonia.[17] In a group of youths receiving psychiatric treatment at a university hospital who were further selected for having a neuropsychiatric diagnosis known to increase risk for catatonia, 17.8% were identified to have catatonia.[5] Catatonia has also been identified in 12%–17% of adolescents with autism.[18,19] The prevalence rate of catatonia in an adult population attributed primarily to medical and not psychiatric disorders was reported at 21%.[10] The prevalence rate of catatonia in pediatric medical conditions is not known because it is often unrecognized.

SCREENING

The most important screening tool for catatonia is awareness of the symptoms and maintaining a high index of suspicion. The symptoms, similar in adults and children, are detailed in Table 13.1 and include the 12 symptoms identified in *DSM-5*,[12] as well as other critical symptoms included in the Bush-Francis Catatonia Rating Scale (BFCRS).[21,22] The threshold for considering the diagnoses of catatonia includes three or more symptoms from DSM-V criteria or two or more symptoms from the BFCRS, the preferred rating scale, given the high interrater reliability and validity.[22] Relying only on DSM-5 criteria is inadequate given that the prevalence rates of symptoms not included in the *DSM*, such as staring and autonomic abnormalities, were found to be 74% and 32%, respectively.[23]

DIAGNOSIS

The diagnosis requires the following:
1. Comprehensive history (medical, neurologic, neuropsychiatric, pharmacotherapy)
2. Physical examination
3. Differentiation from other conditions such as delirium, neuroleptic malignant syndrome (NMS), serotonergic syndrome, and other conditions[4] as listed in Table 13.2
4. Investigation of underlying medical and neuropsychiatric disorders as listed in Table 13.3

TABLE 13.1
Catatonia Symptoms

Motor	*Staring	Fixed gaze, decreased blinking
	*Cataplexy/*posturing	Maintaining regular or odd posture for long periods
	*Posturing	Maintaining constant posture
	*Stereotypy	Repetitive, non–goal-directed activity
	*Mannerisms	Odd, purposeful movements
	*Waxy flexibility	Allows repositioning
	*Grimacing	Odd facial expressions
	*Echopraxia	Mimicking movements
	Rigidity	Rigid position
	Grasp reflex	Automatic closure of palm when touched
Behavior	*Stupor/immobility	Immobile; hypoactive
	*Agitation	
	Excitement	Extreme hyperactivity
	Negativism	Resistant to instructions; contrary behaviors
	Withdrawal	Refusing to eat/drink
	Impulsivity	
	Automatic obedience	Exaggerated cooperation
	Mitgehen	Arm raising with light pressure
	Gegenhalten	Resistance to passive movements
	Ambitendency	Indecisive
	Perseveration	Repeating same topic/movement
	Combativeness	Belligerence, aggression
Speech	*Mutism	Verbally unresponsive; long lag time before responding
	*Echolalia	Mimicking speech
	Verbigeration	Repetition of nonsensical phrases
Dysautonomia	Spinal—sympathetic	Superior cervical ganglion (piloerector muscles, sweat glands, lungs, heart) Celiac gg (liver, stomach, intestine, adrenal medulla). Mesenteric gg (rectum, bladder). Pelvic gg (reproductive organs)
	Cranial—parasympathetic	Cranial nerves III, VII, IX, X Ganglions: ciliary, Sph, SMB, otic, pulmonary, cardiac Stomach Intestine[20]

*These are the twelve symptoms listed in DSM-V. The rest of the list (including the * symptoms) is the Bush-Francis scale
gg, gangllon.
Data from Bush G, Fink M, Petrides G, Dowling F, Francis A. Catatonia. I. Rating scale and standardized examination. *Acta Psychiatr Scand.* 1996;93(2):129–136; Association AP. *Diagnostic and Statistical Manual of Mental Disorders.* 5th ed. Washington, DC: American Psychiatric Association; 2013.

LABORATORY TESTS

Although there are no laboratory tests specific for catatonia, testing for underlying medical or neuropsychiatric disorders should be guided by the medical history and physical examination. These may include blood culture to check for infections or serum panels to test systemic lupus erythematosus (SLE) or D-dimer to check for a coagulopathy.[32] A lumbar puncture may be necessary to obtain cerebral spinal fluid (CSF) if infections or autoimmune disorders such as *N*-methyl-D-aspartate receptor antibodies (NMDA-R) are suspected because serum may give false positives.[33]

TABLE 13.2
Differential Diagnoses

Diagnosis	Definition	Differentiating Factors
Delirium[24,25]	An acute change from baseline with waxing and waning orientation	Motor dysregulation is not typical in delirium
Neuroleptic malignant syndrome[26,27]	Rigidity, hyperthermia, and autonomic dysfunction after exposure to neuroleptic medications	Caused by D2 antagonist History: medication administration with a temporal association to NMS onset Physical examination: fever, tremor, laboratory evidence of muscle injury (CK), leukocytosis Catatonia[28]
Toxic serotonin syndrome[29]	Fever Twitching muscles Tremors Diarrhea Altered sensorium Hyperactive tendon reflexes Myoclonus Catatonia	Caused by excess serotonin Motor symptoms in serotonin syndrome classically do not include waxy flexibility or rigidity
Complex partial seizures[30]	Seizures characterized by change in awareness with a variety of motoric signs	EEG in catatonia should be normal. Both will respond to benzodiazepines, but catatonia should not respond to other antiepileptics
Central nervous system (CNS) infection	Infections of different layers or components of the nervous system, which may affect behavior and consciousness	CNS infections often lack the motor findings classic of catatonia
CNS neoplasm	Variety of pathologies, which may affect awareness and behavior by invasion or mass effect	Focal neurologic deficits should not be present with catatonia
Inborn errors of metabolism[31]	Variety of disorders, including urea cycle defects, MTHFR deficiency, porphyria, Wilson's CTX, and Niemann-Pick	
Paranoia	Increased motor tone	No speech or behavioral symptoms
Pharmacologic sedation	Decreased arousal due to medication administration	Motor features of catatonia are absent

CK, creatine kinase; *CTX,* Cerebrotendinous xanthomatosis; *EEG,* electroencephalogram; *MTHFR,* methylene tetrahydrofolate reductase; *NMS,* neuroleptic malignant syndrome.

ELECTROENCEPHALOGRAM

There are no specific electroencephalogram (EEG) changes associated with catatonia. Low-amplitude background activity[34] has been reported in some cases and high-amplitude slow activity in others.[30] Catatonia has been reported in patients with seizure disorders[30] and in patients where seizures are part of the underlying encephalopathy such as in NMDA-R Ab.[35] Therefore obtaining an EEG may be helpful in the investigation of underlying conditions and in differentiating from delirium.

BRAIN IMAGING

In a computerized tomography and functional magnetic resonance imaging (MRI) study of schizophrenic patients with catatonia, Northoff and colleagues reported enlargement of all inner and outer CSF spaces, mostly pronounced in the left frontal areas and alterations in laterality.[36] Some studies report normal MRI findings.[37] However, in a review of 95 adults with catatonia due to general medical or psychiatric conditions, 31 individuals (37.8%) had some abnormality on MRI

TABLE 13.3
Catatonia—Underlying Medical and Neuropsychiatric Disorders

Encephalitis[10]	Infections	Herpes simplex[66]
		Malaria[67]
		Acquired immune deficiency syndrome[68,69]
		SLE[73,122]
	Autoimmune	NMDA-R-Ab[123,124]
		Hashimoto[10]
		Antiphospholipid syndrome[125]
		PANDAS/PANS[74]
		Epileptic encephalitis[35]
	Seizures	Epileptic encephalitis[35]
Genetic disorders		22q13.3 microdeletion[10]
Hypoventilation		Hypercapnia, hypoxemia[37]
Neurodevelopmental		Dandy-Walker[126]
Neuropsychiatric		Autism[18,127]
		Mood disorders[15,128]
		Schizoaffective disorders[16]
		OCD[129]
Metabolic		G6PD[75]
Thromboembolism		Pulmonary embolism, phlebitis[32,130,131]
Physical trauma		Burns[80]
		Head injury[132,133]
Psychologic trauma		Deprivation, abuse[82]
		Posttraumatic stress disorder[134]
Toxicity		Neuroleptics[26,27]
		Disulfiram[111]
		Steroids[111]
		Antibiotics[111]
		Wellbutrin[111]
		Baclofen[111]
		Recreational drugs[111]
		Venom[135]
Medication withdrawal		Benzodiazepines[136–138]
		Alcohol[139]
		Clozapine[140]
		Antidepressants[141,142]
		Gabapentin[111]

NMDA-R, N-methyl-D-aspartate receptor; *OCD*, obsessive-compulsive disorder; *PANDAS/PANS*, pediatric autoimmune neuropsychiatric disorders associated with streptococcus/pediatric acute-onset neuropsychiatric syndrome; *SLE*, systemic lupus erythematosus.

and 16 individuals (19.5%) had a focal abnormality[10]. This suggests that deciphering brain imaging findings that are related to catatonia or the underlying disorders is challenging.

Data from positron emission tomography (PET) using fluoro-deoxy-glucose (F-18-FDG-PET) indicate deficits in various brain regions. Schizophrenic patients with catatonia showed bilateral thalamic hypermetabolism and bilateral hypometabolism of frontal cortex.[38] In a 19-year-old patient with a static encephalopathy and catatonia, bilateral occipitotemporal and thalamic hypometabolism were reported on FDG-PET.[39] In a 20-year-old patient, where the catatonia and psychiatric symptoms were attributed to hypercapnia/hypoxemia, FDG-PET showed deficits in bilateral thalami, temporal cortices, and cerebellar while frontal and prefrontal cortices were less affected and there were no changes in striatum.[37]

The brain metabolic changes seen with FDG-PET may be secondary to the catatonia or the underlying conditions. Flumazenil (FMZ)-PET changes may be more specific to catatonia, one study showing decreased benzodiazepine receptor binding in the right frontotemporal lobe area where FDG-PET showed glucose metabolism to be preserved.[40] FMZ is a specific antagonist of γ-aminobutyric acid A (GABA$_A$) receptors.[41] Spectroscopy may also offer an even more specific tool because it can observe the combined glutamate and glutamine (glx) peak in vivo.[42]

PATHOPHYSIOLOGY/ETIOLOGY
Animal Models
Some attribute the term *tonic immobility*, the paralysis-like fear response seen in animals, to catatonia.[43] Rather than fight or flight, this mechanism has been described as a third response that comprises behaviors such as the rigidity, waxy flexibility, and catalepsy seen in catatonia.[44] The opossum, *Didelphis virginiana*, spontaneously manifests catatonia-like symptoms, such as immobility, by remaining in an abnormal position for several hours after being stressed.[42]

Neurotransmitters Imbalances
Increasing evidence from animal, neuroimaging, and pharmacologic studies points to neurotransmission imbalances in catatonia, including the following:

Glutamatergic
GABA$_A$ hypoactivity
GABA$_B$ hyperactivity
Glutamate NMDA hyperactivity

Dopaminergic
Dopamine-2 hypoactivity

Serotonergic
Serotonin-2 hyperactivity

Cholinergic
Cholinergic hyperactivity

Glutamate, the principal excitatory neurotransmitter in the brain works through ionotropic (NMDA, AMPA, kainite) and metabotropic receptors.[45] GABA, the main inhibitory neurotransmitter widely distributed throughout the central nervous system, consists of three types of receptors (GABA$_A$, GABA$_B$, and GABA$_C$[46] with GABA$_A$ being the predominant one).[47]

GABAergic dysfunction in the orbitofrontal cortex is thought to be responsible for catatonic affective expression,[48] and frontal lobe dysfunction has also been linked to tonic immobility.[43,49] NMDA-R activation has been shown to increase GABA activity through a variety of processes, including increasing surface GABA$_A$ receptor expression,[50] increasing GABAergic transmission possibly through insertion of GABA$_A$ receptors,[51] increasing GABA$_A$R-mediated spontaneous inhibitory postsynaptic currents,[52] reversing dispersal of GABA$_A$R clusters and increasing in GABA$_A$R lateral movement,[53] and directly triggering presynaptic GABA release for local dendrodendritic feedback inhibition.[54] In NMDA-R Ab encephalopathy, the decreased NMDA-R excitatory activity results in decreased GABA inhibitory activity, resulting in catatonia. Glutamatergic imbalances in the hypothalamic region and the basal ganglia are thought to be responsible for the dysautonomias and motor symptoms, respectively, typical of catatonia.[49,55]

The most effective treatment for catatonia, the benzodiazepines, enhances GABA$_A$ activity by binding to a modulatory site on the GABA$_A$ receptor and prolonging inhibition.[56] On the contrary, GABA$_B$ agonists, such as baclofen, appear to induce, rather than treat, a catatonic state.[44,57] Electroconvulsive therapy (ECT) also balances GABA function, affirming this hypothesis.

Antipsychotics that inhibit dopamine (primarily D$_2$ receptors), other dopamine antagonists, and sudden cessation of dopamine enhancers have been shown to contribute to catatonic motor symptoms. Low serum iron, reported to result in D$_2$ receptor hypofunction,[58] has also been reported in catatonic patients.[59] These observations, in conjunction with the successful treatment of catatonic symptoms via dopamine agonists and ECT, have led scientists to believe that dopamine hypoactivity plays a role in catatonia.[57] Additionally, a decrease in dopamine activity can trigger the release of the excitatory neurotransmitter glutamate, which may, in turn, induce catatonic symptoms.[49] Some dopamine agonists are also NMDA-R antagonists (e.g., amantadine, memantine), blocking NMDA-R and glutamate activity and increasing relative GABA activity can be helpful in decreasing catatonia. However, ketamine, another NMDA-R antagonist, induced catatonic symptoms in healthy subjects.[60]

Increases in serotonin (e.g., through selective serotonergic reuptake inhibitors) have also been linked to catatonia-like reactions,[57] although this connection might be indirect, as serotonin activity can affect both the dopaminergic[61] and GABAergic[62] systems.

Cholinergic hyperactivity has also been hypothesized to be involved because clozapine withdrawal has been associated with catatonia;[63,64] however, serotonergic rebound could also be playing a role[63] and GABAergic activity.[65]

These neurotransmitter systems are interconnected and this complicates teasing out individual effects and processes contributing to catatonia. However, they illustrate a conceptual model of inhibitory and excitatory neurotransmitter imbalances. The respective treatments help to restore balance and subsequently treat and often cure the symptoms of catatonia.

Infectious/Autoimmune

Pediatric catatonia has been reported in a number of infectious and autoimmune disorders, including herpes,[66] malaria,[67] AIDS,[68,69] autoimmune encephalitis,[24,44,70–72] SLE,[73] and PANDAS/PANS (pediatric autoimmune neuropsychiatric disorders associated with streptococcus/pediatric acute-onset neuropsychiatric syndrome).[74] The mechanism by which catatonia results is thought to involve dysregulation of neurotransmitters, as discussed earlier.

Oxidative Damage

Reports of catatonia in patients with G6PD deficiency also raise the possibility that oxidative stress or damage may also confer risk for catatonia.[75]

Genetic Risks

Research focuses primarily on other genetic disorders that can produce catatonia, rather than a genetic basis for catatonia, itself. Science has demonstrated an association between Prader-Willi syndrome (PWS) and catatonia.[70,76] PWS occurs when there is no gene expression on chromosome 15q11-13, and the mechanism is thought to be related to GABAergic and dopaminergic dysregulation.[70,77] The linkage between

schizophrenia and autism with catatonia presents another genetic pathway, involving the neurotransmitter imbalance.[70,78] It is also suggested that catatonia and autism share a common region for genetic susceptibility (15q15-21).[78] MLC1 polymorphisms have also been associated with periodic catatonia in a subgroup of patients with chronic schizophrenia.[79]

Physical and Psychological Trauma

Catatonia has been reported in adult patients who have sustained burn injuries[80,81] and in children and adolescents who have experienced stressful or traumatic life events,[49,82] including cyberbullying.[83]

TREATMENTS

The clinical management of catatonia is complex and needs to be tailored to the individual patient. It includes the following:

1. Treatment of the catatonia
2. Identification and treatment of the underlying medical or neuropsychiatric condition
3. If the catatonia is drug-induced such as in NMS, immediate discontinuation of medication(s) occurs
4. Supportive environment until recovery is achieved. In severe cases, inpatient medical or psychiatric hospitalization may be necessary to manage the underlying medical or neuropsychiatric disorder or drug toxicity

TREATMENTS FOR CATATONIA

Recognizing, diagnosing, and treating catatonia are critical. Failure to treat catatonia early in its course results in increased morbidity and mortality in adults[84] and children.[85] Complications from untreated catatonia can include aspiration pneumonia, muscle contractures, pressure ulcers, malnutrition, severe weight loss, and thromboembolisms.[86]

MEDICATIONS

The first-line medications for catatonia are the benzodiazepines. It was only in the recent past that Fricchione and colleagues successfully used benzodiazepines to treat catatonia secondary to NMS, in four patients that had been unresponsive to all other treatments. Within hours, after receiving 2 mg of intravenous lorazepam, a dramatic improvement occurred.[87] Other reports and open trials with lorazepam[88–90] and other benzodiazepines, including clonazepam,[23,91] diazepam,[92] oxazepam,[93] and zolpidem,[94] further supported efficacy. In a recent study that included 225 adults (aged 18–38 years) treated with benzodiazepines for catatonia, 85% had a significant improvement, 11% partially improved, and 4% did not respond.[23] Withdrawal-induced catatonia has also been reported with benzodiazepines.[2] Effective treatment of catatonia with benzodiazepines appears to be the same regardless of the underlying medical, neurologic, or neuropsychiatric conditions. Anxiety symptoms have been reported to occur either before the catatonic episode or simultaneously;[55] however, it is unlikely that the benzodiazepines treat the catatonia by decreasing anxiety.

Although there are no established clinical guidelines for treatment, expert consensus based on reported cases suggests lorazepam as the first-line treatment.[95] Various doses have been reported, including 1–2 mg lorazepam, as a challenge test to confirm diagnosis and up to 24 mg/day for treatment.[24,96,97] Such high doses appear to be well tolerated and do not result in the sedation or respiratory depression often seen in patients without catatonia.[24] In a naturalistic study that included children and adolescents, 65% improved and dosing range was up to 15 mg of lorazepam.[98] Lower response rates to the benzodiazepines have been reported in adults with catatonia secondary to psychotic and mood disorders and the poor response has been attributed, in part, to inadequate dosing ranges (3–6 mg/day).[99]

There are no established guidelines for dosing or dose titration. The general clinical consensus is to start dosing at 1–2 mg of lorazepam every 4–12 h with dose titration of an additional milligram (every 3–5 days) up to 15 mg if there is none or minimal response to the lower doses.[100] When doses are titrated to the higher levels, monitoring for sedation and respiratory depression is necessary.

Benzodiazepine challenge has also been used to confirm the diagnosis[97] and zolpidem, a GABA receptor modulator.[101] Partial, permanent, or temporary relief of symptoms soon after administration of benzodiazepines is supportive for the diagnosis of catatonia.

Other medications, such as lithium, valproate, memantine, amantadine, and clozapine, can also be helpful with decreasing catatonia.[102] As shown in Table 13.4, these medications increase GABAergic or decrease glutamate. Lithium has been reported to increase GABA[103] and also improve mitochondrial oxidative dysfunction.[104] Lithium has also been reported to be effective in patients with catatonia with low serum iron levels, with poor response to the benzodiazepines.[59]

The role of N-acetyl cysteine (NAC) in catatonia remains to be explored. It is an antioxidant used for the management of acetaminophen overdoses and in one

TABLE 13.4
Medications and Neurotransmission Modulation in Catatonia

Neurotransmitter Imbalance	↑GABA_A	↓Glutamate (NMDA Antagonists)
	Benzodiazepines[56]	
	Zolpidem[94,100,143]	
	Topiramate[144]	
	Valproate[145]	Valproate[145]
	Carbamazepine[146]	
	Lithium[147–149]	Lithium[103]
		Memantine[102]
		Amantadine[102]
		Clozapine[150]

GABA_A, γ-aminobutyric acid A; GABA_B, γ-aminobutyric acid B; NMDA, N-methyl-D-aspartate.

case report the associated catatonia also resolved.[105] As reviewed by Berk and colleagues, NAC increases plasma cysteine levels and this is relevant because cysteine is exchanged for glutamate in glial cells. The increased glutamate stimulates metabotropic glutamate receptors, reducing synaptic release of glutamate and increasing GABA release. NAC also facilitates dopamine release.[106]

ELECTROCONVULSIVE THERAPY

As reviewed by Fink,[96] early reports of successful treatment of catatonia were reported with amobarbital[107] and the induction of grand mal seizures.[108] Subsequently, ECT has been reported to successfully treat catatonia in adult patients[95,97] and in adolescents who have had minimal to partial responses to benzodiazepines.[109] ECT has also been reported to be effective in treating catatonia in youths with neuropsychiatric disorders,[109,110] NMS,[111] and encephalitis.[112] The number of ECT treatments required to achieve full resolution of symptoms is reported to be between 8 and 28.[109]

The mechanism of action for ECT's effect on catatonia is not known. Animal studies have reported increased diazepam binding sites in the cerebral cortex of rats,[113] upregulation of benzodiazepine receptors in frontal cortex,[114] and increased GABA concentration in the striatum.[115,116]

Recurrence of catatonia after effective treatment with either benzodiazepines or ECT[109,117] is very minimal to nonexistent.

It is important to emphasize that the identification and treatment of underlying conditions is essential. In a 20-year-old patient with hypoventilation, the catatonia did not improve with lorazepam (dose not reported), but the catatonia, paranoia, and auditory and visual hallucinations all resolved with adequate ventilation.[37] It is also important to note that treating the underlying condition does not always treat the catatonia. As reported by Fricchione and colleagues, treatment of SLE with intravenous methyl prednisolone and plasma exchange did not improve the catatonia that responded to ECT.[118] In SLE as in other conditions, such as NMDR-Ab encephalitis, the untreated catatonia may mask any improvement that is occurring by treatments for the underlying condition such as steroids, immunotherapy, and plasma exchange.

If antipsychotics are needed, those with low D_2 blockade such as quetiapine or olanzapine or those with partial D_2 agonism such as aripiprazole should be considered.[119]

Implications for Clinical Pediatric Practice

Symptomatology for children and adolescents appears to be similar to those reported in adults; however, there are some important differences.

The GABAergic system and frontal lobe dysfunction have been linked to tonic immobility.[43,49] It is of particular interest that tonic immobility is more common in younger animals because of immature development of the cortical system, thus reflecting that a human pediatric population may be at risk for the same reason.[44] The reemergence of primitive reflexes, such as the grasp reflex, present during early childhood and in only 1% of healthy adults,[120] and other symptoms of catatonia may be due to cortical disinhibition. If we hypothesize that cortical disinhibition, in various brain areas, is one of the pathways, then it may be that children may be more vulnerable in the presence of other risk factors to the development of catatonia than adults.

As noted in Box 13.1, in children the catatonia symptoms may be mistaken for oppositional behaviors. The underlying medical and neuropsychiatric conditions may also differ because some of these may be developmentally specific.

SUMMARY

Catatonia is a constellation of symptoms representing a final common pathway resulting from GABA hypoactivity or glutamate toxicity that can result from many unrelated medical and neuropsychiatric disorders.

Catatonia in children is not rare but frequently remains unrecognized. It has significant morbidity

---

BOX 13.1
Implications for Clinical Pediatric Practice

1. Identifying catatonia
   a. Symptoms are similar for children and adults
      i. In children, focus on motor and language
      ii. Do not attribute behavioral symptoms to an oppositional child unless these were present to the same degree before the acute onset of the catatonia
   b. Screening tools such as the BFCRS are very helpful because in many cases the speech impairment may make it very difficult or impossible to interview the patients
   c. Do not overlook the dysautonomias
2. Identifying underlying medical, neurologic, neuropsychiatric, and medication toxicity/withdrawal
   a. Clinical history and physical examination are essential
   b. EEG, laboratories, and other tests will be guided by clinical presentation
3. First-line treatment for children and adolescents
   a. Benzodiazepines
   b. Nonresponders to benzodiazepines after maximizing dose in a safe setting
      i. Check iron status
      ii. NDMA receptor antagonists
   c. Treatment of underlying medical, neurologic, and neuropsychiatric disorder
4. Importance of timeliness in treatment
   a. Malnutrition
   b. Exhaustion
   c. Self-harm
   d. Fatality (NMS)
   e. Effectiveness of treatment for underlying conditions may be masked by the catatonia. This can lead to more invasive treatments when in fact the less invasive treatment may actually be working.

BFCRS, Bush-Francis Catatonia Rating Scale; *EEG*, electroencephalogram; *NMDA*, N-methyl-D-aspartate; *NMS*, neuroleptic malignant syndrome.

---

and mortality, but because of the lack of recognition in pediatric settings, it frequently goes untreated.

Current treatment guidelines for adults and children, based on clinical reports and expert opinion, indicate that the benzodiazepines are the first-line treatments for catatonia. The large dose ranges reported[24] from 1 mg of lorazepam up to 24° mg suggest variable individual responses and, therefore, dose titration should be considered for the youths not responding to the lower doses. The frequency of dosing when there is a response is also not well established. In our clinical experience, lorazepam appears to confer efficacy for about 4 h with a subsequent return to the catatonic state, concurring with Dhossche and Wachtel's suggestion that lorazepam should be prescribed at regular intervals to maintain improvement.[24]

ECT is also effective; however, this may not be a viable option for younger children where benzodiazepine treatment for catatonia is reported to be underutilized[121] and dose titration not optimized.

Recognizing, diagnosing, and treating catatonia are critical because there are effective treatments. Failure to treat catatonia early in its course results in increased morbidity and mortality in adults[84] and children.[85] As Dhossche and Wachtel report[24] while catatonia has been reported in autoimmune encephalitis, it is usually not assessed or treated in these patients. In younger patients, sluggish responses to immunotherapies are observed and it is possible that the untreated catatonia may be contributing to the prolonged recovery or at the very least masking improvement.

Most of our clinical knowledge of pediatric catatonia is deduced from studies in adults. Although it appears that the clinical manifestations are similar, it will be important to develop and validate pediatric-specific scales. Double-blind, well-controlled studies are also needed to determine effective dosing of benzodiazepines. The few PET studies using FMZ point to dysfunction of the GABAergic system. The development of $GABA_A$ receptor subunit-selective tracers in humans by PET[46] will allow further exploration. Spectroscopy that can allow the investigation of combined glutamate and glutamine (glx) peak in vivo[42] can also help elucidate the pathophysiology and also detect changes resulting from various treatments.

Preventing catatonia is not likely to be a realistic goal given that it has many potential causes. Perhaps, in most cases, catatonia, such as fever, should be regarded as an ally that leads the clinician investigate and identify the underlying cause.

REFERENCES

1. Caroff S, Mann SC, Francis A, Fricchione GL. *Catatonia: From Psychopathology to Neurobiology*. Arlington, VA: American Psychiatric Publishing; 2004.
2. Deuschle M, Lederbogen F. Benzodiazepine withdrawal-induced catatonia. *Pharmacopsychiatry*. 2001;34(1):41–42.
3. Shorter E. Making childhood catatonia visible, separate from competing diagnoses. *Acta Psychiatr Scand*. 2012;125(1):3–10.
4. Saddawi-Konefka D, Berg SM, Nejad SH, Bittner EA. Catatonia in the ICU: an important and underdiagnosed cause of altered mental status. a case series and review of the literature*. *Crit Care Med*. 2014;42(3):e234–e241.
5. Ghaziuddin N, Dhossche D, Marcotte K. Retrospective chart review of catatonia in child and adolescent psychiatric patients. *Acta Psychiatr Scand*. 2012;125(1):33–38.
6. Kahlbaum KL. *Catatonia (Originally Published in 1874)*. Baltimore: John Hopkins University Press; 1973.
7. Kraepelin E. *Dementia Praecox and Paraphrenia*. Chicago: Chicago Medical Book Co.; 1919.
8. Gelenberg AJ. The catatonic syndrome. *Lancet*. 1976; 1(7973):1339–1341.
9. Carroll BT, Anfinson TJ, Kennedy JC, Yendrek R, Boutros M, Bilon A. Catatonic disorder due to general medical conditions. *J Neuropsychiatry Clin Neurosci*. 1994;6(2): 122–133.
10. Smith JH, Smith VD, Philbrick KL, Kumar N. Catatonic disorder due to a general medical or psychiatric condition. *J Neuropsychiatry Clin Neurosci*. 2012;24(2): 198–207.
11. Association AP. *Diagnostic and Statistical Manual of Mental Disorders - 4th Edition (DSM-IV)*. Washington DC: American Psychiatric Association; 1994.
12. Association AP. *Diagnostic and Statistical Manual of Mental Disorders*. 5th ed. Washington, DC: American Psychiatric Association; 2013.
13. Tandon R, Heckers S, Bustillo J, et al. Catatonia in DSM-5. *Schizophr Res*. 2013;150(1):26–30.
14. Taylor MA, Fink M. Catatonia in psychiatric classification: a home of its own. *Am J Psychiatry*. 2003;160(7): 1233–1241.
15. Abrams R, Taylor MA. Catatonia. A prospective clinical study. *Arch Gen Psychiatry*. 1976;33(5):579–581.
16. Rosebush PI, Mazurek MF. Catatonia and its treatment. *Schizophr Bull*. 2010;36(2):239–242.
17. Thakur A, Jagadheesan K, Dutta S, Sinha VK. Incidence of catatonia in children and adolescents in a paediatric psychiatric clinic. *Aust N Z J Psychiatry*. 2003;37(2): 200–203.
18. Wing L, Shah A. Catatonia in autistic spectrum disorders. *Br J Psychiatry*. 2000;176:357–362.
19. Billstedt E, Gillberg IC, Gillberg C. Autism after adolescence: population-based 13- to 22-year follow-up study of 120 individuals with autism diagnosed in childhood. *J Autism Dev Disord*. 2005;35(3):351–360.
20. Espinosa-Medina I, Saha O, Boismoreau F, et al. The sacral autonomic outflow is sympathetic. *Science*. 2016; 354(6314):893–897.
21. Bush G, Fink M, Petrides G, Dowling F, Francis A. Catatonia. I. Rating scale and standardized examination. *Acta Psychiatr Scand*. 1996;93(2):129–136.
22. Sienaert P, Rooseleer J, De Fruyt J. Measuring catatonia: a systematic review of rating scales. *J Affect Disord*. 2011;135(1–3):1–9.
23. Wilson JE, Niu K, Nicolson SE, Levine SZ, Heckers S. The diagnostic criteria and structure of catatonia. *Schizophr Res*. 2015;164(1–3):256–262.
24. Dhossche DM, Wachtel LE. Catatonia is hidden in plain sight among different pediatric disorders: a review article. *Pediatr Neurol*. 2010;43(5):307–315.

25. Hem E, Andreassen OA, Robasse JM, Vatnaland T, Opjordsmoen S. Should catatonia be part of the differential diagnosis of coma? *Nordic J Psychiatry*. 2005;59(6):528–530.

26. White DA, Robins AH. Catatonia: harbinger of the neuroleptic malignant syndrome. *Br J Psychiatry*. 1991;158:419–421.

27. White DA. Catatonia and the neuroleptic malignant syndrome–a single entity? *Br J Psychiatry*. 1992;161:558–560.

28. Lang FU, Lang S, Becker T, Jager M. Neuroleptic malignant syndrome or catatonia? Trying to solve the catatonic dilemma. *Psychopharmacology*. 2015;232(1):1–5.

29. Sternbach H. The serotonin syndrome. *Am J Psychiatry*. 1991;148(6):705–713.

30. Suzuki K, Miura N, Awata S, et al. Epileptic seizures superimposed on catatonic stupor. *Epilepsia*. 2006;47(4):793–798.

31. Sedel F, Baumann N, Turpin JC, Lyon-Caen O, Saudubray JM, Cohen D. Psychiatric manifestations revealing inborn errors of metabolism in adolescents and adults. *J Inherit Metab Dis*. 2007;30(5):631–641.

32. Haouzir S, Lemoine X, Desbordes M, et al. The role of coagulation marker fibrin D-dimer in early diagnosis of catatonia. *Psychiatry Res*. 2009;168(1):78–85.

33. Barry H, Byrne S, Barrett E, Murphy KC, Cotter DR. Anti-N-methyl-D-aspartate receptor encephalitis: review of clinical presentation, diagnosis and treatment. *BJPsych Bull*. 2015;39(1):19–23.

34. Ihara M, Kohara N, Urano F, et al. Neuroleptic malignant syndrome with prolonged catatonia in a dopa-responsive dystonia patient. *Neurology*. 2002;59(7):1102–1104.

35. Wright S, Vincent A. Pediatric autoimmune epileptic encephalopathies. *J Child Neurol*. 2017;32(4):418–428.

36. Northoff G, Waters H, Diekmann S, et al. Left prefrontal cortical progression and alterations of laterality in catatonia: a CT and F-MRI study. *Biol Psychiatry*. 1997;42:164S.

37. Dranovsky A, Needleman JP, Sylvester J, VanHeertum R, Muskin PR. Progressive paranoid psychosis in a 20-year-old with central congenital hypoventilation syndrome. *Pediatrics*. 2014;134(3):e900–e902.

38. Lauer M, Schirrmeister H, Gerhard A, et al. Disturbed neural circuits in a subtype of chronic catatonic schizophrenia demonstrated by F-18-FDG-PET and F-18-DOPA-PET. *J Neural Transm (Vienna)*. 2001;108(6):661–670.

39. Breker D, Bohnen NI. Single case study of brain FDG PET imaging in a patient with catatonia. *Clin Nucl Med*. 2013;38(7):e297–e298.

40. Iseki K, Ikeda A, Kihara T, et al. Impairment of the cortical GABAergic inhibitory system in catatonic stupor: a case report with neuroimaging. *Epileptic Disord*. 2009;11(2):126–131.

41. Olsen RW, McCabe RT, Wamsley JK. GABAA receptor subtypes: autoradiographic comparison of GABA, benzodiazepine, and convulsant binding sites in the rat central nervous system. *J Chem Neuroanat*. 1990;3(1):59–76.

42. Prost RW, Mark L, Mewissen M, Li SJ. Detection of glutamate/glutamine resonances by 1H magnetic resonance spectroscopy at 0.5 tesla. *Magn Reson Med*. 1997;37(4):615–618.

43. Moskowitz AK. "Scared stiff": catatonia as an evolutionary-based fear response. *Psychol Rev*. 2004;111(4):984–1002.

44. Hauptman AJ, Benjamin S. The differential diagnosis and treatment of catatonia in children and adolescents. *Harv Rev Psychiatry*. 2016;24(6):379–395.

45. Mothet JP, Le Bail M, Billard JM. Time and space profiling of NMDA receptor co-agonist functions. *J Neurochem*. 2015;135(2):210–225.

46. Nutt D. GABAA receptors: subtypes, regional distribution, and function. *J Clin Sleep Med*. 2006;2(2):S7–S11.

47. Lee V, Maguire J. The impact of tonic GABAA receptor-mediated inhibition on neuronal excitability varies across brain region and cell type. *Front Neural Circuits*. 2014;8:3.

48. Northoff G. Catatonia and neuroleptic malignant syndrome: psychopathology and pathophysiology. *J Neural Transm (Vienna)*. 2002;109(12):1453–1467.

49. Mazzone L, Postorino V, Valeri G, Vicari S. Catatonia in patients with autism: prevalence and management. *CNS Drugs*. 2014;28(3):205–215.

50. Marsden KC, Beattie JB, Friedenthal J, Carroll RC. NMDA receptor activation potentiates inhibitory transmission through GABA receptor-associated protein-dependent exocytosis of GABA(A) receptors. *J Neurosci*. 2007;27(52):14326–14337.

51. Ouardouz M, Sastry BR. Mechanisms underlying LTP of inhibitory synaptic transmission in the deep cerebellar nuclei. *J Neurophysiol*. 2000;84(3):1414–1421.

52. Xue JG, Masuoka T, Gong XD, et al. NMDA receptor activation enhances inhibitory GABAergic transmission onto hippocampal pyramidal neurons via presynaptic and postsynaptic mechanisms. *J Neurophysiol*. 2011;105(6):2897–2906.

53. Muir J, Arancibia-Carcamo IL, MacAskill AF, Smith KR, Griffin LD, Kittler JT. NMDA receptors regulate GABAA receptor lateral mobility and clustering at inhibitory synapses through serine 327 on the gamma2 subunit. *Proc Natl Acad Sci USA*. 2010;107(38):16679–16684.

54. Chen WR, Xiong W, Shepherd GM. Analysis of relations between NMDA receptors and GABA release at olfactory bulb reciprocal synapses. *Neuron*. 2000;25(3):625–633.

55. Rasmussen SA, Mazurek MF, Rosebush PI. Catatonia: our current understanding of its diagnosis, treatment and pathophysiology. *World J Psychiatry*. 2016;6(4):391–398.

56. Smith GB, Olsen RW. Functional domains of GABAA receptors. *Trends Pharmacol Sci*. 1995;16(5):162–168.

57. Fink M, Taylor M. *Catatonia: A Clinician's Guide to Diagnosis and Treatment*. Cambridge, New York: Cambridge University Press; 2003.

58. Erikson KM, Jones BC, Hess EJ, Zhang Q, Beard JL. Iron deficiency decreases dopamine D1 and D2 receptors in rat brain. *Pharmacol Biochem Behav*. 2001;69(3–4):409–418.

59. Lee JW. Serum iron in catatonia and neuroleptic malignant syndrome. *Biol Psychiatry*. 1998;44(6):499–507.
60. Gouzoulis-Mayfrank E, Heekeren K, Neukirch A, et al. Psychological effects of (S)-ketamine and N,N-dimethyltryptamine (DMT): a double-blind, cross-over study in healthy volunteers. *Pharmacopsychiatry*. 2005;38(6): 301–311.
61. Stahl S. *Stahl's Essential Psychopharmacology: Neuroscientific Basis and Practical Applications*. 3rd ed. Cambridge, New York: Cambridge University Press; 2008.
62. Northoff G. What catatonia can tell us about "top-down modulation": a neuropsychiatric hypothesis. *Behav Brain Sci*. 2002;25(5):555–577. discussion 578–604.
63. Wadekar M, Syed S. Clozapine-withdrawal catatonia. *Psychosomatics*. 2010;51(4):355–355.e352.
64. de Leon J, Stanilla JK, White AO, Simpson GM. Anticholinergics to treat clozapine withdrawal. *J Clin Psychiatry*. 1994;55(3):119–120.
65. Bilbily J, McCollum B, de Leon J. Catatonia secondary to sudden clozapine withdrawal: a case with three repeated episodes and a literature review. *Case Rep Psychiatry*. 2017;2017. 2402731.
66. Raskin DE, Frank SW. Herpes encephalitis with catatonic stupor. *Arch Gen Psychiatry*. 1974;31(4):544–546.
67. Durrant W. Catatonia after malaria. *Br Med J*. 1977;2(6091):893.
68. Volkow ND, Harper A, Munnisteri D, Clother J. AIDS and catatonia. *J Neurol Neurosurg Psychiatry*. 1987;50(1): 104.
69. Prakash O, Bagepally BS. Catatonia and mania in patient with AIDS: treatment with lorazepam and risperidone. *Gen Hosp Psychiatry*. 2012;34(3):321.e325–e326.
70. Dhossche DM, Stoppelbein L, Rout UK. Etiopathogenesis of catatonia: generalizations and working hypotheses. *J ECT*. 2010;26(4):253–258.
71. Dalmau J, Gleichman AJ, Hughes EG, et al. Anti-NMDA-receptor encephalitis: case series and analysis of the effects of antibodies. *Lancet Neurol*. 2008;7(12):1091–1098.
72. Parenti A, Jardri R, Geoffroy PA. How anti-NMDAR encephalitis sheds light on the mechanisms underlying catatonia: the neural excitatory/inhibitory imbalance model. *Psychosomatics*. 2016;57(3):336–338.
73. Grover S, Parakh P, Sharma A, Rao P, Modi M, Kumar A. Catatonia in systemic lupus erythematosus: a case report and review of literature. *Lupus*. 2013;22(6):634–638.
74. Elia J, Dell ML, Friedman DF, et al. PANDAS with catatonia: a case report. Therapeutic response to lorazepam and plasmapheresis. *J Am Acad Child Adolesc Psychiatry*. 2005;44(11):1145–1150.
75. Raj V, Chism K, Minckler MR, Denysenko L. Catatonia and glucose-6-phosphate dehydrogenase deficiency: a report of two cases and a review. *Psychosomatics*. 2014;55(1):92–97.
76. Bartolucci G, Younger J. Tentative classification of neuropsychiatric disturbances in Prader-Willi Syndrome. *J Intellect Disabil Res*. 2008;38(6):621–629.
77. DeJong H, Bunton P, Hare DJ. A systematic review of interventions used to treat catatonic symptoms in people with autistic spectrum disorders. *J Autism Dev Disord*. 2014;44(9):2127–2136.
78. Stober G, Saar K, Ruschendorf F, et al. Splitting schizophrenia: periodic catatonia-susceptibility locus on chromosome 15q15. *Am J Hum Genet*. 2000;67(5): 1201–1207.
79. Selch S, Strobel A, Haderlein J, et al. MLC1 polymorphisms are specifically associated with periodic catatonia, a subgroup of chronic schizophrenia. *Biol Psychiatry*. 2007;61(10):1211–1214.
80. Quinn DK. "Burn catatonia": a case report and literature review. *J Burn Care Res*. 2014;35(2):e135–e142.
81. Zarr ML, Nowak T. Catatonia and burns. *Burns*. 1990; 16(2):133–134.
82. Dhossche DM, Ross CA, Stoppelbein L. The role of deprivation, abuse, and trauma in pediatric catatonia without a clear medical cause. *Acta Psychiatr Scand*. 2012; 125(1):25–32.
83. Goetz M, Kitzlerova E, Hrdlicka M, Dhossche D. Combined use of electroconvulsive therapy and amantadine in adolescent catatonia precipitated by cyber-bullying. *J Child Adolesc Psychopharmacol*. 2013;23(3):228–231.
84. Swartz C, Galang RL. Adverse outcome with delay in identification of catatonia in elderly patients. *Am J Geriatr Psychiatry*. 2001;9(1):78–80.
85. Cornic F, Consoli A, Tanguy ML, et al. Association of adolescent catatonia with increased mortality and morbidity: evidence from a prospective follow-up study. *Schizophr Res*. 2009;113(2–3):233–240.
86. Clinebell K, Azzam PN, Gopalan P, Haskett R. Guidelines for preventing common medical complications of catatonia: case report and literature review. *J Clin Psychiatry*. 2014;75(6):644–651.
87. Fricchione GL, Cassem NH, Hooberman D, Hobson D. Intravenous lorazepam in neuroleptic-induced catatonia. *J Clin Psychopharmacol*. 1983;3(6):338–342.
88. Rosebush PI, Hildebrand AM, Furlong BG, Mazurek MF. Catatonic syndrome in a general psychiatric inpatient population: frequency, clinical presentation, and response to lorazepam. *J Clin Psychiatry*. 1990;51(9):357–362.
89. Wetzel H, Benkert O. Lorazepam for treatment of catatonic symptoms and severe psychomotor retardation. *Am J Psychiatry*. 1988;145(9):1175–1176.
90. Harris D, Menza MA. Benzodiazepines and catatonia: a case report. *Can J Psychiatry*. 1989;34(7):725–727.
91. Benazzi F. Parenteral clonazepam for catatonia. *Can J Psychiatry*. 1991;36(4):312.
92. McEvoy JP, Lohr JB. Diazepam for catatonia. *Am J Psychiatry*. 1984;141(2):284–285.
93. Schmider J, Standhart H, Deuschle M, Drancoli J, Heuser I. A double-blind comparison of lorazepam and oxazepam in psychomotor retardation and mutism. *Biol Psychiatry*. 1999;46(3):437–441.
94. Thomas P, Rascle C, Mastain B, Maron M, Vaiva G. Test for catatonia with zolpidem. *Lancet*. 1997;349(9053):702.

95. Petrides G, Divadeenam KM, Bush G, Francis A. Synergism of lorazepam and electroconvulsive therapy in the treatment of catatonia. *Biol Psychiatry.* 1997;42(5): 375–381.

96. Fink M. Rediscovering catatonia: the biography of a treatable syndrome. *Acta Psychiatr Scand Suppl.* 2013;(441):1–47.

97. Bush G, Fink M, Petrides G, Dowling F, Francis A. Catatonia. II. Treatment with lorazepam and electroconvulsive therapy. *Acta Psychiatr Scand.* 1996;93(2):137–143.

98. Raffin M, Zugaj-Bensaou L, Bodeau N, et al. Treatment use in a prospective naturalistic cohort of children and adolescents with catatonia. *Eur Child Adolescent Psychiatry.* 2015;24(4):441–449.

99. Tibrewal P, Narayanaswamy J, Zutshi A, Srinivasaraju R, Math SB. Response rate of lorazepam in catatonia: a developing country's perspective. *Prog Neuropsychopharmacol Biol Psychiatry.* 2010;34(8):1520–1522.

100. Sienaert P, Dhossche DM, Vancampfort D, De Hert M, Gazdag G. A clinical review of the treatment of catatonia. *Front Psychiatry.* 2014;5:181.

101. Cottencin O, Danel T, Goudemand M, Thomas P, Consoli SM. Catatonia recognition and treatment. *Med Sci Monit.* 2009;15(8): CS129-CS131.

102. Carroll BT, Goforth HW, Thomas C, et al. Review of adjunctive glutamate antagonist therapy in the treatment of catatonic syndromes. *J Neuropsychiatry Clin Neurosci.* 2007;19(4):406–412.

103. Malhi GS, Tanious M, Das P, Coulston CM, Berk M. Potential mechanisms of action of lithium in bipolar disorder. Current understanding. *CNS Drugs.* 2013;27(2): 135–153.

104. Khairova R, Pawar R, Salvadore G, et al. Effects of lithium on oxidative stress parameters in healthy subjects. *Mol Med Rep.* 2012;5(3):680–682.

105. Bestha DP, Padala P. A case of catatonia secondary to polysubstance abuse and acetaminophen overdose. *Prim Care Companion J Clin Psychiatry.* 2010;12(1):PCC 09100790.

106. Berk M, Malhi GS, Gray LJ, Dean OM. The promise of N-acetylcysteine in neuropsychiatry. *Trends Pharmacol Sci.* 2013;34(3):167–177.

107. Bleckwenn W. The production of sleep and rest in psychotic cases. *Arch Neurol Psychiatry.* 1930;24:365–372.

108. Meduna L. Versuche uber die biologische beeinflussung des ablaufes der schizophrenie: camphor and cardiozolkrampfe. *Z Ges Neurol Psychiatr.* 1935;152:235–262.

109. Weiss M, Allan B, Greenaway M. Treatment of catatonia with electroconvulsive therapy in adolescents. *J Child Adolesc Psychopharmacol.* 2012;22(1):96–100.

110. Zaw FK, Bates GD, Murali V, Bentham P. Catatonia, autism, and ECT. *Dev Med Child Neurol.* 1999;41(12):843–845.

111. Fink M, Taylor MA. *Catatonia. A Clinicina's Guide to Diagnosis and Treatment.* Cambridge, UK: Cambridge University Press; 2003.

112. Cohen D, Flament M, Dubos PF, Basquin M. Case series: catatonic syndrome in young people. *J Am Acad Child Adolesc Psychiatry.* 1999;38(8):1040–1046.

113. Paul SM, Skolnick P. Rapid changes in brain benzodiazepine receptors after experimental seizures. *Science.* 1978;202(4370):892–894.

114. Gulati A, Srimal RC, Dhawan BN, Agarwal AK, Seth PK. Upregulation of brain benzodiazepine receptors by electroconvulsive shocks. *Pharmacol Res Commun.* 1986;18(6):581–589.

115. Bowdler JM, Green AR, Minchin MC, Nutt DJ. Regional GABA concentration and [3H]-diazepam binding in rat brain following repeated electroconvulsive shock. *J Neural Transm.* 1983;56(1):3–12.

116. Green AR. Changes in gamma-aminobutyric acid biochemistry and seizure threshold. *Ann N Y Acad Sci.* 1986; 462:105–119.

117. Fink M. Is catatonia a primary indication for ECT? *Convuls Ther.* 1990;6(1):1–4.

118. Fricchione GL, Kaufman LD, Gruber BL, Fink M. Electroconvulsive therapy and cyclophosphamide in combination for severe neuropsychiatric lupus with catatonia. *Am J Med.* 1990;88(4):442–443.

119. Carroll BT, Lee JI, Appiani F, Thomas C. The pharmacotherapy of catatonia. *Prim Psychiatry.* 2010;17(4):41–47.

120. Brown DL, Smith TL, Knepper LE. Evaluation of five primitive reflexes in 240 young adults. *Neurology.* 1998; 51(1):322.

121. Lahutte B, Cornic F, Bonnot O, et al. Multidisciplinary approach of organic catatonia in children and adolescents may improve treatment decision making. *Prog Neuropsychopharmacol Biol Psychiatry.* 2008;32(6):1393–1398.

122. Mon T, L'Ecuyer S, Farber NB, et al. The use of electroconvulsive therapy in a patient with juvenile systemic lupus erythematosus and catatonia. *Lupus.* 2012;21(14): 1575–1581.

123. Dhossche D, Fink M, Shorter E, Wachtel LE. Anti-NMDA receptor encephalitis versus pediatric catatonia. *Am J Psychiatry.* 2011;168(7):749–750.

124. Gulyayeva NA, Massie MJ, Duhamel KN. Anti-NMDA receptor encephalitis: psychiatric presentation and diagnostic challenges from psychosomatic medicine perspective. *Palliat Support Care.* 2014;12(2):159–163.

125. Cardinal RN, Shah DN, Edwards CJ, Hughes GR, Fernandez-Egea E. Psychosis and catatonia as a first presentation of antiphospholipid syndrome. *Br J Psychiatry.* 2009;195(3):272.

126. Kumar S, Sur S, Singh A. Mega cisterna magna associated with recurrent catatonia: a case report. *Biol Psychiatry.* 2011;70(4):e19.

127. Dhossche DM. Autism as early expression of catatonia. *Med Sci Monit.* 2004;10(3):RA31-39.

128. Starkstein SE, Petracca G, Teson A, et al. Catatonia in depression: prevalence, clinical correlates, and validation of a scale. *J Neurol Neurosurg Psychiatry.* 1996;60(3):326–332.

129. Fontenelle LF, Lauterbach EC, Telles LL, Versiani M, Porto FH, Mendlowicz MV. Catatonia in obsessive-compulsive disorder: etiopathogenesis, differential diagnosis, and clinical management. *Cogn Behav Neurol.* 2007;20(1):21–24.

130. Lachner C, Sandson NB. Medical complications of catatonia: a case of catatonia-induced deep venous thrombosis. *Psychosomatics*. 2003;44(6):512–514.

131. McCall WV, Mann SC, Shelp FE, Caroff SN. Fatal pulmonary embolism in the catatonic syndrome: two case reports and a literature review. *J Clin Psychiatry*. 1995;56(1):21–25.

132. James BO, Omoaregba JO, Lawani AO, Ikeji CO, Igbinowanhia NG. Subdural haematoma presenting as catatonia in a 20-year-old male: a case report. *Cases J*. 2009;2:8032.

133. Schwarzbold M, Diaz A, Martins ET, et al. Psychiatric disorders and traumatic brain injury. *Neuropsychiatr Dis Treat*. 2008;4(4):797–816.

134. Shiloh R, Schwartz B, Weizman A, Radwan M. Catatonia as an unusual presentation of posttraumatic stress disorder. *Psychopathology*. 1995;28(6):285–290.

135. Sun Z, Yang X, Ye H, Zhou G, Jiang H. Delayed encephalopathy with movement disorder and catatonia: a rare combination after wasp stings. *Clin Neurol Neurosurg*. 2013;115(8):1506–1509.

136. Parameswaran R, Moore K, Hannan T, Austin M. Catatonia associated with temazepam withdrawal. *Aust N Z J Psychiatry*. 2011;45(11):1006–1007.

137. Sivakumar T, Yadav A, Sood M, Khandelwal SK. Lorazepam withdrawal catatonia: a case report. *Asian J Psychiatr*. 2013;6(6):620–621.

138. Brown M, Freeman S. Clonazepam withdrawal-induced catatonia. *Psychosomatics*. 2009;50(3):289–292.

139. Geoffroy PA, Rolland B, Cottencin O. Catatonia and alcohol withdrawal: a complex and underestimated syndrome. *Alcohol Alcohol*. 2012;47(3):288–290.

140. Yeh AW, Lee JW, Cheng TC, Wen JK, Chen WH. Clozapine withdrawal catatonia associated with cholinergic and serotonergic rebound hyperactivity: a case report. *Clin Neuropharmacol*. 2004;27(5):216–218.

141. Tyrer P. Clinical effects of abrupt withdrawal from tricyclic antidepressants and monoamine oxidase inhibitors after long-term treatment. *J Affect Disord*. 1984;6(1):1–7.

142. Konstantakopoulos G, Kouzoupis AV, Papageorgiou SG, Oulis P. Putative neuroleptic malignant syndrome associated with sertraline withdrawal. *J Clin Psychopharmacol*. 2009;29(3):300–301.

143. Peglow S, Prem V, McDaniel W. Treatment of catatonia with zolpidem. *J Neuropsychiatry Clin Neurosci*. 2013;25(3):e13.

144. McDaniel WW, Spiegel DR, Sahota AK. Topiramate effect in catatonia: a case series. *J Neuropsychiatry Clin Neurosci*. 2006;18(2):234–238.

145. Yoshida I, Monji A, Hashioka S, Ito M, Kanba S. Prophylactic effect of valproate in the treatment for siblings with catatonia: a case report. *J Clin Psychopharmacol*. 2005;25(5):504–505.

146. Rankel HW, Rankel LE. Carbamazepine in the treatment of catatonia. *Am J Psychiatry*. 1988;145(3):361–362.

147. Wald D, Lerner J. Lithium in the treatment of periodic catatonia: a case report. *Am J Psychiatry*. 1978;135(6):751–752.

148. Pheterson AD, Estroff TW, Sweeney DR. Severe prolonged catatonia with associated flushing reaction responsive to lithium carbonate. *J Am Acad Child Psychiatry*. 1985;24(2):235–237.

149. Gjessing LR. Lithium citrate loading of a patient with periodic catatonia. *Acta Psychiatr Scand*. 1967;43(4):372–375. PMID: 5582388.

150. Battegay R, Cotar B, Fleischhauer J, Rauchfleisch U. Results and side effects of treatment with clozapine (leponex R). *Compr Psychiatry*. 1977;18(5):423–428.

CHAPTER 14

Pediatric Inflammatory Brain Disease

PAULA TRAN, MD • JENNIFER FRANKOVICH, MD, MS • HEATHER VAN MATER,
MD, MS • RUSSELL C. DALE, MD • NOGA OR-GEVA, PHD •
ANNE MCHUGH, MD • MARGO THIENEMANN, MD

INTRODUCTION

Pediatric inflammatory brain diseases (PIBDs) vary widely in clinical presentation across neuropsychiatric domains. Emergence of psychiatric symptoms may be initial manifestations of PIBDs. Child psychiatrists who are alert for symptoms of PIBDs can hasten their diagnosis, and prompt referral to immunologic treatment can improve outcomes and lead to symptom resolution.[1] In fact, psychiatric symptoms can fully resolve once the underlying inflammatory disease is controlled—if treatment is started early enough. For example, in cases of autoimmune N-methyl-D-aspartate receptor (NMDAR) encephalitis, 40% of which occur in the pediatric population,[2] 80% of patients recover.[3] Delay or failure in diagnosing PIBDs, on the other hand, can lead to permanent disability.

The child psychiatrist plays an important role in identification and ongoing care of PIBD patients. After PIBD is diagnosed, the child psychiatrist becomes part of the treatment team, providing ongoing psychiatric, behavioral, and supportive care during the PIBD evaluation, illness treatments, and continues later in addressing residual symptoms. His or her knowledge about PIBDs prevents administration of interventions which, while supported by evidence for particular psychiatric symptoms seen in other contexts, could be ineffective and sometimes harmful in PIBD patients. The child psychiatrist's close monitoring and reporting of psychiatric symptoms is essential to direct medical treatment as psychiatric symptoms fluctuate with changes in the patient's inflammatory state. Inflammation of the patient may be retriggered and may recrudesce when immunomodulation is weaned. Thus, close monitoring and reporting symptom changes to the medical team is necessary. The authors hope that this chapter will increase the reader's interest in and knowledge about PIBDs so that the reader will consider PIBDs in their differential diagnosis of patients who present with new emotional, behavioral, cognitive, neurologic and other physical symptoms.

BRAIN IMMUNOLOGY

Local neuroinflammation is apparent in almost all pathologic central nervous system (CNS) conditions, including sterile injuries, chronic neurodegenerative diseases, neurodevelopmental diseases, and even depression. Until recently, the CNS was thought to be protected from the immune system as an evolutionary adaptation to guard it from the harmful and potentially permanent ramifications of local immune activation and infiltration of circulating immune cells. This idea was supported by the anatomical protection of the CNS by the cerebrospinal fluid (CSF), the meninges, and the blood-brain barrier (BBB) and the belief that the CNS lacked both lymphatic drainage and professional antigen-presenting cells.[4,5]

However, it is becoming increasingly clear that the cross-talk between the brain and the immune system is complex, as important roles in maintaining homeostasis and healing are discovered for microglia and other monocyte-derived macrophages, as well as T cells.[6–8] Moreover, discovery of a "glymphatic system" and meningeal lymphatic vasculature—which drain cellular and soluble substances from the CSF into the deep cervical lymph nodes—further demonstrates that CNS substances can be presented in the periphery.[9,10] Thus, neuroimmune cross-talk is highly complex, and CNS immune privilege is being redefined, as we understand the mechanisms that the CNS utilizes to safely benefit from the immune system while minimizing immune and autoimmune disease. It is now believed that it is the dysregulation of these protection mechanisms—caused by pathogens, inflammation, aging, or trauma—that may lead to immune-mediated CNS pathogenesis.

The BBB is a selectively permeable physical interface between the vascular and nervous systems that restricts the entry of factors from the blood such as ions, pathogens, and circulating immune cells into the CNS. The BBB is formed by tight junctions between brain endothelial cells, the basal lamina of these cells, and astrocyte end-feet processes.[11–13] The BBB protection can be compromised when blood-borne factors such as peripheral cytokines or cellular inflammation alter its permeability, thereby allowing entry of peripheral immune cells and antibodies into the CNS.[14,15] Additionally, it is still believed that the brain parenchyma is immune-privileged to some extent, and that infiltration of lymphocytes into it indicates a potentially harmful activation.

Different types of pathologic neuroimmune interactions are thought to cause psychiatric symptoms in patients with PIBD (Table 14.1). For instance, anti-NMDAR encephalitis is characterized by the presence of antibodies against the GluN1 subunit of the NMDAR causing internalization of the receptors and consequent reduction in synaptic signaling, leading to psychiatric symptoms.[16]

Preclinical animal models have also shed light on immune involvement in psychiatric diseases. In one animal study, aimed at determining the ability of Group A *Streptococcus pyogenes* to prime development of autoimmune disease, repeated nasopharyngeal *S. pyogenes* infection led to an abnormal T cell activation, and these T cells ultimately caused disruption of the BBB and neurovascular injury.[22] This scientific finding implicates a subtype of T cells as possible drivers of poststreptococcal basal ganglia autoimmune encephalopathies, including Sydenham chorea and pediatric autoimmune neuropsychiatric disorders associated with streptococcal infections (PANDAS).

CLINICAL PRESENTATION OF INFLAMMATORY BRAIN DISEASE

Symptoms of inflammatory brain disease vary greatly depending on the underlying etiology, which part of the brain is affected, and duration of brain inflammation. Encephalopathies triggered by infection may be preceded by fever and positive indices of infection from laboratory tests. Limbic encephalitis can present as psychosis, movement disorder, altered mental status, and, eventually, seizures. PIBDs that affect the basal ganglia can present as movement disorders, prominent sleep disruption, and sudden onset of obsessions and compulsions. If the amygdala is involved, anxiety may be a prominent symptom. A child's developmental stage can also affect the disease phenotypes or chronology of symptoms of PIBDs. Cognitive deficits, readily detectable in adults upon mental status examination (MSE), may be difficult to detect in children because of the dynamic nature of cognitive development and uncertainty regarding the premorbid state.

DIAGNOSTIC EVALUATION

Given the heterogeneity in the signs and symptoms of the different forms of inflammatory brain disease, it is essential to perform a complete evaluation to ensure an accurate diagnosis. Determining if the primary disease is due to CNS vasculitis versus an autoimmune encephalopathy (AE) is a helpful starting point, as treatments for these conditions differ.[115,126] No single test is sufficient for diagnosing an AE; rather the diagnosis is made when the history, physical examination, and abnormalities on laboratory and imaging studies are consistent with inflammatory brain disease. Autoimmune etiologies for an encephalopathy include both primary disease (without other systemic autoimmune disease) and secondary disease (associated systemic rheumatic/autoimmune disease). Identifying signs and symptoms of systemic disease aids in making the diagnosis and instituting appropriate intervention.

Physical Examination Findings

If PIBD is suspected, the clinical team must pursue a detailed examination (Box 14.1). The hallmark of PIBD

TABLE 14.1
Mechanisms for Immunologic Causes for Abnormal Brain/Neuron Function

Mechanism	Examples
Antibody modulates neuronal receptor[16]	Anti-NMDAR encephalitis Neuromyelitis optica
Cytokine modulates neuron[17]	Interleukin-1 disinhibits GABAergic interneurons Febrile infection–related epilepsy syndrome
Abnormally activated microglial cells[17,18]	Pediatric autoimmune neuropsychiatric disorders associated with streptococcal infections Pediatric acute-onset neuropsychiatric syndrome Obsessive-compulsive disorder Tourette syndrome Depression
Lymphocytes drive inflammation[19]	Multiple sclerosis
Immune system cells or antibodies drive inflammation of blood vessels and BBB[20]	CNS vasculitis Neuropsychiatric lupus
Complement deposition[21]	Neuropsychiatric lupus

BBB, blood-brain barrier; *CNS*, central nervous system; *NMDA*, N-methyl-D-aspartate receptor.

is the *involvement of multiple domains*, including neurologic, cognitive, and psychiatric findings.[47,120,122,127] Though some exam findings are more common in certain types of inflammatory disease (strokes in patients with vasculitis, for example), there is no

---

BOX 14.1
Physical Exam

General Exam:

Systemic: general state, level of alertness, fever (inflammation vs. autonomic instability)

Cardiopulmonary: autonomic instability with hyper- or hypotension, tachycardia, bradycardia (including heart block), heart murmur (i.e., rheumatic fever), rub (pericarditis of lupus)

Rash: erythema marginatum[a] (Sydenham chorea), erythema migrans (Lyme), scarlatiniform (streptococcal infection), livedo reticularis, malar, photosensitivity, petechial, urticarial, folliculitis (Behcet's)

Head, ears, eyes, nose, throat: nasal or oral ulcers, palatal petechiae, pharyngitis, tonsillitis, sinus tenderness

Neck: lymphadenopathy, thyromegaly

Musculoskeletal: arthritis (joint swelling, tenderness, pain on range of motion, loss of range of motion), tenderness at entheseal sites

Ophthalmologic Exam:

Evaluate for uveitis (Behcet's), retinal vasculitis (lupus, antiphospholipid antibody syndrome), optic nerve swelling (multiple sclerosis, neuromyelitis optica [NMO])

Neurologic Exam:

Motor: chorea, dyskinesia, dystonia, nystagmus/abnormal eye movements, ataxia, dysmetria, hypo- or hyperreflexia, hemiparesis, stiffness, tics

Speech: decreased production or loss of language, dysarthria, language regression ("baby talk")

Seizures: partial or generalized, often multifocal

Mental Status Exam:

Behavior: aggression/rages, inappropriate sexual behaviors, panic attacks, compulsive behaviors, irritability, psychomotor retardation, stereotypies, catatonia

Mood/affect: anxiety, fear/terror, depression, emotional lability

Thought process and content: confusion (loss of orientation), non-logical, paranoia, hallucinations, obsessions, compulsions

Insight/judgment: poor judgment, impulsivity

Cognition: memory impairment (especially short term), cognitive impairment (loss of academic skills, activities of daily living), inattentiveness, slowed response time

[a]This is best assessed when patient core temperature is elevated (while in hot bath or heated blankets).

---

single diagnostic exam finding.[99] The physical exam should include a general exam looking for infectious, metabolic, and systemic autoimmune etiologies in addition to autoimmune brain disease. As some of the findings in the General Exam (Box 14.1) may be present before the onset of the psychiatric symptoms (i.e., scarlatiniform rash and palatal petechiae could be seen during active strep infection before presentation of Sydenham chorea or PANDAS), review of records is warranted.

Laboratory Studies

Given the inability to distinguish various forms of autoimmune brain disease from other causes of encephalopathy by history or physical exam findings alone, the initial laboratory workup must be quite broad.[99,121,124] For children with suspected pediatric acute-onset neuropsychiatric syndrome (PANS)/PANDAS presenting with new-onset, mild-moderate psychiatric symptoms associated with infections, the work-up may be more limited and focused on infectious etiologies.[28] However, for patients who present with severe psychiatric symptoms (psychosis/delirium and/or other psychiatric symptoms strongly impacting psychosocial function), encephalopathy, seizures, focal neurologic deficits, and severe movement disorder (other than tics), a thorough evaluation, including lumbar puncture (LP), for autoimmune brain disease is indicated.

Cerebrospinal fluid (CSF) studies should include the standard cell count, protein and glucose, as well as opening pressure, oligoclonal bands and immunoglobulin G (IgG) synthesis index (indicating CNS production of immunoglobulins), and relevant anti-neuronal antibodies. Anti-neuronal antibody testing should be sent on both the serum and CSF, as some relevant antibodies have higher positive rates in the CSF and others in the serum. For example, up to 20% of patients with NMDAR encephalitis have only CSF antibodies, and the diagnosis would be missed if only serum studies were sent.[118] The presence of oligoclonal bands in the CSF may be the only abnormality seen in AE, providing valuable evidence of an autoimmune process. Although basic testing for infectious organisms, metabolic, hematologic, and oncologic diseases may be performed, the extent of testing will vary based on the clinical features and initial test results (Table 14.2).

While anti-neuronal antibody detection is important for the diagnosis of AE, the presence of an antibody alone does not make the diagnosis.[99,117,119] Rather, the diagnosis of AE depends on the combination of a physical exam findings and clinical history

TABLE 14.2
Laboratory Evaluation

Systemic laboratories which may reflect generalized inflammation or metabolic disease	Complete cell count and differential Comprehensive metabolic panel Erythrocyte sedimentation rate, C-reactive protein, ferritin
Autoimmune disease	Autoimmune encephalopathy antibody panel (NMDA, GAD 65 [glutamate decarboxylase], GABA, AMPA [α-amino-3-hydroxy-5-methyl-4-isoxazolepropionic acid receptor: a non-NMDA-type ionotropic transmembrane receptor for glutamate], VGKC [voltage-gated potassium channels]) on serum and CSF Antinuclear antibodies (ANA) Specific ANA (e.g. anti-double-stranded DNA, extractable nuclear antigen antibodies [Smith, Ro, La]) Antiphospholipid antibodies (lupus anticoagulant, anti-cardiolipin, anti-beta-2-glycoprotein 1) Urinalysis and protein/creatinine ratio Thyroid-stimulating hormone, free thyroxine, thyroid autoantibodies (anti–thyroid peroxidase, anti-thyroglobulin, anti-thyroid-stimulating hormone receptor) Celiac panel (TTG [tissue transglutaminase antibody], IgA) Complement (C3, C4) Angiotensin converting enzyme (depending on clinical scenario) von Willebrand factor antigen Quantitative immunoglobulin levels[a]
Infectious disease	Serologic testing for *Mycoplasma*, *Bartonella*, Epstein-Barr virus Nasopharyngeal swab for respiratory viruses and *Mycoplasma* PCR Group A *Streptococcus* culture, ASO (antistreptolysin O), and anti-DNAse B (anti-deoxyribonuclease B) CSF PCR for enterovirus, herpes simplex virus (HSV), and varicella zoster virus Consider consult with Infectious Disease for regional (i.e., Lyme disease), seasonal, and travel-related infectious disease evaluation
Metabolic/toxic	Serum lactate level Vitamin B12 level, vitamin D level Testing for recreational drugs (e.g. marijuana, cocaine) Consider urine organic acids, serum amino acids depending on clinical scenario
Oncology	For children with concern for possible oncologic etiology (based on MRI or suspicion for paraneoplastic disease), consult Hematology/Oncology: Cytology/cytometry (blood and CSF) Chest/abdomen/pelvis MRI (teratoma) Pelvic or testicular ultrasound (teratoma)

[a]Low immunoglobulins may indicate immunodeficiency. Immunodeficiency syndromes predispose autoimmune disease. If immunoglobulins are low, intravenous immunoglobulin (IVIG) will need to be given +/− other immunomodulation.
CSF, cerebrospinal fluid; *GABA*, γ-aminobutyric acid; *MRI*, magnetic resonance image; *NMDA*, N-methyl-D-aspartate; *PCR*, polymerase chain reaction.

consistent with AE, in addition to supporting laboratory, imaging, and electroencephalogram (EEG) findings that together give a diagnosis. Antibody testing should include not only anti-neuronal antibodies but also antibodies associated with systemic autoimmune conditions such as anti-nuclear antibodies, anti-phospholipid antibodies, extractable nuclear antigen antibodies (Ro, La, Smith), and thyroid antibodies (anti-microsomal and anti-thyroglobulin).

Infectious encephalopathies differ in their presenting histories and required initial evaluations. The spectrum of infectious organisms to consider is broad and the mechanism of disease varies; pathology may stem from a primary infection, a post-infectious process, or infections triggering the development of a subsequent autoimmune disease. The most common organisms associated with new-onset neuropsychiatric symptoms include Group A *Streptococcus* (Sydenham chorea PANDAS), *Mycoplasma* (basal ganglia encephalitis, possibly PANS), and influenza virus. A combination of culture or polymerase chain reaction (PCR) for early diagnosis, and serology for later diagnosis, has the highest diagnostic yield.[23] It is important to recognize that initial infectious encephalitis can induce a secondary autoimmune encephalitis. This is best described with herpes simplex virus (HSV) encephalitis triggering anti-NMDAR encephalitis.[120] In these situations, careful consideration of possible infectious agents and mechanisms is required for diagnosis and management.

Imaging

Children presenting with an encephalopathy should have a magnetic resonance image (MRI) with and without contrast to assess for inflammation, as well as diffusion weighted imaging to evaluate for ischemic changes. Finding a normal MRI greatly reduces the possibility of CNS vasculitis, but it does not exclude a diagnosis of AE.[126] Of note, 50% or more of AE cases have a normal brain MRI.[24] An MRI is essential for two reasons: (1) to support a possible autoimmune/inflammatory process and (2) to rule out important mimickers on the differential. The findings on MRI in autoimmune encephalitis vary greatly, from normal to hyperintensities on T2-weighted or fluid-attenuated inversion recovery sequences. Such changes may be focal, such as in the medial temporal lobes, or more diffuse. Some patients have enhancing lesions or abnormalities on diffusion weighted imaging.[113,114] Computerized tomography (CT) scans do not detect the changes seen in inflammatory brain disease. While the role of positron-emission tomography (PET) scans is not well established, they may be useful in cases of suspected inflammatory disease when other studies are normal.[122,125]

Electroencephalogram

EEG can provide further evidence of an encephalopathy with new onset multifocal epilepsy, temporal lobe epilepsy, or diffuse slowing.[114,119] Extreme delta brush, though not a common finding, is more specific for anti-NMDAR encephalitis.[127] A prolonged EEG should be performed, including overnight monitoring to capture awake and asleep periods. Abnormalities on EEG provide further evidence of encephalopathy and help to distinguish patients with inflammatory brain diseases from those with primary psychiatric disease.

Neuropsychiatric Testing

Neuropsychiatric testing provides an objective measure of cognition and memory, two domains impacted by inflammatory brain diseases. This testing quantifies the degree of deficits and can be followed over time to assess response to therapy.

Cognitive function declines in a portion of new-onset primary psychosis patients, but a profound drop in intelligence quotient (IQ) may suggest the presence of a diffuse encephalopathy.[116,123] Obtaining timely testing and the difficulty of the child participating in testing are challenging, but neurocognitive testing may provide key information for diagnosing an encephalopathy in patients with severe cognitive decline who lack classic imaging or CSF changes.

Diagnosis

Currently, pediatric-specific diagnostic criteria have not been developed for many forms of inflammatory brain disease. This is problematic because, in the absence of definitive markers, making the diagnosis of any specific inflammatory brain disease depends on meeting clinical criteria. While these diseases differ in children from adults in certain aspects, the recently developed diagnostic criteria for adult AE provide a useful framework, including those for anti-neuronal antibody–associated encephalitis (anti-NMDAR encephalitis, limbic encephalitis), as well as antibody-negative AE and Hashimoto's/Steroid Responsive Encephalopathy.[117] Many feel that thyroiditis is not required to meet criteria for pediatric Hashimoto's encephalopathy, as most affected children have normal thyroid function.[25] Pediatric and adult presentations for antibody-negative AE differ, as in children, new-onset seizures, especially refractory epilepsy, are important manifestations. Existing pediatric diagnostic criteria for primary CNS vasculitis, acute disseminated encephalomyelitis (ADEM), PANDAS, and PANS are included in Box 14.2, as these inflammatory brain diagnoses are frequently in the differential diagnosis of encephalopathy or new-onset neuropsychiatric symptoms (Box 14.2).

DIFFERENTIAL DIAGNOSIS

Infections and epilepsy themselves may each lead to the acute or subacute development of emotional, behavioral, and/or neurologic symptoms. For example, viral CNS infections such as HSV[30] and enteroviruses[31,32] may result in both acute and chronic neuropsychiatric symptoms. Parasitic infections may also present with neurologic and psychiatric sequelae, as is the case in neurocysticercosis resulting from brain invasion by the parasitic tapeworm *Taenia solium*[33,34] and primary amoebic meningoencephalitis caused by *Naegleria fowleri* infection.[35] Behavior changes may be secondary

BOX 14.2
Current Diagnostic Criteria for Pediatric Encephalopathies and New-Onset Neuropsychiatric Symptoms

DIAGNOSTIC CRITERIA FOR ANTI-NMDAR ENCEPHALITIS
Requires all three of the following criteria
1. Rapid onset (less than 3 months) of at least four of the six following major groups of symptoms:
   - Abnormal (psychiatric) behavior or cognitive dysfunction
   - Speech dysfunction (pressured speech, verbal reduction, mutism)
   - Seizures
   - Movement disorder, dyskinesias, or rigidity/abnormal postures
   - Decreased level of consciousness
   - Autonomic dysfunction or central hypoventilation
2. At least one of the following laboratory study results:
   - Abnormal EEG (focal or diffuse slow or disorganized activity, epileptic activity, or extreme delta brush)
   - CSF with pleocytosis or oligoclonal bands
3. Reasonable exclusion of other disorders
4. Definite NMDAR encephalitis diagnosis if one or more of the six major groups of symptoms and presence of IgG anti-GluN1 antibodies, after reasonable exclusion of other disorders
   Or
   The presence of three of the above groups of symptoms accompanied by a teratoma

DIAGNOSTIC CRITERIA FOR AUTOIMMUNE LIMBIC ENCEPHALITIS
Requires all four of the following criteria:
1. Subacute onset (rapid progression of less than 3 months) of working memory deficits, seizures, or psychiatric symptoms suggesting involvement of the limbic system
2. Bilateral brain abnormalities on T2-weighted fluid-attenuated inversion recovery MRI highly restricted to the medial temporal lobes[†]
3. At least one of the following:
   - CSF pleocytosis (white blood cell count of more than five cells per cubic millimeter)
   - EEG with epileptic or slow-wave activity involving the temporal lobes
4. Reasonable exclusion of alternative causes

DIAGNOSTIC CRITERIA FOR HASHIMOTO'S ENCEPHALOPATHY (MODIFIED*)[25]
Requires all six of the following criteria:
1. Encephalopathy with seizures, myoclonus, hallucinations, or stroke-like episodes
2. *Subclinical or mild overt thyroid disease* (most often normal in children)

3. Brain MRI normal or with non-specific abnormalities
4. Presence of serum thyroid (thyroid peroxidase, thyroglobulin) antibodies
5. Absence of well-characterized neuronal antibodies in serum and CSF
6. Reasonable exclusion of alternative causes

CRITERIA FOR AUTOANTIBODY-NEGATIVE BUT PROBABLE AUTOIMMUNE ENCEPHALITIS (MODIFIED#)[26]
Requires all four of the following criteria:
1. Rapid progression (less than 3 months) of working memory deficits (short-term memory loss), altered mental status, or psychiatric symptoms
2. Exclusion of well-defined syndromes of autoimmune encephalitis (e.g., typical limbic encephalitis, acute disseminated encephalomyelitis)
3. Absence of well-characterized autoantibodies in serum and CSF, and at least two of the following criteria:
   - MRI abnormalities suggestive of autoimmune encephalitis
   - CSF pleocytosis, CSF-specific oligoclonal bands, or elevated CSF IgG index
   - Brain biopsy showing inflammatory infiltrates and excluding other disorders (e.g., tumor)
   - *New-onset seizure or abnormal EEG**
4. Reasonable exclusion of alternative causes

DIAGNOSTIC CRITERIA FOR DEFINITE ACUTE DISSEMINATED ENCEPHALOMYELITIS (ADEM)
Requires all five of the following criteria:
1. A first multifocal, clinical CNS event of presumed inflammatory demyelinating cause
2. Encephalopathy that cannot be explained by fever
3. Abnormal brain MRI:
   - Diffuse, poorly demarcated, large (>1–2 cm) lesions predominantly involving the cerebral white matter
   - T1-hypointense lesions in the white matter in rare cases
   - Deep gray matter abnormalities (e.g., thalamus or basal ganglia) can be present
4. No new clinical or MRI findings after 3 months of symptom onset
5. Reasonable exclusion of alternative causes

DIAGNOSTIC CRITERIA FOR PEDIATRIC ACUTE-ONSET NEUROPSYCHIATRIC SYNDROME (PANDAS)[27]
Requires all six of the following criteria:
1. Prepubertal onset

BOX 14.2
Current Diagnostic Criteria for Pediatric Encephalopathies and New-Onset Neuropsychiatric Symptoms—cont'd

2. Obsessive-compulsive disorder (OCD) and/or a tic disorder
3. Dramatic sudden explosive onset of symptoms
4. Relapsing and remitting course of symptoms that are temporally associated with Group A beta-hemolytic streptococcal (GABHS) infection
5. Presence of other neuropsychiatric abnormalities (hyperactivity, emotional lability, anxiety, or piano-playing choreiform movements)
6. Reasonable exclusion of alternative causes

DIAGNOSTIC CRITERIA FOR PEDIATRIC ACUTE-ONSET NEUROPSYCHIATRIC SYNDROME (PANS)[28]
Requires all of the following criteria:
1. Abrupt, dramatic onset of obsessive-compulsive disorder or severely restricted food intake
2. Concurrent presence of additional neuropsychiatric symptoms, (with similarly severe and acute onset), from at least two of the following seven categories:
   - Anxiety
   - Emotional lability and/or depression

- Behavioral (developmental) regression
- Deterioration in school performance (related to attention deficit hyperactivity disorder–like symptoms, memory deficits, cognitive changes)
- Sensory or motor abnormalities
- Somatic signs and symptoms, including sleep disturbances, enuresis, or urinary frequency
3. Symptoms are not better explained by a known neurologic or medical disorder, such as Sydenham chorea

DIAGNOSTIC CRITERIA FOR PEDIATRIC PRIMARY ANGIITIS OF THE CNS[29]
Requires all of the following criteria:
1. Newly acquired and otherwise unexplained neurologic deficit
2. Classic angiographic and/or histologic features of vasculitis in the CNS
3. Absence of evidence of systemic vasculitis or any condition that could elicit the angiographic or pathologic features

---

†Not required for diagnosis of limbic encephalitis in pediatric population
'Not required for diagnosis of Hashimoto's encephalopathy in pediatric population
#Additional criteria for pediatric diagnosis of AE that is absent in adults
CNS, central nervous system; *CSF,* cerebrospinal fluid; *EEG,* electroencephalogram; *GABA,* γ-aminobutyric acid; *IgG,* immunoglobulin G; *MRI,* magnetic resonance image; *NMDAR,* N-methyl-d-aspartate receptor.

to seizures caused by infectious or noninfectious encephalopathies. Such is the case in electrical status epilepticus in sleep (ESES) syndrome, characterized by cognitive, motor, and behavioral changes in the presence of pathognomonic continuous spike-wave EEG seizure activity during slow-wave or Stage 3 sleep.[36] Therefore, when considering diagnosis in a patient with emotional, behavioral, and/or neurologic changes, the clinician should simultaneously rule out infectious, epilepsy and inflammatory conditions.

As described above, a complete physical examination and thorough history-taking exploring chronology of symptoms and possible exposure to infectious agents can provide important diagnostic clues to identifying an infectious cause or trigger. In particular, *N. fowleri* infection should remain in the differential diagnosis in a pediatric or adolescent patient who has recently gone swimming in warm freshwater areas where the amoeba is endemic. The presence of fever, systemic signs of infection, and lymphocytic pleocytosis in the CSF would support the diagnosis of viral encephalitis.

Medial temporal lobe abnormalities seen on brain MRI should point the clinician toward a diagnosis of HSV encephalitis, which can be confirmed by PCR testing of the CSF. Neurocognitive changes in a young child should raise concern for ESES.

OVERVIEW OF INFLAMMATORY BRAIN DISEASES

The sudden onset of emotional, behavioral, cognitive, and/or neurologic symptoms in a child or adolescent should prompt the clinician to consider the diagnosis of inflammatory brain disease (Table 14.3). Timely diagnosis and treatment of brain inflammation may substantially improve the course of the episode and markedly improve the patient's long-term mental health trajectory. Limiting treatment to usual psychiatric interventions is not only ineffective but also can delay diagnosis and lead to life-threatening symptoms of suicidality and neuroleptic malignant syndrome.

TABLE 14.3
Distinguishing Features of Inflammatory Brain Disease

Inflammatory Brain Disease	Clinical Findings	Common Psychiatric Symptoms
Autoimmune encephalitis	NMDAR encephalitis: Prodrome: nonspecific headache, fever, and flu-like symptoms lasting up to several few weeks Next stage: emergence of psychiatric symptoms and behavioral changes, which can include psychosis, intense anxiety, and sleep disturbance Last stage: sleep difficulties progressively worsen, autonomic instability including hypertension and tachycardia, dyskinesias, impaired consciousness, and seizures may develop	Psychosis, intense anxiety, sleep disturbance
Electrical status epilepticus in sleep syndrome	Pathognomonic "continuous spikes and waves during slow sleep"	Cognitive regression, aggressive behavior, disorganization, hyperactivity[36]
Infection-associated relapsing/remitting CNS disorder (Sydenham chorea, PANDAS, PANS)	Choreiform movements seen on standing and sitting Rhomberg (fingers, arms, legs), rapid eye movement (REM) motor disinhibition, +/– rash +/– arthritis +/– carditis	OCD, anxiety, emotional lability, sleep disturbance, behavior regression, cognitive regression, +/– psychosis +/– tics
Demyelinating inflammatory brain disease[37]	**ADEM** (all are required): • A first polyfocal, clinical CNS event with presumed inflammatory demyelinating cause • An encephalopathy that cannot be explained by fever • No new clinical or MRI findings 3 months or more after onset • Brain MRI is abnormal during the acute (3 months) phase with typically diffuse, poorly demarcated large lesions involving predominantly the cerebral white matter **Pediatric MS:** • Two or more clinically isolated syndromes (CIS) separated by more than 30 days involving more than one area of the CNS • One CIS associated with MRI findings consistent with criteria of dissemination in space (DIS) and in which a follow-up MRI shows at least one new lesion consistent with dissemination in time (DIT) criteria • One ADEM attack followed by one CIS 3 or more months after symptom onset that is associated with new MRI findings consistent with criteria for DIS • A CIS with MRI findings that are consistent with criteria for DIS and DIT (at least one T2 lesion in at least two of four areas: spinal cord, infratentorial, juxtacortical, and periventricular [DIS] associated with a simultaneous presence of asymptomatic gadolinium-enhancing and nonenhancing lesions [DIT] if the patient is ≥12 years old) (revision proposed)	ADEM: Aggression, agitation, auditory hallucinations, catatonic waxy flexibility, delusions, disorganized behavior, disorganized thinking, disorientation, inappropriate laughter, hostility, irritability, mania, mood lability, mutism, paranoia, and personality change[38,39] Psychiatric symptoms can occur as the initial presentation of ADEM before the occurrence of neurologic manifestations or may be associated with neurologic manifestations.[38,40] The psychiatric symptoms may persist after subsidence of the neurologic symptoms or there can be total recovery after treatment with steroids Pediatric MS: Fatigue Cognitive impairment: These involve attention, working memory, processing speech, and executive functioning[41–43] Mood dysfunction: Anxiety, depression, feelings of alienation, irritability, oppositional behavior, and social withdrawal and poor academic performance

TABLE 14.3 Distinguishing Features of Inflammatory Brain Disease—cont'd		
Inflammatory Brain Disease	**Clinical Findings**	**Common Psychiatric Symptoms**
Rheumatologic diseases associated with CNS inflammation	Characterized by multiorgan involvement (rashes, arthritis, nephritis, +/− carditis +/− hepatitis) and often includes constitutional symptoms and signs of systemic inflammation (high ESR, CRP, anemia, and other cytopenias)	Variable but often includes a component of depression and/or psychosis. OCD present at higher rate in patients with lupus[128]
Small-vessel CNS vasculitis	Headache, seizures, movement disorders, vision loss, memory loss, cognitive decline	Behavior changes, hallucinations, loss of higher executive function
Cytokine-associated encephalopathy	Fever followed by frequent seizure activity. Weeks later, the chronic phase emerges, with status epilepticus that is often not responsive antiepileptics. Neuropsychiatric symptoms appear during the chronic phase	Cognitive damage/decline, behavioral difficulties

ADEM, acute disseminated encephalomyelitis; *CNS*, central nervous system; *MRI*, magnetic resonance imaging; *MS*, multiple sclerosis; *PANS*, pediatric acute-onset neuropsychiatric syndrome.

Immune-Mediated Causes

Immune-mediated inflammatory brain diseases can be classified into distinct categories based on underlying etiology and presentation. These include autoimmune encephalitis, demyelinating inflammatory brain disease, rheumatologic diseases that have systemic and CNS inflammation, CNS vasculitis, cytokine-associated encephalopathies and infection-associated relapsing/remitting CNS disorder.

Autoimmune encephalitis

Autoimmune encephalitis describes a group of inflammatory brain diseases caused by autoantibodies erroneously targeting proteins in the brain. To meet the diagnostic criteria for autoimmune encephalitis, a patient must experience a change in psychiatric, mental status, or short-term memory within a 3-month period *and* have new-onset seizures, focal CNS changes, pleocytosis in the CSF, or MRI findings consistent with brain inflammation.[26] Subcategories within the broad category of autoimmune encephalitis describe further details about inflammatory involvement.

Limbic Encephalitis (*N*-Methyl-D-Aspartate Receptor and Others)

Limbic encephalitis, a subcategory of autoimmune encephalitis, affects the amygdala, hypothalamus, and other parts of the limbic system. It is well known to occur in the context of the malignancy ovarian teratoma in young adult women; in pediatric patients, limbic encephalitis can occur with or without an underlying malignancy.[44,45] Anti-NMDAR encephalitis, voltage-gated potassium channel (VGKC) antibody encephalitis, and anti–glutamic acid decarboxylase (GAD) encephalitis are the types of limbic encephalitis. Their names refer to the CNS proteins bound by the pathologic circulating autoantibodies involved.

Identified in 2007 as the first cell-surface antigen implicated in autoimmune encephalitis, NMDAR has been the most studied extracellular protein involved in autoimmune brain inflammation. Research of NMDAR and its encephalitis has greatly expanded the basic science and clinical understanding of the disease process.[46]

Childhood anti-NMDAR encephalitis is a multistage illness that progresses from psychosis, memory deficits, language disintegration, and seizures into a state of unresponsiveness with catatonic features often associated with abnormal movements, and autonomic and breathing instability. Anti-NMDAR encephalitis may be the most common cause of autoimmune encephalitis after acute demyelinating encephalitis. The disease predominantly affects children and young adults, especially females. It was originally discovered to be associated with ovarian teratomas but was later reported that in over 60% of patients the disease is not tumor-related Clinical data and experimental evidence have implicated that cross-reactive anti-NMDAR antibodies contribute to disease process, showing that these antibodies can cause a titer-dependent, reversible decrease of synaptic NMDARs by cross-linking and internalizing them. NMDAR autoantibodies are thought to be produced via molecular mimicry between the receptor and microbial/tumor antigens. Accordingly, most patients are treated with immunosuppressant drugs/therapies (e.g., corticosteroids, cyclophosphamide, anti-CD20, intravenous immunoglobulin [IVIG]). Recovery usually occurs in the inverse order of symptom development and is associated with a decline of antibody titers. Approximately 25% of patients suffer residual brain impairment and patients are known to relapse.

In older pediatric patients and adults, NMDAR encephalitis also evolves in stages. The initial prodrome stage consists of up to several few weeks of nonspecific headache, fever, and flu-like symptoms without psychiatric or behavioral symptoms. The prodrome is followed by the emergence of psychiatric symptoms and behavioral changes, which can include psychosis, intense anxiety, and sleep disturbance. In the last stage, sleep difficulties progressively worsen, and autonomic instability including hypertension and tachycardia, dyskinesias, impaired consciousness, and seizures may develop.

Younger pediatric patients with NMDAR encephalitis frequently display behavioral changes, dyskinesias, and seizures as initial symptoms, unlike older pediatric and adult patients.[24,46] The pediatric disease phenotype almost always involves new and possibly odd behavioral changes, including aggression and agitation.[47,48] Patients with NMDAR encephalitis rarely experience a single isolated neurologic or psychiatric symptom throughout the disease course. Rather, by the first month, three or more distinct categories of neurologic or psychiatric symptoms coexist in more than 90% of patients diagnosed with NMDAR encephalitis.[24,45] Compared with their adult counterparts, pediatric patients with NMDAR encephalitis are also more likely to present with neurologic instead of psychiatric symptoms.[24]

The distinguishing clinical features of psychiatric symptoms, seizures, and subacute short-term memory loss exist in other types of limbic encephalitis but present differently at different ages. VGKC antibody encephalitis involves antibody activity directly against proteins found in neurons, such as epitempin (leucine-rich glioma inactivated-1), that couple with the transmembrane-selective potassium pore: VGKC. In adult cases of VGKC antibody encephalitis, faciobrachial dystonic seizures precede psychiatric and cognitive changes.[48] However, in pediatric patients, CSF-positive VGKC antibodies correlate more generally with encephalitis without a specific phenotypic presentation.[49] GAD antibodies, specifically against GAD-65, may also be present in limbic encephalitis. A 15-year-old male with GAD-65 antibodies presented with fever, headaches, memory difficulties, and leg twitching.[50]

Basal Ganglia Encephalitis

In addition to Sydenham chorea, PANDAS, and PANS described above, other forms of basal ganglia, or striatal, encephalitides may affect pediatric patients. Children with these other types of basal ganglia encephalitis have neurologic manifestations (e.g., parkinsonism, dystonia, or chorea) and psychiatric features such as emotional lability, without significant seizures or aphasia. The causes may be postinfectious from agents such as *Mycoplasma pneumoniae* or idiopathic involving autoantibodies against the dopamine 2 receptor. Encephalitis lethargica in the 1920s has been postulated to follow influenza infection and may have been a postinfectious immune encephalitis.[50,51]

Steroid-Responsive Encephalitis Associated With Thyroiditis (Hashimoto's Encephalitis)

Compared with other types of autoimmune encephalitis, Hashimoto's thyroiditis, also known as encephalopathy associated with autoimmune thyroid disease and steroid-responsive encephalopathy associated with autoimmune thyroiditis (SREAT), is not well understood and the diagnosis is one of exclusion. The median age of diagnosis is 14 years and patients are typically females. Although thyroid antibodies (antithyroglobulin antibody, anti–thyroid peroxidase antibody, and anti-thyroid-stimulating hormone receptor antibody) may be high and decrease with treatment in these patients, thyroid antibodies may be normal. Even when thyroid antibodies are high, the majority of patients with SREAT have normal thyroid function. Presenting concerns may develop insidiously and include unexplained seizures, confusion or hallucinations, altered consciousness, abnormal movements, and behavioral changes such as aggression, bizarre behaviors, or labile mood. Neurologic examination is nonfocal. First-line immunomodulatory treatment with steroids is generally associated with good outcomes.[52]

Based on data gathered from the California Encephalitis Project, 62% of encephalopathies are seronegative.[53] In cases where suspicion of autoimmune encephalitis is high but an autoantibody has yet to be identified, the diagnosis is based on the following constellation of symptoms: (1) changes in psychiatric, mental status, or short-term memory within 3 months; (2) ruling out of other autoimmune encephalitis syndromes; and (3) no serum or CSF autoantibodies but presence of specific MRI, CSF, or brain biopsy findings.[26]

Demyelinating inflammatory brain disease

Because comorbidity of anxiety disorders, mood disorders, and cognitive impairment in pediatric patients with demyelinating brain disease is significant, the child psychiatrist will likely be involved in care of demyelinating inflammatory brain disease.[54–56] As a group, demyelinating inflammatory brain diseases involve damage to the myelin sheath of neurons in the brain and spinal cord, resulting in disruption of interneuron electrical conduction. Examples of these diseases include ADEM, multiple sclerosis (MS), and neuromyelitis optica (NMO), also known as Devic's disease. These diseases often present similarly; therefore, they require careful workup to distinguish between them.

Acute disseminated encephalomyelitis. Exposure to a vaccine or viral pathogen may antecede the acute or subacute encephalopathy and multifocal neurologic deficits seen in ADEM. ADEM, the most common centrally demyelinating condition seen in pediatrics,[57] is a diagnosis of exclusion. Presentation involves impairment in consciousness or marked irritability not accounted for by fever, recent seizure, or systemic illness along with polyfocal neurologic deficits.[58,59] The MRI in ADEM typically demonstrates reversible, ill-defined white matter lesions of the brain and often also the spinal cord, along with frequent involvement of thalami and basal ganglia. CSF analysis may reveal a mild pleocytosis and elevated protein but is generally negative for intrathecal oligoclonal IgG synthesis.

Multiple sclerosis. In MS, the location and development of white matter lesions and neurologic deficits are classically separated by space and time. Pediatric MS appears before 16 years of age, affects girls more than boys, has a relapsing-remitting course,[60,61] and is more likely to present as optic neuritis without other deficits than MS would in adults.[61] In pediatric presentations of NMO, generalized symptoms, including fever, seizures, emesis, and visual and motor symptoms, are the most common first signs of autoimmune disease.[62] Antibodies against aquaporin-4 (AQP-4), a water channel protein found predominantly in the brain, optic nerves, and spinal cord, are present in up to 68%–91% of patients with NMO and have a specificity as high as 98%.[63] In those individuals with NMO or symptoms along the NMO spectrum without AQP-4 antibodies, myelin oligodendrocyte glycoprotein (MOG) antibodies may be detected. MOG antibodies exist more commonly in younger patients, male patients, and in patients with both optic neuritis and transverse myelitis occurring closely in time. NMO patients positive for MOG antibodies have better clinical trajectories than those positive for AQP-4 antibodies.[63,64]

Central nervous system vasculitis and rheumatologic diseases associated with central nervous system inflammation

Neuropsychiatric symptoms may accompany generalized rheumatologic diseases such as pediatric systemic lupus erythematosus, antiphospholipid syndrome, Behcet's disease, and sarcoidosis. Suspicion of a rheumatologic disease requires a comprehensive physical examination and thorough laboratory workup by a pediatric rheumatologist.

Central Nervous System Vasculitis

CNS vasculitis presents variably, with headaches, behavioral changes, cognitive decline, and even stroke. Neurologic abnormalities are common if large blood vessels are involved but less common in small-vessel vasculitis. The size and location of CNS blood vessels involved are reflected in the nature of symptoms. CNS vasculitis may be primary, in which only blood vessels in the CNS are inflamed (primary angiitis of the central nervous system of childhood [cPACNS]), or secondary, in which blood vessels within and outside the CNS are affected. Childhood primary angiitis of the CNS is further categorized by vessel size and disease course. Categories include angiography-positive, large-medium-vessel progressive and nonprogressive cPACNS, and angiography-negative, small-vessel CNS vasculitis (SVcPACNS).[65–67]

Small-vessel disease can present with generalized neuropsychiatric symptoms that often mimic other inflammatory brain diseases. SVcPACNS may cause refractory headaches, behavioral changes, seizures, regression, cognitive decline, school difficulties, and hallucinations.[66] Angiography in SVcPACNS is by definition normal; a brain biopsy is the gold standard for diagnosis.[68]

MRI can often detect changes in both small- and large-medium-vessel vasculitis; MRI was abnormal in more than 95% of pediatric patients with primary vasculitis in one study cohort.[69]

The most common cause of secondary CNS vasculitis in children includes systemic lupus erythematosus (SLE), antiphospholipid antibody syndrome (APS), and Behcet's disease, but others (such as Hashimoto's encephalopathy) are also associated with CNS vasculitis.[70,71] Both primary and secondary CNS vasculitis require treatment with immunomodulating therapies and antithrombotics.

Systemic Lupus Erythematosus and Antiphospholipid Antibody Syndrome

The prevalence of neuropsychiatric symptoms is variable in pediatric SLE and generally higher (25%–35%) than that seen in adult SLE.[72,73] Psychotic symptoms, most commonly visual hallucinations, are seen in 22% and 36%.[72–74] Between 30% and 60% of pediatric SLE patients demonstrate cognitive and memory deficits.[72] Depression is and obsessive-compulsive disorder (OCD) are also quite frequent[72,128]. Unexplained constitutional symptoms such as fever, fatigue, and lymphadenopathy may be the first presenting signs in SLE patients. Pediatric SLE patients usually have more severe disease course than adult SLE patients and more often develop nephritis and CNS disease within the first few years of diagnosis.[72] Patients with SLE may also have APS, immunologic thrombocytopenia, autoimmune hemolytic anemia, skin lesions (including Raynaud's phenomenon), arthritis, pulmonary hypertension, and heart valve vegetations.

Antiphospholipid syndrome can be primary or secondary to an autoimmune disease, most frequently SLE. Depression and cognitive/memory deficits are common (REF). Antiphospholipid antibodies (aPLs) in the CNS most typically cause thrombotic disease, resulting in ischemic stroke or cerebral sinus vein thrombosis.[75,76] Nonthrombotic neurologic symptoms, thought to be due to an immunologic effect of aPLs beyond their typical thrombotic effect, are migraines (7%), chorea (4%), and epilepsy (3%).[77] The cause of psychiatric symptoms may be due to either thrombotic or nonthrombotic mechanisms.

Behcet's Disease

Behcet's disease is a vasculitis that can affect arteries and veins and is characterized by the development of recurrent oral and/or genital aphthous ulcers along with cutaneous, ocular, articular, gastrointestinal, and/or CNS inflammatory lesions.[78] Behcet's disease can be difficult to diagnose in children, as patients often do not meet full diagnostic criteria until adulthood. The most common associated CNS disorder in children is cerebral venous sinus thrombosis and it presents as headaches. When present, the typical behavioral symptoms described are euphoria, loss of insight, disinhibition, indifference to their disease, psychomotor

retardation and agitation, paranoid attitudes, and obsessive concerns.[77,79,80]

Sjogren's Syndrome and Sarcoidosis

Sjogren's syndrome can involve the peripheral nervous system and/or CNS. In one French cohort of 392 patients, the prevalence of CNS disease in pediatric Sjogren's patients was 18.9%.[81] Cognitive impairment, movement disorders, seizures, neuropathies, and chronic meningitis have been described.[82]

Children can have neurosarcoidosis and have been reported to present with seizures, hypothalamic dysfunction, and space-occupying lesions, while less commonly having cranial nerve palsies.[83]

Cytokine-associated encephalopathy

Febrile infection–related epilepsy syndrome (FIRES), a rare condition, is recognized as an epileptic encephalopathy that follows an episode of febrile illness. Its other names include devastating epilepsy of school-aged children and acute encephalitis with refractory, repetitive partial seizures. FIRES most commonly occurs in school-aged children. Inflammatory or infection-induced mechanisms are thought to cause seizures and cooccurring neuropsychiatric symptoms.[84,85] The course is often described as biphasic. In the acute phase of FIRES, frequent seizure activity usually appears days after fever, with fever more often than not remitting upon seizure onset. Weeks later, the chronic phase emerges, with status epilepticus that is often not responsive to concurrent administration of multiple antiepileptics. Neuropsychiatric symptoms appear during the chronic phase. The prognosis of FIRES is dismal, with up to 30% of children affected dying. Most patients who survive suffer from permanent cognitive damage.[84,85] As the disease progresses, cerebral atrophy and hippocampal sclerosis worsen.[86]

Infection-associated relapsing/remitting central nervous system disorder: neuropsychiatric symptoms that follow infections outside of the brain

Patients presenting with Sydenham chorea, PANDAS, and PANS may first seek help from mental health professionals; therefore, it is imperative that psychiatrists recognize these syndromes and coordinate the evaluation.

Amongst these, Sydenham chorea, an infection-associated relapsing/remitting CNS syndrome, has the most scientific evidence and understanding of this category of illnesses to date. Sydenham chorea is caused by an inflammatory reaction to Group A β-hemolytic *Streptococcus* (GABHS) and is recognized as one of the secondary diagnostic criteria for acute rheumatic fever (ARF). Chorea consists of involuntary writhing of the face, arms, and legs, and hypotonia. Most patients with Sydenham chorea demonstrate the psychiatric symptoms of OCD, mood dysregulation, emotional incongruence, and sometimes psychosis. Patients may or may not have other manifestations of ARF, including carditis, erythema marginatum, and migratory polyarthritis of large joints. In ARF, antibodies produced to combat GABHS infection cross-react with the heart, joint, and basal ganglia tissue and cause inflammation. Basal ganglia inflammation produces movement and emotional symptoms seen in Sydenham's chorea.

Obsessions and compulsions in patients with Sydenham chorea often precede chorea, with a severity as debilitating as the choreic motor dysfunction.[87] In the process of studying pediatric onset OCD, researchers noted that a subpopulation of early-onset OCD had symptoms that started abruptly. Further investigation found that these children demonstrated additional neurologic and psychiatric symptoms and that the onset had a temporal relationship to GABHS exposure or infection, such as Sydenham chorea. This observation led to the development of research/diagnostic criteria (Table 14.2) for pediatric autoimmune neuropsychiatric disorders associated with streptococcal infections (PANDAS).[88] In addition to sharing psychiatric symptoms, PANDAS and Sydenham chorea both demonstrate similar antineuronal antibodies[78,89–91] and have symptoms that respond well to immunomodulation.[75,76,78]

Because a causal relationship between GABHS infection and the abrupt onset of OCD cannot be established for individual patients and because other infections have been reported to precede abrupt-onset OCD, criteria for PANS were developed. PANS is agnostic for a particular presumed trigger (i.e., preceding infection). Despite the paucity of research in this area, preliminary retrospective studies suggest an association with concurrent and familial autoimmune/inflammatory disease[92,93] and response to immunomodulation.[94–96]

The onset of PANS is dramatic, with OCD or eating restriction and two other neuropsychiatric symptoms (such as separation anxiety, motor or vocal tics, and urinary changes) manifesting almost overnight[97] (Table 14.2). Individuals with PANS often experience relapses that correlate with inflammatory triggers and remissions or partial remission of neuropsychiatric symptoms associated with treatment of infection, inflammation, and time. Most patients meeting PANS criteria have at least several additional neuropsychiatric symptoms,[98] although only two additional neuropsychiatric symptoms are required by the criteria.

TREATMENT

Immunomodulation is necessary to treat PIBD. Delay in giving immunomodulation (in all inflammatory disorders) leads to more tissue injury. Intravenous corticosteroids are commonly used as first line because they work fast and can expedite remission. Steroids work on suppressing both the innate and adaptive immune systems; therefore, in diseases where the mechanism is not well understood, steroids are used as first line. Most inflammatory brain disease conditions (especially if the patient had long-standing disease or frequent relapses) will relapse once the steroids are discontinued; therefore, steroid-sparing agents are commonly used (IVIG, mycophenolate, rituximab, etc.). Steroid use often increases psychiatric symptoms initially and temporarily. In general, psychiatric symptoms in PIBD may worsen before they improve and warrant intense management by psychiatry.

Three principles of treating inflammatory brain disease[92,99,126]:
1. Patients *given immunotherapy* do better and relapse less than patients given no treatment.
2. Patients given *early treatment* do better than patients treated late.
3. *When patients fail* first-line therapy, second-line therapy improves outcomes and reduces relapses.

THREE PEDIATRIC ACUTE-ONSET NEUROPSYCHIATRIC SYNDROME CONSENSUS GUIDELINES: A POSSIBLE MODEL FOR PEDIATRIC INFLAMMATORY BRAIN DISEASES

In 2017, expert clinicians and researchers in PANS published a set of three clinical treatment guidelines focused on psychiatric and behavioral interventions,[100] immunomodulatory therapies,[92] and treatment and prevention of infections.[101] As is required in clinical practice treating PIBDs, treatment recommendations were generated from available research, extrapolation from evidence in similar conditions, and clinical experience, with input from many individuals with various areas of expertise.

ROLE OF PSYCHIATRIST IN MANAGING INFLAMMATORY BRAIN DISORDER

As many presenting symptoms of pediatric inflammatory brain disorders are psychiatric, child psychiatrists (and other mental healthcare providers) may be the first clinicians to encounter and evaluate affected children. It is critical for psychiatrists to maintain vigilance for and consider inflammatory brain disorders in their differential diagnoses when psychiatric symptoms emerge or change. Inflammatory brain disorder patients are often first seen in emergency departments, hospitalized on psychiatric units, and sometimes sent to residential treatment, which has sadly delayed diagnosis and treatment and frequently led to the introduction of ineffective and possibly exacerbating interventions.

Recognition

By paying attention to the type and timing of onset, course, and comorbidities of psychiatric illnesses, the child psychiatrist will be ready to recognize inflammatory brain diseases. Considering the comorbidity of psychiatric, neurologic, and physical symptoms is important. A child who develops headaches or seizures and exhibits emotional, cognitive, and behavioral changes must be evaluated for inflammatory brain disease. Fever, joint pains, ulcers, and weakness each also point to a possible inflammatory brain disease. Children with new emotional and behavioral symptoms along with movement abnormalities need evaluation that includes workup for inflammatory brain disorder.

Children presenting with a panoply of psychiatric symptoms emerging abruptly, especially with such symptoms as handwriting deterioration and frequent urination, should be considered for a PANS diagnosis.

When psychiatric symptoms emerge at an atypical age or have an atypical disease course, the odd timing can provide clues to etiology. For example, in PANS, symptoms fluctuate and age of onset differs from idiopathic conditions. Idiopathic anxiety disorders begin during predictable developmental stages and persist, whereas in PANS, separation anxiety can emerge suddenly for the first time at age 7–11 years. Mood disorders are rare before puberty, but in PANS they suddenly emerge before puberty. Early-onset OCD compared with PANS has a waxing and waning course versus an abrupt sawtooth pattern.

Worsening of psychiatric symptoms, despite conventional treatment, warrants suspicion of inflammatory brain disease. If symptoms remit and relapse, the same is true. Psychotic symptoms in any youth warrant a thorough medical evaluation, as do signs and symptoms of cognitive decline.

Psychiatric Evaluation

In cases of inflammatory brain disease, the child psychiatrist is responsible for monitoring psychiatric symptoms to assist the medical team to track response to therapies.

He/she must obtain records from the pediatrician, the school, and other health professional therapists to integrate records. Integrating the information, with attention to relationships between illnesses, stressors, and psychiatric symptoms, is key to making the correct diagnosis. The history may give clues to the trigger of emotional and behavioral changes. In addition to the standard psychiatric review of systems, the child psychiatrist needs to ask about all organ systems. Family histories may direct questioning for infectious, psychiatric, neurologic, and rheumatologic illnesses. Inquiry should be made about recent travel and illnesses in close contacts. Documenting the mental status exam (MSE) will provide anchor points from which progress of the disease or treatment may be measured. Although abnormalities in the MSE may vary, particular deficits may point toward particular illnesses, such as memory difficulties in VGKC antibody encephalitis. A neurologic examination during the visit might reveal abnormalities, such as focal deficits, which may be seen after *Mycoplasma* infection or sensory abnormalities in pediatric MS.

Consultation with other specialists will be necessary. Early laboratory evaluation will likely require blood and urine tests, LP, MRI, and EEG. Inpatient admission facilitates and hastens getting these accomplished. Medical treatment requires input from a variety of specialists, which might include neurology, rheumatology, dermatology, ophthalmology, sleep, and otolaryngology. The child psychiatrist, family, and primary care taker will need to work together to coordinate evaluation, treatment, and communication.

Once the diagnosis of an inflammatory brain disorder has been made, child psychiatrists need to address emotional and behavioral symptoms, so that the child may cooperate with diagnostic procedures and treatment of the underlying cause, as well as to alleviate suffering and hasten recovery of function. Early psychologic and behavioral treatments may serve as rehabilitation and improve outcome, as they do in other brain injuries.[102–106] The child psychiatrist's skills make him/her well-equipped to support and educate families about the illness and necessary actions.

Symptom presentations vary between the different inflammatory brain disorders, vary among patients with the same diagnoses, and change over time. Therapeutic teams will need to tailor and adjust interventions to meet each child's specific needs. For example, when children are unable to cooperate with phlebotomy, LPs, MRIs, and other invasive diagnostic and treatment procedures may require sedation, whereas calmer children may only need emotional and environmental support. Needs for and type of psychologic, behavioral, and psychopharmacologic interventions will require reassessment over the course of illness.

The diagnostic evaluation should identify symptoms that compromise safety, such as impulsivity, physical violence or aggression, refusal to eat or drink, and suicidality. We have difficulty finding inpatient facilities able to contain and address dangerous behaviors, *and* provide medical treatment while allowing parents' vigil. Unsettlingly, in the course of treatment, a child might be transferred between some combination of an emergency department, an intensive care unit, a psychiatric unit, a general pediatrics unit, an infusion unit, and home to accomplish containment, diagnosis, and treatment.

The emotional and behavioral symptoms of inflammatory brain disorders burden patients and their families. In patients themselves, symptoms have been found to disrupt activities of daily living, math, handwriting, extracurricular activities, free play, organized sports, community and family social participation, higher-level thinking, attention, memory, sequencing, emotional coping, and energy and drive.[107] Parents often require leave from work to find and coordinate medical care, interact with schools, and continue to care for siblings. Families describe themselves as traumatized by the illness and fear its recurrence. In the context of remarkable challenge and stress, families must attempt to continue to use effective parenting strategies, including setting necessary limits, reinforcing desirable behaviors, and ignoring or punishing unwanted behaviors (except dangerous ones) by removing privileges, all in the new world of a child's new (hopefully temporary) debilitation and the rest of the family's reactions. Parents involved in a pilot of a parenting skills group for parents of PANS patients found the support and skill training useful. Many parents find remarkable support from online resources, but, of course, they may find misinformation, too. The Autoimmune Encephalitis Alliance (https://aealliance.org/patient-support/resources/) and the PANDAS Network (http://www.pandasnetwork.org) are examples of community-supported organizations that provide information and can point families to useful resources.

During the acute phase of illness, the child may not be ready to participate in psychotherapies because of overwhelming agitation, anxiety, sensory discomfort, emotional lability, and/or cognitive impairments. It is, nonetheless, helpful when parents learn strategies to "hold the line" and prevent symptoms from further worsening through their inadvertent accommodation to the child's dysfunctional behaviors. They can apply skills acutely and be prepared to use them as necessary in the future. Using psychotherapeutic tools of differential reinforcement of desired behaviors, distraction, behavioral modification, activity planning, mindfulness techniques, cognitive behavioral therapy (CBT), and dialectical behavior therapy (DBT) skills will decrease distress and interference from symptoms in the short and long terms.[108] In our clinical experience, when parents applied DBT skills of distress tolerance, mindfulness, chain analysis, radical acceptance and addressing effectiveness of their interpersonal interactions, they found that their sense of burden and anxiety diminished.

Controlled trials of psychopharmacologic interventions for inflammatory brain disorders have not been completed. Conducting such studies would be complicated by the rarity of the illnesses and concurrence of many changing variables: changing psychopharmacologic medications, introducing medical treatments and fluctuating course of the illnesses. Clinical experience suggests that some psychiatric symptoms of inflammatory brain disorders can either be exacerbated by or respond to psychopharmacotherapy.

Inflammatory brain disorder patients appear to be very sensitive to adverse effects of psychotropic medications.[102] In anti-NMDAR antibody encephalitis, approximately half of patients treated with either typical or atypical neuroleptics demonstrated features of neuroleptic malignant syndrome,[109] potentially dangerous and possibly confusing the encephalitis and side effect symptoms.[110] Indeed, in another study, nearly half of patients with anti-NMDAR antibody encephalitis were transferred from a psychiatric unit to a medical/intensive care unit for treatment of antipsychotic intolerance and suspected neuroleptic malignant syndrome.[102] As is the case for antipsychotic medications, SSRI side effects can match targeted symptoms. SSRI use in children with PANDAS resulted in behavioral activation, including hyperactivity, mania, disinhibited behavior, worsening OCD behavior, aggression, irritability, agitation, and suicidality in 37%.[111] A case report of a patient with PANS described development of suicidal behaviors when treated with 5 mg/day of fluoxetine, cessation of the suicidal behaviors on fluoxetine discontinuation, and tolerance and improvement of OCD symptoms when fluoxetine was reintroduced at a dose of 2 mg/day.[111] As is the case for antipsychotic medications, SSRI side effects can match targeted symptoms. Careful attention to the course of symptoms and their relationships to medication dose and other interventions is critical. Clinicians are advised to "start low and go slow" in prescribing these medications—beginning with dosages one-fourth (or less) of typical and using an extended upward titer at a rate no faster than every 2 weeks. Benzodiazepines may be a good first treatment, as they may address anxiety, agitation, aggression, insomnia, and other symptoms, but they risk paradoxical disinhibition. Clonidine and guanfacine have also been used in treating agitated children with benefit, with the clonidine patch an alternative to oral medication.

After the acute phase of illness, children can continue to suffer from emotional, cognitive, and physical symptoms. Although some children's OCD, tics, anxiety, mood disorder symptoms, and attentional problems resolve, others do not. Some are left with ongoing emotional, processing, attentional, and fine motor difficulties. Some are left with ongoing pain and poor muscle tone.

Ongoing troubles require standard symptom-specific interventions, such as CBT, family therapy, DBT skills training, educational interventions, occupational therapy, and physical therapy.

Some children report that they have little memory of their time in flares, but others remember them and have reported feeling traumatized by their symptoms, disrupted family interaction, multiple doctor visits, and painful medical interventions. Several PANS/PANDAS children have described their desperate families unsuccessfully trying the practice of exorcism to help them. Children and adolescents can feel ashamed, angry, resentful, and confused about their medical condition and their futures. A study of youth with SLE reported that their identity formation, sense of independence, and self-confidence were adversely affected by having been ill.[112] Age-appropriate psychoeducation, social support, and deemphasis on identifying themselves as ill people were suggested.

Most children with inflammatory brain disorders require school accommodation for psychiatric, behavioral, cognitive difficulties and absence. Designing accommodations for illness conditions that require variable degrees of accommodation at different times challenges traditional classroom design and staffing. Writing the plans with the most difficult days in mind will assure that the child can receive adequate accommodations without revisiting the 504 or Individualized Education Program (IEP) process often.

Management of psychiatric symptoms should cleave as close to the evidence base as possible. Because empirically supported psychotherapies for inflammatory brain disorders are few, in general, management of psychiatric and behavioral symptoms of inflammatory brain disorder closely mirrors that of childhood mental illness of idiopathic etiology. Mainstays of treatment include psychoeducational, psychotherapeutic, behavioral, family, school-based, and generally postflare (and to a lesser degree), pharmacologic interventions. Psychiatric intervention reduces suffering and improves functioning until the immunologic and infectious processes are addressed. Fortunately, many patients with inflammatory brain disorders will recover completely and symptomatic treatments can be discontinued. Others are less fortunate and have ongoing symptoms that require continuous intervention and accommodation. The child psychiatrist can affect the course of the illness by suspecting the diagnoses, referring promptly to medical specialists, educating families, schools, and other healthcare professionals, aiding in coordinating care, and providing supportive and other evidence-based psychotherapies.

REFERENCES

1. Twilt M, Benseler SM. Childhood inflammatory brain diseases: pathogenesis, diagnosis and therapy. *Rheumatology.* 2014;53(8):1359–1368.
2. Florance NR, Davis RL, Lam C, et al. Anti-N-methyl-D-aspartate receptor (NMDAR) encephalitis in children and adolescents. *Ann Neurol.* 2009;66(1):11–18.
3. Titulaer MJ, McCracken L, Gabilondo I, et al. Treatment and prognostic factors for long-term outcome in patients with anti-NMDA receptor encephalitis: an observational cohort study. *Lancet Neurol.* 2013;12(2):157–165.
4. Wayne Streilein J. Transplantation immunobiology in relation to neural grafting: lessons learned from immunologic privilege in the eye. *Int J Dev Neurosci.* 1988;6(6):497–511.
5. Klein RS, Hunter CA. Protective and pathological immunity during central nervous system infections. *Immunity.* 2017;46(6):891–909.
6. Schwartz M, Baruch K. Breaking peripheral immune tolerance to CNS antigens in neurodegenerative diseases: boosting autoimmunity to fight-off chronic neuroinflammation. *J Autoimmun.* 2014;54:8–14.
7. Louveau A, Harris TH, Kipnis J. Revisiting the mechanisms of CNS immune privilege. *Trends Immunol.* 2015; 36(10):569–577.
8. Schwartz M, Raposo C. Protective autoimmunity: a unifying model for the immune network involved in CNS repair. *Neuroscientist.* 2014;20(4):343–358.
9. Louveau A, Plog BA, Antila S, Alitalo K, Nedergaard M, Kipnis J. Understanding the functions and relationships of the glymphatic system and meningeal lymphatics. *J Clin Invest.* 2017;127(9):3210–3219.

10. Jessen NA, Munk ASF, Lundgaard I, Nedergaard M. The glymphatic system: a beginner's guide. *Neurochem Res.* 2015;40(12):2583–2599.

11. Obermeier B, Verma A, Ransohoff RM. The blood-brain barrier. *Handb Clin Neurol.* 2016;133:39–59.

12. Ransohoff RM, Kivisäkk P, Kidd G. Three or more routes for leukocyte migration into the central nervous system. *Nat Rev Immunol.* 2003;3(7):569–581.

13. Bentivoglio M, Kristensson K. Tryps and trips: cell trafficking across the 100-year-old blood-brain barrier. *Trends Neurosci.* 2014;37(6):325–333.

14. Engelhardt B, Ransohoff RM. Capture, crawl, cross: the T cell code to breach the blood–brain barriers. *Trends Immunol.* 2012;33(12):579–589.

15. Takeshita Y, Ransohoff RM. Inflammatory cell trafficking across the blood-brain barrier: chemokine regulation and in vitro models. *Immunol Rev.* 2012;248(1):228–239.

16. Dalmau J. NMDA receptor encephalitis and other antibody-mediated disorders of the synapse: the 2016 Cotzias lecture. *Neurology.* 2016;87(23):2471–2482.

17. Frick L, Pittenger C. Microglial dysregulation in OCD, tourette syndrome, and PANDAS. *J Immunol Res.* 2016; 2016:8606057.

18. Najjar S, Pearlman DM, Alper K, Najjar A, Devinsky O. Neuroinflammation and psychiatric illness. *J Neuroinflammation.* 2013;10(1). https://doi.org/10.1186/1742-2094-10-43.

19. Steinman L. Immunology of relapse and remission in multiple sclerosis. *Annu Rev Immunol.* 2014;32(1):257–281.

20. Cellucci T, Benseler SM. Central nervous system vasculitis in children. *Curr Opin Rheumatol.* 2010;22(5):590–597.

21. Tsokos GC, Lo MS, Costa Reis P, Sullivan KE. New insights into the immunopathogenesis of systemic lupus erythematosus. *Nat Rev Rheumatol.* 2016;12(12):716–730.

22. Platt MP, Agalliu D, Cutforth T. Hello from the other side: how autoantibodies circumvent the blood-brain barrier in autoimmune encephalitis. *Front Immunol.* 2017;8:442.

23. Waites KB, Balish MF, Prescott Atkinson T. New insights into the pathogenesis and detection of *Mycoplasma pneumoniae* infections. *Future Microbiol.* 2008;3(6):635–648.

24. Armangue T, Petit-Pedrol M, Dalmau J. Autoimmune encephalitis in children. *J Child Neurol.* 2012;27(11):1460–1469.

25. Zhou JY, Xu B, Lopes J, Blamoun J, Li L. Hashimoto encephalopathy: literature review. *Acta Neurol Scand.* 2017;135(3):285–290.

26. Graus F, Titulaer MJ, Balu R, et al. A clinical approach to diagnosis of autoimmune encephalitis. *Lancet Neurol.* 2016;15(4):391–404.

27. Swedo SE, Leonard HL, Garvey M, et al. Pediatric autoimmune neuropsychiatric disorders associated with streptococcal infections. *Focus.* 2004;2(3):496–506.

28. Chang K, Frankovich J, Cooperstock M, et al. Clinical evaluation of youth with pediatric acute-onset neuropsychiatric syndrome (PANS): recommendations from the 2013 PANS Consensus Conference. *J Child Adolesc Psychopharmacol.* 2015;25(1):3–13.

29. Calabrese LH, Furlan AJ, Gragg LA, Ropos TJ. Primary angiitis of the central nervous system: diagnostic criteria and clinical approach. *Cleve Clin J Med.* 1992;59(3):293–306.

30. Więdłocha M, Marcinowicz P, Stańczykiewicz B. Psychiatric aspects of herpes simplex encephalitis, tick-borne encephalitis and herpes zoster encephalitis among immunocompetent patients. *Adv Clin Exp Med.* 2015;24(2):361–371.

31. Rhoades RE, Tabor-Godwin JM, Tsueng G, Feuer R. Enterovirus infections of the central nervous system. *Virology.* 2011;411(2):288–305.

32. Jain S, Patel B, Bhatt GC. Enteroviral encephalitis in children: clinical features, pathophysiology, and treatment advances. *Pathog Glob Health.* 2014;108(5):216–222.

33. Tejado Lde A, Pozo KT, Palomino CB, de Dios de Vega JL. Psychiatric manifestations of neurocysticercosis in paediatric patients. *BMJ Case Rep.* 2012:2012. https://doi.org/10.1136/bcr.03.2010.2840.

34. Carabin H, Ndimubanzi PC, Budke CM, et al. Clinical manifestations associated with neurocysticercosis: a systematic review. *PLoS Negl Trop Dis.* 2011;5(5):e1152.

35. Barnett ND, Kaplan AM, Hopkin RJ, Saubolle MA, Rudinsky MF. Primary amoebic meningoencephalitis with *Naegleria fowleri*: clinical review. *Pediatr Neurol.* 1996;15(3):230–234.

36. Yilmaz S, Serdaroglu G, Akcay A, Gokben S. Clinical characteristics and outcome of children with electrical status epilepticus during slow wave sleep. *J Pediatr Neurosci.* 2014;9(2):105–109.

37. Waldman A, Ness J, Pohl D, et al. Pediatric multiple sclerosis: clinical features and outcome. *Neurology.* 2016;87(9 suppl 2):S74–S81.

38. Matsuda M, Miki J, Tabata K-I, Ikeda S-I. Severe depression as an initial symptom in an elderly patient with acute disseminated encephalomyelitis. *Intern Med.* 2001;40(11):1149–1153.

39. Bachmann S, Schröder J. Catatonic syndrome related to acute disseminated encephalomyelitis (ADEM). *Schizophr Res.* 2006;87(1–3):336–337.

40. Patel SP, Friedman RS. Neuropsychiatric features of acute disseminated encephalomyelitis: a review. *J Neuropsychiatry Clin Neurosci.* 1997;9(4):534–540.

41. MacAllister WS, Christodoulou C, Milazzo M, Krupp LB. Longitudinal neuropsychological assessment in pediatric multiple sclerosis. *Dev Neuropsychol.* 2007;32(2):625–644.

42. Amato MP, Goretti B, Ghezzi A, et al. Cognitive and psychosocial features of childhood and juvenile MS. *Neurology.* 2008;70(20):1891–1897.

43. Wang CX, Greenberg BM. Pediatric multiple sclerosis. *Neurol Clin.* 2018;36(1):135–149.

44. Haberlandt E, Bast T, Ebner A, et al. Limbic encephalitis in children and adolescents. *Arch Dis Child.* 2010;96(2):186–191.

45. Armangue T, Titulaer MJ, Málaga I, et al. Pediatric anti-N-methyl-d-aspartate receptor encephalitis—clinical analysis and novel findings in a series of 20 patients. *J Pediatr.* 2013;162(4). 850–856.e2.

46. Dalmau J, Tüzün E, Wu H-Y, et al. Paraneoplastic anti-*N*-methyl-D-aspartate receptor encephalitis associated with ovarian teratoma. *Ann Neurol.* 2007;61(1):25–36.

47. Wright S, Hacohen Y, Jacobson L, et al. *N*-methyl-D-aspartate receptor antibody-mediated neurological disease: results of a UK-based surveillance study in children. *Arch Dis Child.* 2015;100(6):521–526.

48. Goldberg EM, Titulaer M, de Blank PM, Sievert A, Ryan N. Anti-*N*-methyl-D-aspartate receptor-mediated encephalitis in infants and toddlers: case report and review of the literature. *Pediatr Neurol.* 2014;50(2):181–184.

49. Wright S, Vincent A. Pediatric autoimmune epileptic encephalopathies. *J Child Neurol.* 2017;32(4):418–428.

50. Bigi S, Hladio M, Twilt M, Dalmau J, Benseler SM. The growing spectrum of antibody-associated inflammatory brain diseases in children. *Neurol Neuroimmunol Neuroinflamm.* 2015;2(3):e92.

51. Dale RC, Brilot F. Autoimmune basal ganglia disorders. *J Child Neurol.* 2012;27(11):1470–1481.

52. Lee J, Yu HJ, Lee J. Hashimoto encephalopathy in pediatric patients: homogeneity in clinical presentation and heterogeneity in antibody titers. *Brain Dev.* 2017. https://doi.org/10.1016/j.braindev.2017.07.008.

53. Glaser CA, Gilliam S, Schnurr D, et al. In search of encephalitis etiologies: diagnostic challenges in the California Encephalitis Project, 1998-2000. *Clin Infect Dis.* 2003;36(6):731–742.

54. Weisbrot D, Charvet L, Serafin D, et al. Psychiatric diagnoses and cognitive impairment in pediatric multiple sclerosis. *Mult Scler.* 2014;20(5):588–593.

55. Weisbrot DM, Ettinger AB, Gadow KD, et al. Psychiatric comorbidity in pediatric patients with demyelinating disorders. *J Child Neurol.* 2010;25(2):192–202.

56. Pakpoor J, Goldacre R, Schmierer K, Giovannoni G, Waubant E, Goldacre MJ. Psychiatric disorders in children with demyelinating diseases of the central nervous system. *Multiple Scler J.* 2017. https://doi.org/10.1177/1352458517719150.

57. Lee YJ. Acute disseminated encephalomyelitis in children: differential diagnosis from multiple sclerosis on the basis of clinical course. *Korean J Pediatr.* 2011;54(6):234–240.

58. Krupp LB, Tardieu M, Amato MP, et al. International Pediatric Multiple Sclerosis Study Group criteria for pediatric multiple sclerosis and immune-mediated central nervous system demyelinating disorders: revisions to the 2007 definitions. *Mult Scler.* 2013;19(10):1261–1267.

59. Pohl D, Alper G, Van Haren K, et al. Acute disseminated encephalomyelitis: updates on an inflammatory CNS syndrome. *Neurology.* 2016;87(9 suppl 2):S38–S45.

60. Duquette P, Murray TJ, Pleines J, et al. Multiple sclerosis in childhood: clinical profile in 125 patients. *J Pediatr.* 1987;111(3):359–363.

61. Renoux C, Vukusic S, Confavreux C. The natural history of multiple sclerosis with childhood onset. *Clin Neurol Neurosurg.* 2008;110(9):897–904.

62. Chitnis T, Ness J, Krupp L, et al. Clinical features of neuromyelitis optica in children: US Network of Pediatric MS Centers report. *Neurology.* 2016;86(3):245–252.

63. Jarius S, Paul F, Franciotta D, et al. Mechanisms of disease: aquaporin-4 antibodies in neuromyelitis optica. *Nat Clin Pract Neurol.* 2008. https://doi.org/10.1038/ncpneuro0764.

64. Kitley J, Waters P, Woodhall M, et al. Neuromyelitis optica spectrum disorders with aquaporin-4 and myelin-oligodendrocyte glycoprotein antibodies: a comparative study. *JAMA Neurol.* 2014;71(3):276–283.

65. Lanthier S, Lortie A, Michaud J, Laxer R, Jay V, deVeber G. Isolated angiitis of the CNS in children. *Neurology.* 2001;56(7):837–842.

66. Benseler SM, Silverman E, Aviv RI, et al. Primary central nervous system vasculitis in children. *Arthritis Rheum.* 2006;54(4):1291–1297.

67. Twilt M, Benseler SM. Central nervous system vasculitis in adults and children. In: *Handbook of Clinical Neurology.* 2016:283–300.

68. Benseler SM, deVeber G, Hawkins C, et al. Angiography-negative primary central nervous system vasculitis in children: a newly recognized inflammatory central nervous system disease. *Arthritis Rheum.* 2005;52(7):2159–2167.

69. Cellucci T, Tyrrell PN, Sheikh S, Benseler SM. Childhood primary angiitis of the central nervous system: identifying disease trajectories and early risk factors for persistently higher disease activity. *Arthritis Rheum.* 2012;64(5):1665–1672.

70. Elbers J, Benseler SM. Central nervous system vasculitis in children. *Curr Opin Rheumatol.* 2008;20(1):47–54.

71. Gowdie P, Twilt M, Benseler SM. Primary and secondary central nervous system vasculitis. *J Child Neurol.* 2012;27(11):1448–1459.

72. Mina R, Brunner HI. Pediatric lupus–are there differences in presentation, genetics, response to therapy, and damage accrual compared with adult lupus? *Rheum Dis Clin North Am.* 2010;36(1):53–80, vii–viii.

73. Benseler SM, Silverman ED. Review: neuropsychiatric involvement in pediatric systemic lupus erythematosus. *Lupus.* 2007;16(8):564–571.

74. Yu H-H, Lee J-H, Wang L-C, Yang Y-H, Chiang B-L. Neuropsychiatric manifestations in pediatric systemic lupus erythematosus: a 20-year study. *Lupus.* 2006;15(10):651–657.

75. Perlmutter SJ, Leitman SF, Garvey MA, et al. Therapeutic plasma exchange and intravenous immunoglobulin for obsessive-compulsive disorder and tic disorders in childhood. *Lancet.* 1999;354(9185):1153–1158.

76. Garvey MA, Snider LA, Leitman SF, Werden R, Swedo SE. Treatment of Sydenham's chorea with intravenous immunoglobulin, plasma exchange, or prednisone. *J Child Neurol.* 2005;20(5):424–429.

77. Avcin T, Cimaz R, Silverman ED, et al. Pediatric antiphospholipid syndrome: clinical and immunologic features of 121 patients in an international registry. *Pediatrics.* 2008;122(5):e1100–e1107.

78. Kirvan CA, Cox CJ, Swedo SE, Cunningham MW. Tubulin is a neuronal target of autoantibodies in Sydenham's chorea. *J Immunol.* 2007;178(11):7412–7421.

79. Siva A, Altintas A, Saip S. Behçet's syndrome and the nervous system. *Curr Opin Neurol.* 2004;17(3):347–357.

80. Patel P, Steinschneider M, Boneparth A, Lantos G. Neuro-Behçet disease presenting with acute psychosis in an adolescent. *J Child Neurol.* 2013;29(9):NP86–NP91.

81. Carvajal Alegria G, Alegria GC, Guellec D, et al. Epidemiology of neurological manifestations in Sjögren's syndrome: data from the French ASSESS Cohort. *RMD Open.* 2016;2(1):e000179.

82. Lvovich S, Goldsmith DP. Neurological complications of rheumatic disease. *Semin Pediatr Neurol.* 2017;24(1):54–59.

83. Baumann RJ, Robertson Jr WC. Neurosarcoid presents differently in children than in adults. *Pediatrics.* 2003;112(6 Pt 1):e480–e486.

84. Van Baalen A, Häusler M, Boor R, et al. Febrile infection-related epilepsy syndrome (FIRES): a nonencephalitic encephalopathy in childhood. *Epilepsia.* 2010;51(7):1323–1328.

85. Kramer U, Chi C-S, Lin K-L, et al. Febrile infection-related epilepsy syndrome (FIRES): pathogenesis, treatment, and outcome: a multicenter study on 77 children. *Epilepsia.* 2011;52(11):1956–1965.

86. Rivas-Coppola MS, Shah N, Choudhri AF, Morgan R, Wheless JW. Chronological evolution of magnetic resonance imaging findings in children with febrile infection-related epilepsy syndrome. *Pediatr Neurol.* 2016;55:22–29.

87. Swedo SE, Leonard HL, Schapiro MB, et al. Sydenham's chorea: physical and psychological symptoms of St Vitus dance. *Pediatrics.* 1993;91(4):706–713.

88. Swedo SE. Sydenham's chorea. A model for childhood autoimmune neuropsychiatric disorders. *JAMA.* 1994;272(22):1788–1791.

89. Kirvan CA, Swedo SE, Heuser JS, Cunningham MW. Mimicry and autoantibody-mediated neuronal cell signaling in Sydenham chorea. *Nat Med.* 2003;9(7):914–920.

90. Kirvan CA, Swedo SE, Kurahara D, Cunningham MW. Streptococcal mimicry and antibody-mediated cell signaling in the pathogenesis of Sydenham's chorea. *Autoimmunity.* 2006;39(1):21–29.

91. Kirvan CA, Swedo SE, Snider LA, Cunningham MW. Antibody-mediated neuronal cell signaling in behavior and movement disorders. *J Neuroimmunol.* 2006;179(1–2):173–179.

92. Frankovich J, Swedo S, Murphy T, et al. Clinical management of pediatric acute-onset neuropsychiatric syndrome: part II—use of immunomodulatory therapies. *J Child Adolesc Psychopharmacol.* 2017. https://doi.org/10.1089/cap.2016.0148.

93. Lougee L, Perlmutter SJ, Nicolson R, Garvey MA, Swedo SE. Psychiatric disorders in first-degree relatives of children with pediatric autoimmune neuropsychiatric disorders associated with streptococcal infections (PANDAS). *J Am Acad Child Adolesc Psychiatry.* 2000;39(9):1120–1126.

94. Spartz EJ, Freeman Jr GM, Brown K, Farhadian B, Thienemann M, Frankovich J. Course of neuropsychiatric symptoms after introduction and removal of nonsteroidal anti-inflammatory drugs: a pediatric observational study. *J Child Adolesc Psychopharmacol.* 2017;27(7):652–659.

95. Brown K, Farmer C, Farhadian B, Hernandez J, Thienemann M, Frankovich J. Pediatric acute-onset neuropsychiatric syndrome response to oral corticosteroid bursts: an observational study of patients in an academic community-based PANS clinic. *J Child Adolesc Psychopharmacol.* 2017. https://doi.org/10.1089/cap.2016.0139.

96. Brown KD, Farmer C, Freeman Jr GM, et al. Effect of early and prophylactic nonsteroidal anti-inflammatory drugs on flare duration in pediatric acute-onset neuropsychiatric syndrome: an observational study of patients followed by an academic community-based pediatric acute-onset neuropsychiatric syndrome clinic. *J Child Adolesc Psychopharmacol.* 2017;27(7):619–628.

97. Swedo E, Swedo SE. From research subgroup to clinical syndrome: modifying the PANDAS criteria to describe PANS (pediatric acute-onset neuropsychiatric syndrome). *Pediatr Ther.* 2012;02(02). https://doi.org/10.4172/2161-0665.1000113.

98. Swedo SE, Frankovich J, Murphy TK. Overview of treatment of pediatric acute-onset neuropsychiatric syndrome. *J Child Adolesc Psychopharmacol.* 2017;27(7):562–565.

99. Dale RC, Gorman MP, Lim M. Autoimmune encephalitis in children: clinical phenomenology, therapeutics, and emerging challenges. *Curr Opin Neurol.* 2017;30(3):334–344.

100. Thienemann M, Murphy T, Leckman J, et al. Clinical management of pediatric acute-onset neuropsychiatric syndrome: part I–Psychiatric and behavioral interventions. *J Child Adolesc Psychopharmacol.* 2017. https://doi.org/10.1089/cap.2016.0145.

101. Cooperstock MS, Swedo SE, Pasternack MS, Murphy TK, PANS PANDAS Consortium. Clinical management of pediatric acute-onset neuropsychiatric syndrome: Part III—treatment and prevention of infections. *J Child Adolesc Psychopharmacol.* 2017. https://doi.org/10.1089/cap.2016.0151.

102. Lejuste F, Thomas L, Picard G, et al. Neuroleptic intolerance in patients with anti-NMDAR encephalitis. *Neurol Neuroimmunol Neuroinflamm.* 2016;3(5):e280.

103. Turner-Stokes L, Pick A, Nair A, Disler PB, Wade DT. Multidisciplinary rehabilitation for acquired brain injury in adults of working age. *Cochrane Database Syst Rev.* 2015;20(3).

104. Liguz-Lecznar M, Kossut M. Influence of inflammation on poststroke plasticity. *Neural Plast.* 2013;2013:258582.

105. Prosperini L, Piattella MC, Giannì C, Pantano P. Functional and structural brain plasticity enhanced by motor and cognitive rehabilitation in multiple sclerosis. *Neural Plast.* 2015;2015:481574.

106. Ellis MJ, Leddy J, Willer B. Multi-Disciplinary management of athletes with post-concussion syndrome: an evolving pathophysiological approach. *Front Neurol.* 2016;7. https://doi.org/10.3389/fneur.2016.00136.

107. Tona JT, Bhattacharjya S, Calaprice D. Impact of PANS and PANDAS exacerbations on occupational performance: a mixed-methods study. *Am J Occup Ther*. 2017;71(3):7103220020P1–P7103220020P9.

108. Nadeau JM, Jordan C, Selles RR, et al. A pilot trial of cognitive-behavioral therapy augmentation of antibiotic treatment in youth with pediatric acute-onset neuropsychiatric syndrome-related obsessive-compulsive disorder. *J Child Adolesc Psychopharmacol*. 2015;25(4):337–343.

109. Oldham M. Autoimmune encephalopathy for psychiatrists: when to suspect autoimmunity and what to do next. *Psychosomatics*. 2017;58(3):228–244.

110. Gable M, Glaser C. Anti-*N*-methyl-ᴅ-aspartate receptor encephalitis appearing as a new-onset psychosis: disease course in children and adolescents within the California encephalitis project. *Pediatr Neurol*. 2017;72:25–30.

111. Murphy TK, Storch EA, Strawser MS. Selective serotonin reuptake inhibitor-induced behavioral activation in the PANDAS subtype. *Prim Psychiatry*. 2006;13(8):87–89.

112. Tunnicliffe DJ, Singh-Grewal D, Chaitow J, et al. Lupus means sacrifices: perspectives of adolescents and young adults with systemic lupus erythematosus. *Arthritis Care Res*. 2016;68(6):828–837.

113. Albert DV, Pluto CP, Weber A, et al. Utility of neurodiagnostic studies in the diagnosis of autoimmune encephalitis in children. *Pediatr Neurol*. February 2016;55:37–45.

114. Brenton JN, Goodkin HP. Antibody-mediated autoimmune encephalitis in childhood. *Pediatr Neurol*. July 2016;60:13–23.

115. Clare H, Jorina E, William H, et al. Treatment of small vessel primary CNS vasculitis in children: an open-label cohort study. *Lancet Neurol*. 2010;9:1078–1084.

116. Fitzgerald D, Lucas S, Redoblado MA, et al. Cognitive functioning in young people with first episode psychosis: relationship to diagnosis and clinical characteristics. *Aust N Z J Psychiatry*. 2004;38(7):501–510.

117. Graus F, Titulaer M, Balu R, et al. A clinical approach to diagnosis of autoimmune encephalitis. *Lancet Neurol*. 2016;15(4):391–404.

118. Gresa-Arribas N, Titulaer MJ, Torrents A, et al. Antibody titres at diagnosis and during follow-up of anti-NMDA receptor encephalitis: a retrospective study. *Lancet Neurol*. 2014;13:167–177.

119. Hacohen Y, Wright S, Waters P, et al. Paediatric autoimmune encephalopathies: clinical features, laboratory investigations and outcomes in patients with or without antibodies to known central nervous system autoantigens. *J Neurol Neurosurg Psychiatry*. 2013;84(7):748–755.

120. Hacohen Y, Deiva K, Pettingill P, et al. N-methyl-D-aspartate receptor antibodies in post-herpes simplex virus encephalitis neurological relapse. *Mov Disord*. 2014;29(1):90–96.

121. Lancaster E. The diagnosis and treatment of autoimmune encephalitis. *J Clin Neurol (Seoul, Korea)*. 2016;12(1):1–13.

122. Newey CR, Sarwal A, Hantus S. [(18)F]-Fluoro-deoxy-glucose positron emission tomography scan should be obtained early in cases of autoimmune encephalitis. *Autoimmune Dis*. 2016;2016:9450452.

123. Peleikis DE, Varga M, Sundet K, Lorentzen S, Agartz I, Andreassen OA. Schizophrenia patients with and without post-traumatic stress disorder (PTSD) have different mood symptom levels but same cognitive functioning. *Acta Psychiatr Scand*. 2013;127(6):455–463.

124. Pillai SC, Hacohen Y, Tantsis E, et al. Infectious and autoantibody-associated encephalitis: clinical features and long-term outcome. *Pediatrics*. 2015;135(4).

125. Probasco JC, Solnes L, Nalluri A, et al. Abnormal brain metabolism on FDG-PET/CT is a common early finding in autoimmune encephalitis. *Neurol Neuroimmunol Neuroinflamm*. 2017;4(4):e352.

126. Van Mater H. Pediatric inflammatory brain diseases: a diagnostic approach. *Curr Opin Rheumatol*. 2014;26(5):553–561.

127. Veciana M, Becerra JL, Fossas P, et al. EEG extreme delta brush: an ictal pattern in patients with anti-NMDA receptor encephalitis. *Epilepsy Behav*. August 2015;49:280–285.

128. Slattery MJ, Dubbert BK, Allen AJ, et al. Prevalence of obsessive-compulsive disorder in patients with systemic lupus erythematosus. *J Clin Psychiatry*. 2004;65(3):301–306.

FURTHER READING

1. Aviv RI, Benseler SM, DeVeber G, et al. Angiography of primary central nervous system angiitis of childhood: conventional angiography versus magnetic resonance angiography at presentation. *AJNR Am J Neuroradiol*. 2007;28(1):9–15.

CHAPTER 15

Disruptive Mood Dysregulation Disorder

DALE ZHOU, BS • STEFANIE SEQUEIRA, BS • DAVID DRIVER, MD • SHARI THOMAS, MD

INTRODUCTION

Irritability is a symptom, which is found in several pediatric psychiatric illnesses, from depression to bipolar disorder (BD) to oppositional defiant disorder (ODD). Until recently, it was not studied outside of these illnesses. However, the description of irritability in these illnesses does not capture the impairment that is caused by severe nonepisodic irritability. The increased incidence and prevalence of BD[1,2,10] seems to be in some part driven by the need to recognize and treat nonepisodic irritability as it is severely debilitating. One of the most troublesome implications of diagnosing more and more children with BD is the increased use of antipsychotic medications as mood stabilizers. Given the potency of these agents, their potential for deleterious side effects and the widespread use of the medications in young children,[11] there has been investigation into the prescribing trends in the United States.

Research aimed at elucidating the relationship between irritability and BD led to the definition of SMD, an illness defined for study protocols but not found in the *DSM*.[10] The diagnostic criteria capture those patients who have chronic nonepisodic irritability and emotional reactivity. Longitudinal follow-up studies showed that patients with SMD did not have an increased incidence of mania compared with counterparts with narrowly defined BD.[3] However, irritability does increase risk for anxiety, depression,[5–8] and suicidality.[12] The introduction of DMDD allows clinicians to target nonepisodic irritability and has spurred research to investigate novel interventions, which can alleviate symptoms and protect against long-term sequelae.

Disruptive mood dysregulation disorder (DMDD) is defined as severe nonepisodic (chronic) irritability and exaggerated emotional reactivity, which lasts for at least 12 months, with breaks no longer than 3 months, in children ages 6–18 years. Irritability is defined as intolerance of and excessive reactivity to negative emotional stimuli often resulting in anger, frustration, and aggression.[13] Although aggression may stem from irritability, it is important to distinguish between them. Irritability is a trait, and aggression is a behavior. Traits are defined as being both stable and heritable.[14] The heritability of irritability has been shown to be 0.3–0.4, and it is a trait that is stable over time.[14]

Even mild irritability can disrupt daily functioning.[15] Because of its shared presentation in BD, depression, and ODD,[16,17] identification of the features of irritability, such as time course and severity, is integral in differentiating DMDD from other disorders. The heterogeneity in the presentation of irritability demonstrates that there are different mechanisms in these illnesses which can cause the phenotype. This is supported by the fact that some treatments for these illnesses are diametrically opposed.

Irritability is also one of the primary targets of treatment, as it is often the most debilitating aspect of those illnesses. Armed with the data from longitudinal studies of SMD, the development of DMDD was shaped by the hypothesis that the illness is more etiologically similar to depression, anxiety, and attention deficit hyperactivity disorder (ADHD). Convincing evidence from longitudinal and family aggregation studies of children diagnosed with DMDD supports this conceptualization.[16,18a] Thus, DMDD is listed under depressive disorders in *Diagnostic and Statistical Manual of Mental Disorders*, 5th ed. (*DSM-5*), whereas symptoms of BD, such as manic and hypomanic episodes, are exclusionary criteria.

Because of the disorder's new nosologic status, recommendations for treatment interventions are emerging. The body of evidence does reveal that treatment algorithms for disorders, which share biologic pathways, are relevant in treating DMDD. Further there are novel approaches, developed because of the understanding of the neurobiologic correlates of irritability[4], which are promising and have led to an improvement in functioning and altered circuitry.

TABLE 15.1
Disruptive Mood Dysregulation Disorder Diagnostic Criteria

Symptoms	Type/Duration	Context
Exaggerated emotional reactivity: Excessive episodes of anger outbursts or aggression that are grossly disproportionate to the stimulus or provocation	On average, at least three times per week	Severe presentation observable in at least two settings (at home, school, or with peers) by multiple people (parents, teachers, peers, etc.)
Chronic irritability: Between episodes, mood is persistently and pervasively irritable, which may manifest affectively as anger or behaviorally as aggression	For most of the day, between episodes, and chronic (occurs every day)	Severe presentation observable in at least two settings (at home, school, or with peers) by multiple people (parents, teachers, peers, etc.)
Inappropriate for developmental stage: These episodes are inconsistent with normative developmental levels		Normative developmental levels refer to maturing cognitive and emotional regulatory systems

TABLE 15.2
Disruptive Mood Dysregulation Disorder Exclusionary Criteria

Exclusionary Criteria	Notes
Manic or hypomanic episode	Are symptoms better explained by bipolar disorder?
Observations of qualifying behaviors that exclusively occur during episodes of depression, that can be attributable to effects of substance use, or that can be better explained by other neurologic, medical, or psychiatric conditions	Are symptoms better explained by depression, substance use, or other conditions?
Coexistence of ODD or intermittent explosive disorder	If meeting criteria for both DMDD and ODD, the former should be diagnosed.

DMDD, disruptive mood dysregulation disorder; *ODD*, oppositional defiant disorder.

DEFINITION/SYMPTOM CRITERIA

According to the *DSM-5*[18b], the following diagnostic criteria (see Tables 15.1 and 15.2) must occur for at least 12 months with no more than 3 months symptom-free. Diagnosis must be made between ages 6 and 18 years to accommodate the typical developmental trajectory of irritability. The onset of symptoms must occur before 10 years of age.

PREVALENCE/EPIDEMIOLOGY

DMDD occurs in 0.8–3.3% of the population.[19] Affected children exhibit greater rates of service use, school suspension, social impairments, and poverty.[19] There were no significant sex differences in 3-month prevalence rates in community samples, except that the number of settings in which symptoms were observed was higher in boys than in girls. However, prevalence for children in clinics has been predominantly male.[5,16]

The frequency of tantrums and negative mood tends to decrease with age, aligning with developmental studies, suggesting that the peak of temper tantrums and irritability occurs during early childhood and then wanes in adolescence.[20,21] Of those who met criteria for severe, chronic irritability, half no longer did so after 1 year.[5] Although a community study of preschoolers aged 2–5 years had greater prevalence rates of DMDD symptoms than older children aged 9–17 years,[19] the *DSM-5* precludes diagnosis before age 6 years owing to concerns of pathologizing normal behavior. DMDD cooccurs with another disorder 62%–92% of the time, most often with depressive disorders and ODD.[19]

ETIOLOGY/PATHOPHYSIOLOGY

Research has shown that there are four major processes which undergird the symptoms of DMDD: (1) impaired regulation of emotion and attention[4,22,23] (2) misinterpretation of social, emotional, and threat

TABLE 15.3
Disorders that Share Symptoms With DMDD

	Bipolar Disorder	ODD	ADHD
Differences with DMDD	• Episodic, instead of chronic, irritability • Manic or hypomanic episodes, instead of consistent anger and irritability	• Outbursts occur less frequently (once instead of three/week) • Shorter duration (6 instead of 12 months)	• Although aggressive outbursts and irritability are common symptoms, they are not required for diagnosis and are episodic rather than consistent
Common behavioral rating scales	• Kiddie Schedule for Affective Disorders and Schizophrenia • Young Mania Rating Scale	• Interview for Antisocial Behavior • ODD Rating Scale • Connors Rating Scales (parent and teacher versions) • Buss-Perry Aggression Questionnaire • Parent Daily Report	• ADHD Rating Scale-IV • Child Behavior Checklist • Connors Rating Scales (parent and teacher versions) • Vanderbilt ADHD Diagnostic Parent and Teacher Scales

ADHD, attention deficit hyperactivity disorder; *DMDD*, disruptive mood dysregulation disorder; *ODD*, oppositional defiant disorder.

stimuli[4,24,25] (3) impaired context sensitivity[26,27] and (4) reward system dysfunction. The dysfunction in these domains mediates the inappropriate emotional and behavioral responses to frustration and blocked goal attainment.[16,17,28] In patients with DMDD, functional magnetic resonance imaging studies suggest disrupted engagement of subcortical brain regions associated with emotion and reward (such as the amygdala, caudate, and nucleus accumbens), frontal regions associated with executive function (such as the prefrontal cortex), and associational areas (such as the parietal cortex and anterior cingulate cortex).

Although both individuals with DMDD symptoms and BD exhibit abnormalities in social and emotional cue interpretation, individuals with DMDD symptoms demonstrate lower amygdala activity than patients with BD or ADHD during face emotion processing.[4] Amygdala hypoactivity during face emotion processing is also seen in patients with depression,[20] suggesting a common pathway that contributes to the increased risk for depression in patients with chronic irritability.[5,6] Those with DMDD have deficits in early attention processes, which parallel similar findings in ADHD.[29] The common pathways and phenotypes between DMDD and both depression and ADHD have led to the investigation of treatments for the latter two illnesses to be explored as interventions for DMDD. Although definitive neuroimaging biomarkers remain elusive, these studies provide models for future research on pathophysiology and treatment.

DIFFERENTIAL DIAGNOSES AND DIAGNOSTIC DILEMMAS

The *DSM-5* provides detailed decision trees for distinguishing between irritable mood and aggressive behaviors (see Table 15.3 for a comparison of disorders with similar or shared symptoms).[30] Differentiating between DMDD and BD rests on elucidating the chronicity of irritability. Episodic irritability points to BD. Furthermore, any present or past manic episodes rule out DMDD. Manic or hypomanic episodes suggest a form of BD. If irritability only occurs during periods of depressed mood, this suggests a depressive disorder. Discerning if ODD is the cause of irritability depends on the severity and pervasiveness of anger outbursts and irritability, with more extreme requirements for DMDD.[31] Furthermore, if anger outbursts and irritability occur in association with argumentativeness, defiance, and vindictiveness, it suggests ODD. If they occur in association with volatile interpersonal relationships, unstable self-image, and marked impulsivity, it suggests maladaptive coping skills/traits. Finally, if they occur in association with the disregard for the rights of others, it suggests conduct disorder.

WORKUP

Individuals must meet the DSM-5 diagnostic criteria, and screening may be conducted using instruments derived from the *DSM*. Irritability can be measured, and there are validated scales,[10] which are reasonable to use in clinical settings. The Affective Reactivity Index is a short questionnaire, which allows the youth, parent, and teacher to report on irritability. The K-SADS DMDD module is a tool, which was developed by Leibenluft and colleagues at the National Institute of Mental Health and was revised to be concise enough for clinical settings. The Multidimensional Assessment of Preschool Disruptive Behavior questionnaire facilitates the assessment of preschool-age children. Of note, to meet diagnostic criteria for DMDD, irritability must be present in two settings. It is imperative to ascertain if irritability is experienced by the child and observed by others. In a study comparing self- and parent-reported irritability, parents consistently rated higher irritability.[32] It is unclear if this is due to deficits in attention, which affect monitoring of emotions and/or limited ability to label and process emotions. A complete understanding of the severity and scope of the symptoms is essential in devising a treatment plan.

Because irritability cuts across several diagnostic categories, it is incumbent on the clinician to assess for the presence of a number of different psychiatric illnesses such as anxiety, depression, BD, ODD, and conduct disorder. To identify psychiatric disorders, which may be presenting as irritability and anger outbursts, the Schedule for Affective Disorders and Schizophrenia for School-Age Children, Child Behavior Checklist-Juvenile Bipolar Disorder profiler, Child and Adolescent Psychiatric Assessment, and the Preschool Age Psychiatric Assessment may be administered. A thorough history and physical examination must be obtained to rule out other medical conditions and medications contributing to symptoms. No biologic tests, including imaging or genetics workup, are currently helpful in diagnosis.

TREATMENT

As in most pediatric psychiatric illnesses, the combination of different interventions may yield the best outcome for patients with DMDD. Current pharmacologic treatment recommendations are based on existing treatments for similar symptoms of anger outbursts and irritability in ADHD, ODD, and depressive disorders. The use of medications alone is not recommended. Because irritability is a response to threat and frustrative nonreward,[10] these two stimuli have been used to elucidate the neurobiologic correlates of DMDD. These studies also engendered two treatments, which aim to alter the circuitry by shifting responses to the stimuli. Computer training aimed at hostile interpretation bias has shown efficacy in improving mood and altering responses in the amygdala and prefrontal cortex.[33] Similarly, treatment using exposures to elicit frustration has led to increased tolerance to aversive stimuli and more adaptive coping strategies.[12]

Potential pharmacologic treatment can include stimulants,[33,34] anticonvulsants,[2,35] antidepressants,[36-38] antipsychotics,[39,40] and mood stabilizers.[41] There are several clinical trials underway to evaluate the efficacy of medications to target irritability and DMDD, but currently there is little evidence available. Because DMDD shares biologic pathways with ADHD[42] and depression[9] and is often comorbid with these illnesses, it is prudent to first consider agents that will treat the comorbidities. As such, stimulants and selective serotonin reuptake inhibitors (SSRIs) are often used in the treatment of DMDD.

As expected, studies evaluating the use of stimulants in youth have been done in those with ADHD. Two symptoms often associated with ADHD are irritability and aggression. Consequently, metaanalyses have been done to understand the effect of stimulants on aggression and have shown large effect sizes.[34] The popular lore that stimulants can worse irritability has been disproven.[43,44]

Although there is a robust body of evidence, which verifies the benefits of using SSRIs to treat irritability in adults with depression,[45] a recent review of the literature[38] showed small effect sizes for SSRIs on irritability in children and adolescents. The presence of severe irritability may concern some clinicians about using an SSRI and inducing an iatrogenic mood switch, but two studies in 2009 demonstrated that irritability is not associated with SSRI-triggered mania.[46,47]

Risperidone and aripiprazole have FDA approval for the treatment of irritability in autism spectrum disorders. There is also evidence for olanzapine. Krieger et al. showed that risperidone is efficacious in the treatment of SMD in patients without autism.[48] The use of this class of agents must be done cautiously, given the significant side effects and resulting medical sequelae. Olanzapine and risperidone are the two second-generation antipsychotics with the most propensity for causing weight gain. The risk of extrapyramidal symptoms, particularly in neuroleptic-naïve patients, must be considered. Although aripiprazole is a partial agonist at the dopamine receptor, it also confers risk for metabolic syndrome.

Anecdotal evidence for the use of anticonvulsants to treat irritability and aggression can be found in the literature, but the only trial that demonstrated efficacy for valproic acid occurred when the agent was combined with stimulants to treat aggression in ADHD. A placebo-controlled trial for lithium did not demonstrate beneficial effects. Because of significant side effects of antidepressants,[49,50] stimulants, antipsychotics,[39,40] and mood stabilizers,[41] drugs should be considered in this order.

Conceptualizing irritability as a response to threat akin to anxiety has led to the study of cognitive behavioral therapy (CBT) and exposure and response prevention (ERP) therapy in the treatment of DMDD. CBT focuses on monitoring and relabeling distorted perceptions, and developing coping skills. There are CBT manuals, which target irritability and anger. Treatment with exposures to a frustrating situation can help teach an irritable child strategies to reduce reactivity and to employ coping skills. Ongoing research is investigating the efficacy of computer-based training for correcting impaired emotional recognition, which may contribute to anger and irritability.[51] Preliminary evidence shows that there are sustained improvements in mood and changes in key circuits that connect emotion and attention. Treatment must also address psychosocial stressors, such as conflict at home or bullying.

Treating youth effectively is predicated on understanding the context in which a child lives. As such, interventions that equip parents and teachers with tools are essential. Parent management training (PMT) teaches parents to use their responses to increase the frequency of desired behaviors and extinguish maladaptive behaviors.[52] Research shows that this intervention is particularly effective in disruptive behavior disorders. There are also limited data, which support a group intervention for parents.[53] In school, a behavior report card should reward positive behaviors. Teacher rating scales can aid in monitoring the patient's symptoms and responses to treatment.

RISK FACTORS

Specific risk factors in the development of DMDD are still being investigated, but studies looking at irritability have shown that genetics, developmental trajectory, environment, and family history all influence the emergence and severity of the trait. Several candidate genes have been identified to have effects on negative affect and irritability.[13] Children who have been diagnosed with ADHD and ODD at age 3 years and those with a difficult temperament are more likely to later be diagnosed with DMDD.[54] Parental hostility increases the

likelihood of severe irritability.[54] This mirrors data that established associations between parental depression, maternal warmth, paternal laxness, and the development of ODD.[19,55] Early family and caregiving factors may be especially important in assessing risk for DMDD in childhood.[56]

Given the genetic link between irritability and depression,[8] a family history of depression may confer increased risk for DMDD. However, a recent study found that the parents of children with DMDD did not differ from parents of children without DMDD in terms of current diagnosis or history of depression, BD, anxiety, or psychotic disorders.[57] Furthermore, in a study on DMDD in preschoolers, those with chronic irritability and frequent temper outbursts did not differ from those without DMDD in parental psychopathology or parental stress.[56] Thus, the question of how exactly family history plays a role in the development of DMDD remains unanswered.

One controversial issue that may make studying the antecedents of DMDD difficult is the age at which DMDD first presents. Currently, the age of onset criterion states that DMDD may not be diagnosed before age 6 years.[58] However, in a recent study examining symptoms of DMDD in preschoolers, 45.3% presented with frequent temper outbursts and chronic irritability.[56] These children also demonstrated more aggression, higher emotional reactivity, lower receptive language skills, and increased rates of ODD and ADHD.[56] Furthermore, in a separate sample of 2- to 5-year-old children, 3.3% were identified as meeting full criteria for DMDD, with high comorbidity of ODD, ADHD, and depressive disorders.[19] This latter prevalence rate aligns with those found in older children, suggesting that the lower age limit in the onset criterion for DMDD may not be justified.[56] However, assessing DMDD in preschoolers is challenging because it presents a need to distinguish emerging DMDD symptoms from developmentally appropriate emotional displays.[56] Nonetheless, these findings suggest that the earliest expressions of DMDD may occur in preschool-age children.[56] If these early expressions are valid, research on the genetic, neuroimaging, and behavioral markers of DMDD in this age group may help elucidate the nuances in the development of DMDD.

POTENTIAL OUTCOMES

In addition to potential risk factors of DMDD, potential outcomes associated with symptoms of DMDD in childhood are also currently being investigated. Controlling for all psychiatric disorders and demographic confounds, DMDD at age 6 years was predictive for a current DMDD diagnosis, current and lifetime depressive disorder, and current and lifetime ADHD diagnosis at age 9 years.[59] In addition, parent-reported symptoms of DMDD at age 3 years have been associated with enhanced reward processing in preadolescence,[60] adding to the understanding of the pathophysiology of DMDD and the predictive validity of DMDD even in preschool. There is little research done in the presentation of irritability in middle childhood, but cross-sectional data show that DMDD wanes after early childhood. In a study by Deveney et al., most children with DMDD do not meet criteria for the illness 4 years later.[61] If irritability persists into adolescence, it is predictive for severe psychiatric illness (i.e., major depressive disorder, generalized anxiety disorder, and dysthymia) 20 years later[22] and functional impairment in health, legal, financial, educational, and social spheres.[54] Chronic irritability in adolescence, however, did not predict the development of BD or Axis II disorders in adulthood.[22]

COMORBIDITIES

As is the case with most childhood psychiatric disorders, DMDD has been found to cooccur with several other disorders, especially behavioral disorders such as ODD, ADHD, and conduct disorder.[41,54,57,60,62] This may in some part be due to the overlap in symptoms between DMDD and these disorders. Findings on the comorbidity of DMDD and emotional disorders, such as depression and anxiety, are more mixed.[19,57,63] In the largest study of DMDD to date, combining data from three separate community samples, involving over 3000 participants ages 2–17 years, researchers found that DMDD cooccurred with all common psychiatric disorders (i.e., depression, anxiety, ODD, conduct disorder, ADHD) but cooccurred most strongly with depressive disorders and ODD.[19] The rates of comorbidity were very high, with the likelihood of DMDD cooccurring with at least one other psychiatric disorder ranging from 62% to 92%, depending on the sample. Furthermore, ODD specifically cooccurred with DMDD 57%–71% of the time.[19] A second study, which examined DMDD diagnoses retrospectively, reported that children ages 6–12 years who met criteria for DMDD had significantly higher rates of ODD, conduct disorder, and ADHD than children who did not meet criteria for DMDD. However, these groups did not differ in rates of anxiety disorders, depression, or BD.[57] Similarly, a study with 6- to 18-year-olds found that DMDD

significantly cooccurred with ODD, conduct disorder, and ADHD but did not significantly cooccur with any depressive disorder.[63]

Although the magnitudes of the associations differ depending on the study, DMDD has repeatedly been found to cooccur especially strongly with ODD, leading some to question whether DMDD is a disorder distinct from ODD[63,64] or would be better served as a specifier for ODD.[65] A recent study of DMDD symptoms in a population sample of children ages 6–12 years found that 92% of children with DMDD symptoms were diagnosed with ODD and 66% of children with ODD had symptoms of DMDD.[64] However, on the continuum of irritability, children with DMDD have more severe irritability than irritable children with ODD. Consequently, children with DMDD ultimately have more morbidity and utilize more services.[15] The overlap in both genetic associations and risk for suicidality between DMDD and depression underscores the mood component of DMDD.[66]

IMPLICATIONS FOR CLINICAL PRACTICE

DMDD appeared in the *DSM-5* largely because of concerns about over diagnosing BD in children and adolescents.[67] In the United States, incidence of BD in children increased as much as 40 fold between 1994 and 2003.[58] International data did not show a similar increase, and risk factors had not changed,[68] suggesting that the incidence rate of pediatric BD was not actually increasing but that diagnostic errors or changing diagnostic criteria best explained the increase in BD diagnoses.[65] Cooccurring with this increase in incidence rate was an increase in prescribing antipsychotic medications,[40] which led to concerns that children were not only being overdiagnosed but also being given potentially harmful and unnecessary medications.[67] Research into SMD established that severe chronic irritability was not in fact a form of pediatric BD and that chronic irritability must be understood as separate from the episodic mood changes that are characteristic of BD.[16]

It is critical to distinguish between chronic irritability and BD[16] because the treatment of these two constellations of symptoms is vastly different. Children with severe nonepisodic irritability are not at increased risk for BD,[16] and a randomized controlled trial (RCT) in children with SMD found no benefit of lithium over placebo.[40] Importantly chronic nonepisodic irritability in youth is associated with an increased risk for anxiety and unipolar depression in adulthood[16] and significant functional impairment.[7]

The investigation into the etiology and the course of chronic nonepisodic irritability has established the need for the diagnosis of DMDD. This change in nosology will likely lower the incidence and prevalence rates of BD in youth and will allow for more nuanced diagnosis and prognostication. Although there is a dearth of RCTs to define the most effective pharmacologic interventions for DMDD,[69] the understanding of the neurobiologic correlates of the disease process points to sensible medication options. PMT and CBT allow patients and their families to reinforce prosocial behaviors and identify and label maladaptive coping mechanisms. Novel therapeutic interventions such as graduated exposures to frustrative nonreward situations and computer-based training aimed at hostile interpretation bias are promising.

DMDD and chronic irritability predict greater clinical and functional impairment longitudinally making it imperative to target irritability in treatment. DMDD predicts depressive disorders at age 6 years and ADHD at age 9 years, after controlling for all psychiatric disorders at age 6 years.[59] Functionally, DMDD at age 6 years also predicts poorer interviewer-rated peer relations at school, greater peer victimization, and greater teacher-reported relational aggression and peer exclusion at age 9 years.[59] Chronic irritability in adolescence predicted major depressive disorder, generalized anxiety disorder, and dysthymia in adulthood (20 years later).[22] Chronic irritability is also negatively correlated with educational attainment and income in adulthood.[22] With the advent of validated scales for irritability, increased understanding of the biologic pathways, and the potential for significant morbidity, it is incumbent on clinicians to be well versed in recognizing DMDD and to design multimodal treatment plans for patients and their families.

REFERENCES

1. Blader JC, Carlson GA. Increased rates of bipolar disorder diagnoses among U.S. child, adolescent, and adult inpatients. *Biol Psychiatry*. 1996–2004;62:107–114.
2. Moreno C, Laje G, Blanco C, Jiang H, Schmidt AB, Olfson M. National trends in the outpatient diagnosis and treatment of bipolar disorder in youth. *Arch Gen Psychiatry*. 2007;64(9):1032–1039.
3. Stringaris A, Baroni A, Haimm C, et al. Pediatric bipolar disorder versus severe mood dysregulation: risk for manic episodes on follow-up. *J Am Acad Child Adolesc Psychiatry*. 2010;49:397–405.
4. Brotman MA, Rich BA, Guyer AE, et al. Amygdala activation during emotion processing of neutral faces in children with severe mood dysregulation versus ADHD or bipolar disorder. *Am J Psychiatry*. 2010;167(1):61–69.
5. Brotmanm MA, Schmajuk M, Rich BA, et al. Prevalence, clinical correlates, and longitudinal course of severe mood dysregulation disorder in children. *Biol Psychiatry*. 2006;60:991–997.
6. Stringaris A, Cohen P, Pine DS, Leibenluft E. Adult outcomes of youth irritability: a 20 year prospective community-based study. *Am J Psychiatry*. 2009;166:1048–1054.
7. Copeland WE, Shanahan L, Egger H, Angold A, Costello EJ. Adult diagnostic and functional outcomes of DSM-5 disruptive mood dysregulation disorder. *Am J Psychiatry*. 2014;171:668–674.
8. Stringaris A, Zavos H, Leibenluft E, Maughan B, Eley TC. Adolescent irritability: phenotypic associations and genetic links with depressed mood. *Am J Psychiatry*. 2012;169:47–54.
9. Savage J, Verhulst B, Copeland W, Althoff RR, Lchtenstein P, Roberson-Nay R. A genetically informed study of the longitudinal relation between irritability and anxious/depressed symptoms. *J Am Acad Child Adolesc Psychiatry*. 2014;54:377–384.
10. Stringaris A, Vidal-Ribas P, Brotman MA, Leibenluft E. Practitioner review: definition, recognition, and treatment challenges of irritability in young people. *J Child Psychol Psychiatry*. 2017.
11. Lohr WD, Chowning RT, Stevenson MD, Williams PG. Trends in atypical antipsychotics prescribed to children six years of age or less on Medicaid in Kentucky. *J Child Adolesc Psychopharmacol*. 2015;35:440–443.
12. Pickles A, Aglan A, Collishaw S, Messer J, Rutter M, Maughan B. Predictors of suicidality across the life span: the Isle of Wight study. *Psychol Med*. 2010;40:1453–1466.
13. Leibenluft E, Stoddard J. The developmental psychopathology of irritability. *Dev Psychopathol*. 2013;25(4 Pt 2):1473–1487.
14. Cocccaro EF, Bergerman CS, Kavoussi RJ, Seroczynski AD. Heritability of aggression and irritability: a twin study of the Buss-Durkee aggression scales in adult male subjects. *Biol Psychiatry*. 1997;41:273–284.
15. Copeland WE, Brotman MA, Costello EJ. Normative irritability in youth: developmental findings from the Great Smoky Mountains Study. *J Am Acad Child Adolesc Psychiatry*. 2015;54(8):635–642.
16. Leibenluft E. Severe mood dysregulation, irritability, and the diagnostic boundaries of bipolar disorder in youths. *Am J Psychiatry*. 2011;168(2):129–142.
17. Brotman MA, Kircanski K, Stringaris A, Pine DS, Leibenluft E. Irritability in youths: a translational model. *Am J Psychiatry*. 2017;174(6):520–532.
18a. Brotman MA, Kassem L, Reising MM, et al. Parental diagnoses in youth with narrow phenotype bipolar disorder or severe mood dysregulation. *Am J Psychiatry*. 2007;164(8):1238–1241.

18b. Association AP. *Diagnostic and Statistical Manual of Mental Disorders*. 5th ed. Arlington, VA: American Psychiatric Publishing; 2013.

19. Copeland WE, Angold A, Costello EJ, Egger H. Prevalence, comorbidity, and correlates of DSM-5 proposed disruptive mood dysregulation disorder. *Am J Psychiatry*. 2013;170(2):173–179.

20. Christopher JA. Handbook of disruptive behavior disorders. *Behav Interv*. 2002;17(1):54–56.

21. Egger HL, Angold A. Common emotional and behavioral disorders in preschool children: presentation, nosology, and epidemiology. *J Child Psychol Psychiatry*. 2006;47(3–4):313–337.

22. Rich BA, Schmajuk M, Perez-Edgar KE, Fox NA, Pine DS, Leibenluft E. Different psychophysiological and behavioral responses elicited by frustration in pediatric bipolar disorder and severe mood dysregulation. *Am J Psychiatry*. 2007;164(2):309–317.

23. Rich BA, Holroyd T, Carver FW, et al. A preliminary study of the neural mechanisms of frustration in pediatric bipolar disorder using magnetoencephalography. *Depress Anxiety*. 2010;27(3):276–286.

24. Rich BA, Grimley ME, Schmajuk M, Blair KS, Blair RJ, Leibenluft E. Face emotion labeling deficits in children with bipolar disorder and severe mood dysregulation. *Dev Psychopathol*. 2008;20(2):529–546.

25. Crick NR, Dodge KA. A review and reformulation of social information-processing mechanisms in childrens social-adjustment. *Psychol Bull*. 1994;115(1):74–101.

26. Blair RJ. Psychopathy, frustration, and reactive aggression: the role of ventromedial prefrontal cortex. *Br J Psychol*. 2010;101(Pt 3):383–399.

27. Dickstein DP, Nelson EE, McClure EB, et al. Cognitive flexibility in phenotypes of pediatric bipolar disorder. *J Am Acad Child Adolesc Psychiatry*. 2007;46(3):341–355.

28. Dickstein DP, Finger EC, Brotman MA, et al. Impaired probabilistic reversal learning in youths with mood and anxiety disorders. *Psychol Med*. 2010;40(7):1089–1100.

29. Jonkman LM, Kemner C, Verbaten MN, et al. Attentional capacity, a probe ERP study: differences between children with attention-deficit hyperactivity disorder and normal control children and effects of methylphenidate. *Psychophysiology*. 2000;37(3):334–346.

30. Boland RJ. DSM-5 (R) handbook of differential diagnosis. *J Psychiatr Pract*. 2015;21(2):171–173.

31. Roy AK, Lopes V, Klein RG. Disruptive mood dysregulation disorder: a new diagnostic approach to chronic irritability in youth. *Am J Psychiatry*. 2014;171(9):918–924.

32. Stoddard J, Stringaris A, Brotman MA, Montville D, Pine DS, Leibenluft E. Irritability in child and adolescent anxiety disorders. *Depress Anxiety*. 2014;31:566–573.

33. Waxmonsky J, Pelham WE, Gnagy E, et al. The efficacy and tolerability of methylphenidate and behavior modification in children with attention-deficit/hyperactivity disorder and severe mood dysregulation. *J Child Adolesc Psychopharmacol*. 2008;18(6):573–588.

34. Connor DF, Glatt SJ, Lopez ID, Jackson D, Melloni Jr RH. Psychopharmacology and aggression. I: a meta-analysis of stimulant effects on overt/covert aggression-related behaviors in ADHD. *J Am Acad Child Adolesc Psychiatry*. 2002;41(3):253–261.

35. Donovan SJ, Stewart JW, Nunes EV, et al. Divalproex treatment for youth with explosive temper and mood lability: a double-blind, placebo-controlled crossover design. *Am J Psychiatry*. 2000;157(5):818–820.

36. Halbreich U, O'Brien PM, Eriksson E, Backstrom T, Yonkers KA, Freeman EW. Are there differential symptom profiles that improve in response to different pharmacological treatments of premenstrual syndrome/premenstrual dysphoric disorder? *CNS Drugs*. 2006;20(7):523–547.

37. Landen M, Nissbrandt H, Allgulander C, Sorvik K, Ysander C, Eriksson E. Placebo-controlled trial comparing intermittent and continuous paroxetine in premenstrual dysphoric disorder. *Neuropsychopharmacol*. 2007;32(1):153–161.

38. Kim S, Boylan K. Effectiveness of antidepressant medications for symptoms of irritability and disruptive behaviors in children and adolescents. *J Child Adolesc Psychopharmacol*. 2016;26(8):694–704.

39. Scotto Rosato N, Correll CU, Pappadopulos E, et al. Treatment of maladaptive aggression in youth: CERT guidelines II. Treatments and ongoing management. *Pediatrics*. 2012;129(6):e1577–e1586.

40. Carlson GA, Potegal M, Margulies D, Basile J, Gutkovich Z. Liquid risperidone in the treatment of rages in psychiatrically hospitalized children with possible bipolar disorder. *Bipolar Disord*. 2010;12(2):205–212.

41. Dickstein DP, Towbin KE, Van Der Veen JW, et al. Randomized double-blind placebo-controlled trial of lithium in youths with severe mood dysregulation. *J Child Adolesc Psychopharmacol*. 2009;19(1):61–73.

42. Riglin L, Eyre O, Cooper M, et al. The genetic nature of early irritability: investigation associations with ADHD and depression risk alleles. *Transl Psychiatry*. 2017;7:e1241.

43. Ahmann PA, Waltonen SJ, Olson KA, Theye FW, Van Erem AJ, LaPlant RJ. Placebo-controlled evaluation of Ritalin side effects. *Pediatrics*. 1993;91:1101–1106.

44. Manos MJ, Brams M, Childress AC, Findling RL, Lopez FA, Jensen PS. Changes in emotions related to medications used to treat ADHD. Part I: literature Review. *J Atten Disord*. 2011;15:101–112.

45. Coccaro EF, Lee RJ, Kavoussi RJ. A double-blind, randomized, placebo-controlled trial of fluoxetine in patients with intermittent explosive disorder. *J Clin Psychiatry*. 2009;70:653–662.

46. Frye MA, Helleman G, McElroy SL, et al. Correlates of treatment-emergent mania associated with antidepressant treatment in bipolar depression. *Am J Psychiatry*. 2009;166:164–172.

47. Perlis RH, Fava M, Trivedi MH, et al. Irritability is associated with anxiety and greater severity, but not bipolar spectrum features, in major depressive disorder. *Acta Psychiatr Scand.* 2009;119:282–289.

48. Krieger FV, Pheula CF, Coelho R, et al. An open-label trial of risperidone in children and adolescents with severe mood dysregulation. *J Child Adolesc Psychopharmacol.* 2001;21:237–243.

49. Martin A, Young C, Leckman JF, Mukonoweshuro C, Rosenheck R, Leslie D. Age effects on antidepressant-induced manic conversion. *Arch Pediatr Adolesc Med.* 2004;158(8):773–780.

50. Safer DJ, Zito JM. Treatment-emergent adverse events from selective serotonin reuptake inhibitors by age group: children versus adolescents. *J Child Adolesc Psychopharmacol.* 2006;16(1–2):159–169.

51. Stoddard J, Sharif-Askary B, Harkins E, et al. An open-pilot study of training hostile interpretation bias to treat disruptive mood dysregulation disorder. *J Child Adolesc Psychopharmacol.* 2016;26:49–57.

52. Barkley RA. *Taking Charge of ADHD: The Complete Authoritative Guide for Parents.* New York: Guilford Press; 2013.

53. Waxmonsky JG, Waschbuusch DA, Belin P, et al. A randomized clinical trial of an integrative group therapy for children with severe mood dysregulation. *J Am Acad Child Adolesc Psychiatry.* 2016;55:196–207.

54. Dougherty LR, Smith VC, Bufferd SJ, et al. DSM-5 disruptive mood dysregulation disorder: correlates and predictors in young children. *Psychol Med.* 2014;44(11):2339–2350.

55. Harvey E, Metcalfe L. The interplay among preschool child and family factors and the development of ODD symptoms. *J Clin Child Adolesc Psychol.* 2012;41:458–470.

56. Martin SE, Hunt JI, Mernick LR, et al. Temper loss and persistent irritability in preschoolers: implications for diagnosing disruptive mood dysregulation disorder in early childhood. *Child Psychiatry Hum Dev.* 2017;48(3):498–508.

57. Axelson D, Findling RL, Fristad MA, et al. Examining the proposed disruptive mood dysregulation disorder diagnosis in children in the Longitudinal Assessment of Manic Symptoms Study. *J Clin Psychiatry.* 2012;73(10):1342–1350.

58. Washburn JJ, West AE, Heil JA. Treatment of Pediatric Bipolar Disorder: A Review. *Minerva Psichiatr.* 2011;52(1):21–35.

59. Dougherty LR, Smith VC, Bufferd SJ, Kessel EM, Carlson GA, Klein DN. Disruptive mood dysregulation disorder at age six and clinical and functional outcomes three years later. *Psychol Med.* 2016;46(5):1103–1114.

60. Kessel EM, Dougherty LR, Kujawa A, Hajcak G, Carlson GA, Klein DN. Longitudinal associations between preschool disruptive mood dysregulation disorder symptoms and neural reactivity to monetary reward during preadolescence. *J Child Adolesc Psychopharmacol.* 2016;26:131–137.

61. Deveney CM, Hommer RE, Stringaris A, et al. A prospective study of severe irritability in youths: 2-and 4-year follow-up. *Depress Anxiety.* 2015;32:364–372.

62. Sparks GM, Axelson DA, Yu H, et al. Disruptive mood dysregulation disorder and chronic irritability in youth at familial risk for bipolar disorder. *J Am Acad Child Adolesc Psychiatry.* 2014;53(4):408–416.

63. Freeman AJ, Youngstrom EA, Youngstrom JK, Findling RL. Disruptive mood dysregulation disorder in a community mental health clinic: prevalence, comorbidity and correlates. *J Child Adolesc Psychopharmacol.* 2016;26(2):123–130.

64. Mayes SD, Waxmonsky JD, Calhoun SL, Bixler EO. Disruptive mood dysregulation disorder symptoms and association with oppositional defiant and other disorders in a general population child sample. *J Child Adolesc Psychopharmacol.* 2016;26(2):101–106.

65. Lochman JE, Evans SC, Burke JD, et al. An empirically based alternative to DSM-5's disruptive mood dysregulation disorder for ICD-11. *World Psychiatry.* 2015;14:30–33.

66. Vidal-Ribas P, Brotman MA, Valdivieso I, Leibenluft E, Stringaris A. The status of irritability in psychiatry: a conceptual and quantitative review. *J Am Acad Child Adolesc Psychiatry.* 2016;55:556–570.

67. Krieger FV, Stringaris A. Bipolar disorder and disruptive mood dysregulation in children and adolescents: assessment, diagnosis and treatment. *Evid Based Ment Health.* 2013;16:93–94.

68. Parens E, Johnston J. Controversies concerning the diagnosis and treatment of bipolar disorder in children. *Child Adolesc Psychiatry Ment Health.* 2010;4:9. https://doi.org/10.1186/1753-2000-4-9.

69. Benarous X, Consoli A, Guilé JM, et al. Evidence-based treatments for youths with severely dysregulated mood: a qualitative systematic review of trials for SMD and DMDD. *Eur Child Adolesc Psychiatry.* 2017;26(1):5–23.

CHAPTER 16

Pediatric Bipolar Disorder

ADELAIDE S. ROBB, MD

INTRODUCTION

The recognition, diagnosis, and treatment of pediatric bipolar disorder have undergone a number of changes over the last 30 years in the field of child and adolescent psychiatry. In a review of the history of pediatric bipolar disorder, Glovinsky noted descriptions of mania and melancholy that go all the way back to ancient Greece.[1] However, it was the French in the 1670s who described melancholicus mania, which evolved into the folie circulaire in 1854 under the team at the La Salpetriere hospital. Kraepelin in Germany described manic depressive illness. The US definition of bipolar disorder did not become prominent until the 1950s, and the concept of bipolar disorder in children did not become widely recognized until decades later when child psychiatry separated from psychoanalysis and embraced the field of biologic psychiatry. While people did have clinical descriptions of bipolar disorder in isolated children in the literature, the first case series was a 1920s collection of 10 children out of 5000 consecutive admissions.[2] After Kanner's 1935 textbook, little was said in American psychiatry until much later in the century due to the psychoanalytic influence on the field.[3] Even today with excellent diagnostic criteria and treatment protocols for both medication and therapy, controversy surrounds the diagnosis of pediatric bipolar disorder. The field has ranged over the last 30 years from underdiagnosis in the 1990s to increasing awareness and then claims of overdiagnosis. Several authors have examined this controversy and claim that children with chronic irritability are misdiagnosed as bipolar when they actually have disruptive mood disorder with dysthymia (see Chapter 4). One review by James and colleagues compared the rates of diagnosis at discharge in England and the United States from 2000 to 2010 in pediatric patients aged 1–19 years.[4] The rates of pediatric bipolar disorder at discharge were 12.5-fold higher in the United States, whereas adult bipolar rates were 7.2-fold higher and other pediatric diagnoses at discharge were 3.9-fold higher in England. The authors postulated the difference was due to disparate diagnostic practices between the two countries.

DIAGNOSTIC AND STATISTICAL MANUAL OF MENTAL DISORDERS, FIFTH EDITION DEFINITION

In *Diagnostic and Statistical Manual of Mental Disorders, Fifth Edition* (*DSM-5*), to meet criteria for bipolar disorder one must have met criteria for at least one manic episode.[5] This includes an elevated, expansive, or irritable mood for most of the day nearly every day for at least a week or for any duration if hospitalized. While in the altered mood state, one must have at least three or four (if mood is primarily irritable) of the following symptoms: inflated self-esteem or grandiosity, decreased need for sleep (not insomnia), more talkative or pressured speech, flight of ideas or racing thoughts, distractibility, increase in goal-directed activity or psychomotor agitation, and excessive involvement in activities that have a high potential for painful consequences. The mood must cause impairment in social or occupational (school for kids) functioning or require hospitalization or have psychotic features. The episode cannot be due to the effects of a substance or another medical condition. One departure from DSM-IV-TR is that if mania merges with antidepressant treatment (medication or electroconvulsive therapy (ECT)) and persists at full syndromal level after the effects of treatment are gone, the individual is in a real manic episode and meets criteria for bipolar I disorder (BPI). Hypomania has the same criteria but requires only 4 days of symptoms without hospitalization, the mood and functioning changes are observable by others, and the functioning is not severely disturbed. If a person with suspected hypomania has psychotic features, they are by definition manic and not hypomanic.

Several symptoms of bipolar disorder can overlap with more common childhood disorders, such as attention deficit hyperactivity disorder (ADHD). To help clinicians distinguish pediatric bipolar disorder from the much more common childhood disorder, Dr Barbara Geller and colleagues conducted a large study comparing the frequency of different DSM-IV symptoms in both disorders.[6] They determined that five cardinal symptoms were much more common in youth with bipolar disorder than in those with ADHD or normal controls. These cardinal symptoms were elation, grandiosity, flight of ideas/racing thoughts, decreased need for sleep, and hypersexuality. They noted that irritability, hyperactivity, accelerated speech, and distractibility were common in both groups.

DIFFERENTIAL DIAGNOSIS

The differential diagnosis of bipolar disorder in children and adolescents is similar to that seen in adults. It is described in both *DSM-5* and Kaplan and Sadock's *Synopsis of Psychiatry*.[5,7] The differential includes multiple medical and psychiatric illnesses, including the effects of prescription medications (steroids, antiepileptic drugs, antidepressants, stimulants); illicit drugs (ketamine, phencyclidine, amphetamines, lysergic acid diethylamide); medical illnesses (lupus, brain tumor, hyperthyroidism); and psychiatric differential, including psychotic disorders, oppositional defiant disorder, conduct disorder, anxiety disorders, ADHD, mood disorders due to a medical condition, and substance-induced mood disorder.

EPIDEMIOLOGY AND GENETICS

The prevalence of BPI in the general population is approximately 1% and when one expands to the bipolar spectrum (bipolar II [BPII] and cyclothymia) the rate increases to 4%–6% of the population.[8] The majority of adult patients remember a pediatric onset, including prepubertal episodes.[9] In examining adults with bipolar disorder using retrospective interviews, approximately 30% had a very early onset and 40% had an adolescent onset.[9] A metaanalysis of pediatric bipolar disorder yielded a rate of 1.8% of the US population.[10]

Bipolar disorder runs in families and having a parent or sibling with the disease increases the risk. The risks of bipolar disorder range from 15%–30% with one affected parent to 50%–75% when both parents have the disorder.[11] For siblings and dizygotic twins the rate is similar, from 15% to 25%, whereas the concordance rates in monozygotic twins range from 60% to 80%.

One large genetic investigation examined participants from the Treatment of Early Age Mania (TEAM) study and adult samples of those with early-onset bipolar disorder versus normal controls in a genetic risk score analysis.[12,13] They examined 8 candidate SNPs in the 69 TEAM subjects, 732 adult patients with early-onset BPI, and 776 controls and found that the CACNA1C (calcium channel, voltage-dependent, L type, α 1C subunit)

haplotype was associated with early-onset bipolar disorder. The same group examined brain-derived neurotrophic factor and found an association with the rs6265 minor allele in the TEAM and early-onset bipolar groups.

COMMON COMORBIDITY

A variety of illnesses can cooccur with bipolar disorder in adults and children. Some of the more common comorbid psychiatric disorders include ADHD, anxiety disorders, substance use disorders (SUD), and alcohol dependence. A recent review of 167 studies between 1990 and 2014 noted that pediatric bipolar disorder had common comorbidities, including anxiety disorders (54%), followed by ADHD (48%), disruptive behavior disorders (oppositional defiant disorder or conduct disorder) (31%), and SUD (31%).[14] The team also noted that having comorbid anxiety disorder or ADHD had a negative impact on symptoms and clinical course, neurocognitive profile, and overall functioning. The youth with both bipolar disorder and ADHD did respond in controlled trials to both stimulants and atomoxetine over placebo.

Substance Use Disorders

Several studies have examined rates of substance use in pediatric bipolar disorder. The Longitudinal Assessment of Manic Symptoms study examined children 6–12.9 years of age for a score higher than 10 on the General Behavior Inventory manic scale.[15] In those youth over the age of 9 years at entry, 34.9% used alcohol with 11.9% being regular users. In the same study, rates of substance use were 30.1% with 16.2% being regular users. The predictors for regular alcohol use over the first 24 months of follow-up were parental marital status, age, and sustained mania symptoms. Predictors of regular drug use were parental marital status, stressful life events, and baseline disruptive behavior disorder diagnosis. Medications at baseline decreased the risk of regular drug use. They further suggested that children in single parent or remarried households and those with disruptive behavioral disorders at baseline be targeted as high risk for the prevention of SUD and alcohol use disorder. In a separate study, Wilens and colleagues examined the prospective risk of developing substance use and smoking disorders in youth with bipolar disorder and conduct disorder.[16] At the 5-year follow-up, youth with bipolar disorder had higher rates of SUD 49% versus 26% in normal controls and cigarette use 49% versus 17%. The youth with comorbid conduct disorder had higher rates of SUD and nicotine dependence than those with bipolar alone or controls.

Anxiety Disorders

In a long-term study of bipolar disorder, the Course and Outcome of Bipolar Youth (COBY) study examined 413 youth aged 7–17 years with BPI (244), BPII (28), or BP-Not Otherwise Specified (BP-NOS) (141) and followed them longitudinally. After 5 years, they received a longitudinal follow-up interview.[17] At both intake and follow-up, the rates of comorbid anxiety disorders were high with 62% having at least one anxiety disorder and 50% having two or more anxiety disorders. Those with anxiety had more time in depressive episodes and longer median times to recovery. The youth with two or more anxiety disorders spent less time without mood symptoms and more time cycling. The most common anxiety disorders seen were separation anxiety disorder (46%) and generalized anxiety disorder (43%). Other anxiety disorders in decreasing prevalence were social anxiety disorder (28%); obsessive-compulsive disorder (OCD) (23%); panic disorder (19%); posttraumatic stress disorder (19%); anxiety NOS (17%), and agoraphobia (7%). The rates of comorbid anxiety disorder in another large pediatric bipolar disorder trial, the TEAM study, showed similar comorbidity frequencies among the 279, 6- to 16-year-old, study participants.[18] The overall anxiety prevalence was 71%, with specific phobia 56.6%; social phobia 25.4%; separation anxiety 24.7%; generalized anxiety 14.0%; panic attack 12.9%; OCD 11.1%; and panic disorder without agoraphobia 5.4%. In a study of OCD and bipolar disorder, Tonna and colleagues discussed findings from their metaanalysis.[19] In their pooled analysis of 345 youth with bipolar disorder, the rate of OCD was 23.2%, which is above the adult comorbid OCD rate of 12.6%. The presentation of the two disorders most frequently begins with OCD (60%), but they can begin simultaneously (25%) or with bipolar (15%). For many of those individuals, the treatment included mood stabilizers; over 40% needed more than one mood stabilizer and one-tenth needed an antipsychotic medication. Some of these individuals only had OCD symptoms during depressive episodes of the bipolar illness with OCD remission during euthymia and mania.

Attention Deficit Hyperactivity Disorder and Disruptive Behavior Disorders

The TEAM study reported high rates of disruptive behavioral disorders with a total rate of Disruptive Behavior Disorder (DBD) at 98.6% of all the participants.[18] More specifically, 92.8% had ADHD, 90.0%

had oppositional defiant disorder, and 15.8% had conduct disorder. Thirty-two percent of the participants used a stable dose of stimulants throughout the 8-week trial, and outcomes were not different for those on and off stimulant medication.

Learning Disabilities

In a recent review of cognitive impairment in euthymic youth with bipolar disorder, Elias and colleagues examined specific learning difficulties in this population.[20] The study analyzed 24 other studies of youth with bipolar disorder in a euthymic mood state and normal controls. The learning issues with moderate to large effect sizes (0.76–0.99) comprised verbal learning, verbal memory, working memory, visual learning, and visual memory. They did not find problems in attention/vigilance reasoning, problem solving, or processing speed. They noted some youth had comorbid anxiety and ADHD, which were treated with medications and ADHD or anxiety disorder and their treatments could also impact cognitive performance. Many clinicians know that youth who are experiencing a manic or depressive episode can struggle with academic functioning. What this study shows is that youth with bipolar disorder will continue to need academic support even when their mood is stabilized and problematic mood symptoms are not present. Knowing these findings can help clinicians and families advocate for psychoeducational testing and appropriate academic placement and supports (Individual Education Plan (IEP) or 504 plans) to help support academic progress and avoid destabilization because of school difficulties. The authors suggested that these cognitive deficits could be targets of pharmacologic and psychotherapeutic treatments.

A second article by Dickstein and colleagues examined the cognitive functioning among youth with BPI, BPII, or BP-NOS plus TDC (typically developing controls) in the National Institute of Mental Health (NIMH) COBY study.[21] In the trial, 175 youth completed the Cambridge Neuropsychological Test Automated Battery (CANTAB). Their findings revealed that BPI/II youth took more trials to complete a shifting task, and all BP youth (I, II, and NOS) had impairments in sustained attention and information processing for emotionally valenced words.

Suicide

Up to half of those with bipolar disorder have a lifetime suicide attempt. In a review of suicide rates in pediatric studies, Hauser noted the rates of current and lifetime suicidal ideation were 50% and 57%, respectively.[22] The suicide attempt rates ranged from 21% to 25%, and up to 8% of youth with bipolar disorder had multiple attempts. Hauser also noted in the adult literature that up to 20% of patients with bipolar disorder died from suicide. Their team emphasizes that suicide in bipolar should be a focus of treatment and that early diagnosis, treatment, and intervention may help mitigate the long-term suicide risk.

Medical Comorbidity

The authors of a large study of US inpatient discharges in 2009 using the Kids' Inpatient Database examined the rates of anxiety, depression, and bipolar disorder among youth whose primary ICD9 discharge diagnosis was sickle cell disease, type 1 or 2 diabetes mellitus, asthma, or ADHD.[23] Although some illnesses had low rates of bipolar disorder, such as specifically 0.1% in asthma, 0.3% in sickle cell, and 0.6% in Type 2 Diabetes Mellitus (DM2), other disorders had higher rates, including 2.3% in Type 1 Diabetes Mellitus (DM1) and 33.2% in ADHD. Rates of anxiety and depression were also elevated in these disorders. Depression was the highest among those with ADHD, sickle cell disease, and type 1 diabetes. Anxiety was most prevalent in ADHD and type 1 diabetes.

Treatment

The American Academy of Child and Adolescent Psychiatry has a practice parameter for the treatment of pediatric bipolar disorder.[24] The practice parameter includes the history of bipolar disorder in the field of child psychiatry and emphasizes the necessity of making an accurate diagnosis. They gave a series of 11 recommendations for practitioners who treat youth with bipolar disorder (see Tables 16.1–16.3). The recommendations cover making an accurate diagnosis and then discuss treatment that consists of both medication and psychotherapy.

Pharmacology, immediate and long-term

Pharmacotherapy is the cornerstone of the treatment of pediatric bipolar disorder. Some medications were originally "grandfathered in" by the FDA, such as lithium, whereas many others were used off-label based on results in adult studies. With the advent of the Best Pharmaceuticals for Children Act, pharmaceutical companies began testing medication for bipolar disorder in children and adolescents. The federal government also funded two trials of medication in pediatric bipolar disorder: TEAM, an NIMH trial, and collaborative lithium trial (CoLT), an National Institute of Child Health and Development (NICHD) trial. The results of the different short-term industry and federal trials are discussed below. The trials used the

TABLE 16.1	
Practice Parameter Recommendations	
1	Assessments for youth should include screening questions for bipolar (BP) disorder
2	DSM criteria, including duration, should be followed for diagnosis of mania/hypomania
3	Bipolar NOS should be in youth with manic symptoms lasting hours and less than 4 days or those with chronic manic–like symptoms as their baseline
4	Youth with suspected bipolar should be evaluated for suicidality, comorbid disorder, psychosocial stressors, and medical problems
5	Use caution when applying the diagnosis to preschool children
6	For mania in bipolar I disorder, pharmacotherapy is the primary treatment
7	Most youth will require ongoing medication to prevent relapse and some will need lifelong treatment
8	Psychopharmacologic treatment requires baseline and follow-up symptom, side effect, and laboratory monitoring
9	In severely impaired youth, ECT may be used if medications are not helpful or cannot be tolerated
10	Psychotherapeutic interventions are an important component of comprehensive treatment
11	Treatment of BP-NOS involves psychopharmacology and behavioral/psychosocial interventions

Young Mania Rating Scale (YMRS) as the primary outcome measure unless otherwise noted below. A large metaanalysis of 29 open-label and 17 randomized trials conducted between 1989 and 2010 reported on the various agents that have been tested for pediatric bipolar disorder.[25]

Failed or Negative Trials

The majority of failed and negative trials involve the antiepileptic drugs used as mood stabilizers in adults.

The valproic acid extended-release trial consisted of a double-blind, short-term trial, and a longer open-label extension trial in 150 youth aged 10–17 years with BPI titrated to a serum level of 80–125 mcg/mL.[26] The change in YMRS was 8.8 on divalproex and 7.9 on placebo. The most common adverse events (AEs) were headache and vomiting, and there was no difference in AEs between drug and placebo.

TABLE 16.2
Medications to Treat Mixed or Manic Bipolar Disorder in Placebo-Controlled Trials

Medication	N	Age (years)	Daily Dose (mg)	YMRS (drug(s)/pbo)	AE
Aripiprazole	296	10–17	10, 30	16, 19/10	EPS somnolence
Asenapine	403	10–17	5, 10, 20	12.8, 14.9, 15.8/12.8	Somnolence, sedation, oral hypesthesia, oral paresthesia, increased appetite, weight gain
Olanzapine	167	13–17	2.5–20, mean 10.7	17.65/9.99	Appetite increase, weight increase, somnolence, sedation
Risperidone	169	10–17	0.5–2.5; 3–6	18.5, 16.5/9.1	Somnolence, headache, fatigue
Quetiapine	277	10–17	400, 600	14.25, 15.60/9.04	Somnolence, dizziness, fatigue, increased appetite, nausea, vomiting, dry mouth, tachycardia, and weight gain
Ziprasidone	237	10–17	40–160	13.83/8.61	Sedation, somnolence, headache, fatigue, and nausea
Lithium	81	7–17	600–2400, mean C/A 1292/1716	11.7/7/7	Nausea, vomiting, increased thirst, frequent urination, tremor, and elevated thyroid-stimulating hormone
Valproic acid ER	150	10–17	15–35 mg/k/d, mean 1286	8.8/7.9	Headache, vomiting
Oxcarbazepine	116	7–18	900–2400, mean 1515	10.90/9.79	Dizziness, nausea, somnolence, diplopia, fatigue, and rash
Topiramate	56	6–17	50–400, mean 278	9.7/4.7	Decreased appetite, nausea, diarrhea, and paresthesia

AE, adverse events; *C/A*, child/adolescent; *EPS*, extrapyramidal symptoms; *N*, number in trial; *YMRS*, young mania rating scale.
Not approved: ziprasidone, valproic acid, oxcarbazepine, topiramate; negative trials: valproic acid, oxcarbazepine, topiramate.

References in order of lines: Findling RL, Nyilas M, Forbes RA, et al. Acute treatment of pediatric bipolar I disorder, manic or mixed episode, with aripiprazole: a randomized, double-blind, placebo-controlled study. *J Clin Psychiatr*. 2009;70(10):1441–1451; Findling RL, Landbloom RL, Szegedi A, et al. Asenapine for the acute treatment of pediatric manic or mixed episode of bipolar I disorder. *J Am Acad Child Adolesc Psychiatr*. 2015;54(12):1032–1041; Tohen M, Kryzhanovskaya L, Carlson G, et al. Olanzapine versus placebo in the treatment of adolescents with bipolar mania. *Am J Psychiatr* 2007;64(10):1547–1556; Haas M, Delbello MP, Pandina G, et al. Risperidone for the treatment of acute mania in children and adolescents with bipolar disorder: a randomized, double-blind, placebo-controlled study. *Bipolar Disord*. 2009;11(7):687–700; Pathak S, Findling RL, Earley WR, et al. Efficacy and safety of quetiapine in children and adolescents with mania associated with bipolar I disorder: a 3-week, double-blind, placebo-controlled trial. *J Clin Psychiatr*. 2013;74(1):e100–e109; Findling RL, Cavuş I, Pappadopulos E, et al. Efficacy, long-term safety, and tolerability of ziprasidone in children and adolescents with bipolar disorder. *J Child Adolesc Psychopharmacol*. 2013;23(8):545–557; Findling RL, Kafantaris V, Pavuluri M, et al. Post-acute effectiveness of lithium in pediatric bipolar I disorder. *J Child Adolesc Psychopharmacol*. 2013;23(2):80–90; Findling RL, Chang K, Robb A, et al. Adjunctive maintenance lamotrigine for pediatric bipolar I disorder: a placebo-controlled, randomized withdrawal study. *J Am Acad Child Adolesc Psychiatr*. 2015;54(12):1020–1031; Wagner KD, Redden L, Kowatch RA, et al. A double-blind, randomized, placebo-controlled trial of divalproex extended-release in the treatment of bipolar disorder in children and adolescents. *J Am Acad Child Adolesc Psychiatr*. 2009;48(5):519–532; Wagner KD, Kowatch RA, Emslie GJ, et al. A double-blind, randomized, placebo-controlled trial of oxcarbazepine in the treatment of bipolar disorder in children and adolescents. *Am J Psychiatr* 2006;163(7):1179–1186; Delbello MP, Findling RL, Kushner S, et al. A pilot controlled trial of topiramate for mania in children and adolescents with bipolar disorder. *J Am Acad Child Adolesc Psychiatr*. 2005;44(6):539–547.

TABLE 16.3
Medications to Treat Depressed Bipolar Disorder in Placebo-Controlled Trials

Medication	N	Age (years)	Dose (mg)	CDRS (drug(s)/pbo)	AE
Olanzapine/ fluoxetine	291	10–17	6/25–12/50	28.4/23.4	Weight gain, increased appetite, somnolence
Lurasidone	471	10–17	20–80		

AE, adverse events; CDRS, child depression rating scale; N, number in trial.
Not approved: none but lurasidone pending.
References in order of lines: Detke HC, DelBello MP, Landry J, et al. Olanzapine/Fluoxetine combination in children and adolescents with bipolar I depression: a randomized, double-blind, placebo-controlled trial. *J Am Acad Child Adolesc Psychiatr*. 2015;54(3):217–224; Delbello MP, Goldman R, Phillips D et al. Efficacy and safety of lurasidone in children and adolescents with bipolar I depression: a double-blind, placebo-controlled study. *J Am Acad Child Adolesc Psychiatr*. 2017;56(12):1015–1025.

The trial of oxcarbazepine versus placebo examined 116 youth aged 7–18 years with BPI and dosed the medication at 900–2400 mg/day.[27] The mean dose was 1515 mg/day, and the mean reduction in the YMRS on drug was not significantly different than placebo 10.90 versus 9.79. They noted both groups had more psychiatric side effects, primarily worsening of bipolar symptoms, while the oxcarbazepine group had elevated rates of dizziness, nausea, somnolence, diplopia, fatigue, and rash.

A registration trial of topiramate in pediatric bipolar disorder was ended early when the adult trials failed to separate from placebo, while lithium did (negative not failed trial).[28] In the 56, 6- to 17-year-olds, results showed a difference between the slope of the YMRS but not the actual YMRS scores (9.7 vs. 4.7). AEs included decreased appetite, nausea, diarrhea, and paresthesia.

Positive Double-Blind Trials

Findling and colleagues examined the use of 10 and 30 mg of aripiprazole compared with placebo in 296 youth aged 10–17 years with mixed or manic mood episodes.[29] The YMRS change scores at 4 weeks were 16 and 19 points for 10 and 30 mg aripiprazole doses, respectively, compared with only 10 points on placebo. The most common AEs were extrapyramidal disorder and somnolence, both with higher rates on 30 mg than 10 mg.

In a double-blind trial of asenapine, investigators compared placebo with asenapine 2.5, 5, and 10 mg BID in 403 youth aged 10–17 years with bipolar disorder for change in YMRS at 21 days.[30] The YMRS scores on drug were 3.2–6.2 points larger improvement than the placebo arm. AEs seen more commonly on drug included somnolence, sedation, oral hypesthesia, oral paresthesia, increased appetite, and weight gain.

A 6-week trial of lurasidone for pediatric bipolar depression compared lurasidone and placebo for a reduction in the Child Depression Rating Scale-Revised (CDRS-R).[31] The trial compared placebo and lurasidone flexibly dosed from 20 to 80 mg daily over 6 weeks. The mean daily dose was 32.6 mg. The mean reduction in CDRS was 21.0 on lurasidone and 15.3 on placebo, yielding an effect size of 0.45. Response but not remission rates were also statistically significant on lurasidone compared with placebo. Common side effects included nausea, somnolence, increased weight, and insomnia.

Tohen and colleagues examined the effects of flexibly dosed olanzapine compared with placebo in 167 adolescents aged 13–17 years with bipolar disorder.[32] The mean dose of olanzapine was 10.7 mg. The YMRS change was 17.65 on olanzapine and 9.99 on placebo with mean weight gain of 3.7 kg. Other AEs included appetite increase, weight increase, somnolence, and sedation.

The risperidone bipolar trial compared placebo with two dose ranges, 0.5–2.5 and 3–6 mg/day, of risperidone in 169 youth aged 10–17 years with bipolar mixed or manic episodes.[33] The mean reduction in YMRS on placebo was 9.1, on low dose 18.5, and on high dose 16.5. The common AEs on risperidone included somnolence, headache, and fatigue.

Pathak and colleagues reported on the multisite trial of quetiapine 400 or 600 mg versus placebo in 277 youth aged 10–17 years with bipolar disorder.[34] The mean change in YMRS on placebo was 9.04 compared with 14.25 and 15.60 on 400 and 600 mg of quetiapine, respectively. The most common drug-related AEs were somnolence, dizziness, fatigue, increased appetite, nausea, vomiting, dry mouth, tachycardia, and weight gain.

The ziprasidone trial was positive but had methodological errors in the trial execution with dosing and did not lead to FDA labeling, unlike the other positive trials described in this section.[35,36] In the trial, 237, 10- to 17-year-olds were given 40–160 mg daily based on the subject's weight (40–80 mg/d < 45 kg and 80–160 > 45 kg). The mean change in YMRS was 13.83 on drug and 8.61 on placebo. The most common side effects were sedation, somnolence, headache, fatigue, and nausea. A second trial is currently underway across the United States.

Positive Open-Label Trials

Two different open-label trials examined carbamazepine in pediatric bipolar disorder.[37,37a] The Joshi trial studied carbamazepine extended release up to 788±252 mg/d in pediatric bipolar spectrum and monitored changes in 27 participants. Two participants had to discontinue because of rash, and only 16 subjects/patients completed the 8-week trial. Although the mean change was 10.1 points on the YMRS, the participants still had elevated mania scores at the end of the trial at 21.8. Other symptoms did improve, including depressive, ADHD, and psychotic symptoms. The Findling trial examined 10- to 17-year-olds and titrated from 200 to 1200 mg daily over 5 weeks with a 21-week extension. The study comprised 157 children and teenagers for an average of 109 days, and the mean reduction in the YMRS was 14.8 points. Because of AEs, including rash, decreased WBC, nausea, and vomiting, 26 people dropped out. The most common side effects were headache, somnolence, nausea, dizziness, and fatigue.

Federal Treatment Trials

The first large pediatric trial funded by the NIMH was the TEAM.[18] The trial examined 279 youth aged 6–15 years with bipolar mixed or manic episodes who were randomized to lithium titrated up to 1.4 mEq/L, risperidone titrated up to 4 mg daily, or divalproex sodium titrated up to 125 μg/mL.[18] The primary outcome was the blind rater's score on the clinical global impression-bipolar-improvement-mania (CGI-BP-I-M) after 8 weeks of treatment. Mean doses and levels were 1.09 mEq/L of lithium, 2.57 mg of risperidone, and 113.6 μg/mL of divalproex sodium. The response rates were risperidone 68.5%, lithium 35.6%, and divalproex sodium 24.0%. Several follow-up papers presented additional findings from the study. Vitiello reported on mediators and moderators noting that study site, presence of ADHD, and obesity were all moderators.[38] Participants with comorbid ADHD had a better response on risperidone than lithium, and nonobese patients responded better to risperidone than lithium. Older age and less severe symptoms were associated with better response on the Kiddie Mania Rating Scale (similar to the YMRS). In an examination of the depression and suicidality outcomes on the trial, they found the same pattern of response rates on the clinical global impression-bipolar-improvement-depression (CGI-BP I-D) with risperidone 60.7% versus lithium 42.2% versus divalproex sodium 35.0%.[39] By week 8, all patients had similar reductions in the CDRS, but those in the risperidone group had more significant early improvement in depressive symptoms at week 1, which continued through the trial. The level of suicidality in the trial was low and did not differ among the three treatments. The TEAM trial had a second 8-week phase for the 89 nonresponders and the 65 partial responders.[40] Nonresponders were randomized to one of the other two treatments, whereas partial responders remained on the initial drug with a second agent added on to the first study drug. For those children switched to risperidone, 47.6% responded, compared with those switched to lithium (12.8%) or divalproex (17.2%). The response rate for partial responders who added risperidone was 53.3% compared with those who added divalproex sodium (0%) or lithium (26.7%). They concluded that risperidone was most useful for partial or nonresponders to lithium in an initial trial of a bipolar medication. The common side effects for risperidone were weight gain, increased appetite, increased prolactin level, and drowsiness; for lithium, weight gain nausea, vomiting, excessive thirst, and abdominal pain; and for divalproex, increased appetite, weight gain, difficulty waking up, and drowsiness.

The second large pediatric trial in bipolar disorder was a series of trials examining the use of lithium carbonate in youth aged 7–17 years with bipolar disorder in a mixed or manic episode. Findling describes the CoLT study design, including diagnosis and pharmacokinetics (PK).[41] The first trial, CoLT I, would examine an 8-week open-label dose escalation trial followed by a 16-week long-term effectiveness phase and a 28-week discontinuation phase (blinded randomization to lithium or placebo to see if symptoms recurred). The CoLT I trial reported long-term outcomes in all those who demonstrated at least a partial response at 8 weeks of open-label lithium and allowed up to two adjunctive medications.[36] The 41 participants received lithium for 14.9 weeks, and 68.3% had response defined as a 50% reduction in YMRS and CGI-I of much or very much improved. People who responded in the acute study maintained the response, whereas those with a partial response did not receive additional improvement despite the option to receive adjunctive medications.

The CoLT I trial established the optimal dosing strategy based on PK data.[42] The 39 children aged 7–17 years received a single dose of 600 mg or 900 mg and had serial serum lithium samples drawn over 24 h. The single-dose PK study yielded a half-life of 2.4 h and a terminal phase of up to 27 h. With simulation, QD dosing yielded a half-life of 13.1 h, 14.0 for BID dosing, and 15.1 h for TID dosing. Further examination of the youth in the CoLT I study yielded a recommendation to dose by weight.[43] In the findings from 61 youth, the optimal initial dosing was 300 mg BID for those less than 30 kg and 300 mg TID for youth at or above 30 kg. Over half (58%) of the 61 youth in the trial had a response defined as a 50% decrease in the YMRS and a CGI of much or very much improved.

The CoLT II study was an 8-week double-blind, placebo-controlled trial, a 16- to 24-week open-label trial, a 28-week double-blind discontinuation trial, and an 8-week restabilization trial. In the CoLT II double-blind efficacy trial of lithium versus placebo in youth aged 7–17 years with bipolar I mixed or manic episodes, participants were titrated up to maximum tolerability, 40 mg/k/day, or a level of ≤1.4 mEq/L.[44] At 8 weeks, the change in YMRS was significantly better on lithium than on placebo, with similar improvements in CGI-I. The commonly seen side effects included nausea, vomiting, increased thirst, frequent urination, tremor, and elevated thyroid-stimulating hormone.

Combination Trials

A large multisite placebo-controlled trial of olanzapine/fluoxetine was conducted for youth aged 10–17 years with bipolar depression. All participants had CDRS scores ≥40 and YMRS scores ≤15, ensuring they were in a depressed rather than mixed mood episode.[45] At the end of 8 weeks, the olanzapine/fluoxetine combination was superior to placebo in reducing the depressive symptoms. The findings led to FDA approval for this combination medication in the treatment of adolescent bipolar depression; the most commonly used dose was olanzapine 12 mg and fluoxetine 50 mg daily. The most frequent AEs were weight gain, increased appetite, and somnolence.

A double-blinded combination trial was the lamotrigine add-on trial where youth aged 10–17 years with bipolar manic, hypomanic, or depressed episodes had open-label lamotrigine added on to their previous medication.[46] After reaching response and dose stabilization over 18 weeks, participants entered the blinded discontinuation phase and were randomized to remain on lamotrigine or switch to placebo. In the original analysis of all participants, there was no statistically significant difference in time to relapse. When separated into children (10–12 years) and adolescents (13–17 years), the teens had a statistically significant difference in time to relapse on lamotrigine. Although the FDA did not approve lamotrigine for pediatric bipolar disorder because of the negative findings on the primary combined age group analysis, this study shows lamotrigine is a safe and effective add-on medication for both bipolar manic and depressed episodes in adolescents. In the lamotrigine treatment arms (open and blinded), common AEs were headache, abdominal pain, nausea, oropharyngeal pain, and dermatologic events.

Long-term trial

In a 6-month open-label valproic acid trial of 66 youth aged 10–17 years with BPI disorder, the mean reduction in manic symptoms on the YMRS was 2.2 points relative to baseline.[26] Dorfman conducted a review of the long-term treatment studies for pediatric bipolar disorder, including both medication and therapies.[47] The paper noted that atypical antipsychotics, aripiprazole, quetiapine, and ziprasidone, as well as mood stabilizers lithium and carbamazepine, had some demonstration of efficacy in up to 6-month trials. The paper also discussed long-term psychotherapy trials, which are noted in the next section as a possibly efficacious add-on treatment to pharmacotherapy in pediatric bipolar disorder. Asenapine has since been shown to have benefit in long-term open-label treatment.[48]

Psychotherapy

Several different types of therapy have been studied in pediatric bipolar disorder, including dialectical behavioral therapy (DBT), cognitive behavioral therapy (CBT), and family-focused therapy (FFT). For a more extensive review of the various family therapies tried in pediatric bipolar disorder, the review by Young and Fristad is comprehensive.[49] What is crucial to recognize about therapy trials for adolescents with bipolar disorder is that all the trials add therapy onto stable pharmacologic treatment to determine if therapy adds benefit to symptom improvement and/or quality of life (QOL) and functioning above that provided by medication.

Goldstein et al.[50] studied DBT versus treatment as usual (TAU) in teens with bipolar disorder. The youth had psychopharmacologist-titrated medication and those in DBT had 18 adolescent sessions and 18 family skills sessions, whereas TAU was eclectic therapy with supportive psychoeducational and cognitive therapy (but not formal CBT). Those in DBT attended more sessions, had less depression, and exhibited greater improvement in suicidality. There were no group differences in manic or emotional dysregulation symptoms.

Miklowitz and colleagues conducted some of the earliest randomized trials of family-focused therapy for adolescents (FFT-A) versus brief psychoeducation (labeled EC or enhanced care).[51] Those in EC had three psychoeducational sessions, whereas those in FFT-A had 21 sessions over 9 months. Those in FFT-A had more rapid improvement of depression, less time in depressive episodes, more time in depression free, and greater improvement in depressive symptoms over 2 years. In the same trial comparing FFT-A versus EC, the authors followed self-reported QoL for 2 years.[52] Two-year overall QoL did not differ between the two groups. However, youth on FFT reported improved family relationships and physical health in their QoL measures.

West and colleagues adapted the FFT-A for children with bipolar disorder and reported their findings.[53] Their child- and family-focused CBT (CFF-CBT) was compared with psychotherapy as usual (TAU) as 12 weekly sessions and 6 monthly booster sessions over a period of 9 months. As with the adolescent studies, those in CFF had greater attendance and satisfaction with treatment. They also reported reductions in parent-reported mania and depressive symptoms at post-treatment (month 9).

MacPherson and colleagues further examined the randomized trial of CFF-CBT for pediatric bipolar disorder to determine if there were mediators of treatment response.[54] This trial examined the addition of CFF-CBT or TAU to pharmacotherapy. CFF-CBT led to greater improvements in mania, depression, and overall functioning. Several parent and family factors improved in CFF-CBT and mediated these mood changes, including parenting skills, parental coping, family flexibility, and positive reframing. No child coping changes were associated with mediator effects. The team also performed/conducted a moderator analysis to identify factors that altered response to the same intervention.[55] The CFF-CBT impact on youth depressive symptoms was greater in families where parents had more severe baseline depression, lower income, and higher cohesion (marginal effect). TAU was less effective in youth with less severe (not worse) depression and less effective for mania in youth with higher self-esteem. Lower depression and higher self-esteem in youth did not impact response to CFF-CBT.

A Swedish group led by Knutsson wanted to expand on FFT by using it to treat families in a group format rather than one family at a time as was done in the US trials described previously.[56] The Swedes wanted to improve symptoms, psychosocial functioning, knowledge, and coping skills and decrease family-expressed emotion. They delivered 12 sessions to two multifamily groups and found such a format was feasible and led to improvements similar to those seen when the treatment was delivered to individual families.

CONCLUSIONS

Pediatric bipolar disorder remains an illness that affects children as early as in elementary school and increases in prevalence across puberty and into young adulthood. Accurate diagnosis requires a good clinical interview, which should include family history, development, onset of symptoms, previous psychiatric diagnoses and treatment, medical history and treatments, and mental status examination. The clinician should look for the DSM-5 diagnostic criteria with special attention paid to Geller's cardinal symptoms. Once a diagnosis has been made, treatment should be initiated to prevent consequences of untreated mania, which include hospitalization, development of comorbid disorders, psychotic symptoms, and adverse psychosocial sequelae. Treatment as per American Academy of Child and Adolescent Psychiatry (AACAP) practice parameters should consist of mood-stabilizing medications, many of which are now FDA approved, in combination with psychotherapy and educational support. Early diagnosis and treatment may be effective in reducing both medical and psychiatric long-term consequences seen in adults with bipolar disorder.

REFERENCES

1. Glovinsky I. A brief history of childhood-onset bipolar disorder through 1980. *Child Adolesc Psychiatr Clin N Am.* 2002;11:443–460.
2. Strecker EA. The prognosis in manic-depressive psychosis. *NY Med J.* 1921;114:209–211.
3. Kanner L. *Child Psychiatry.* Springfield (IL): CC Thomas; 1935.
4. James A, Hoang U, Seagroatt V, et al. A comparison of American and English hospital discharge rates for pediatric bipolar disorder, 2000 to 2010. *J Am Acad Child Adolesc Psychiatr.* 2014;53(6):614–624.
5. American Psychiatric Association. Bipolar and related disorders. In: *Diagnostic and Statistical Manual of Mental Disorders Fifth Edition.* Washington DC: American Psychiatric Publishing; 2013:123–154.

6. Geller B, Zimerman B, Williams M, et al. DSM-IV mania symptoms in a prepubertal and early adolescent bipolar disorder phenotype compared to attention-deficit hyperactive and normal controls. *J Child Adolesc Psychopharmacol.* 2002;12(1):11–25.

7. Pataki CS, Sussman N. Mood disorders. In: Sadock BJ, Sadock VA, Ruiz P, eds. *Kaplan and Sadock's Brief Synopsis of Psychiatry Behavioral Sciences/Clinical Psychiatry.* 11th ed. Philadelphia: Wolter Kluwer; 2015. 8.1.

8. Judd LL, Akiskal HS. The prevalence and disability of bipolar spectrum disorders in the US population: reanalysis of the ECA database taking into account subthreshold cases. *J Affect Disord.* 2003;73:123–131.

9. Perlis RH, Miyahara S, Marangell LB, et al. Long-term implications of early onset in bipolar disorder data from the first 1000 participants in the systematic treatment enhancement program for bipolar disorder (SEP-BD). *Biol Psychiatr.* 2004;55:875–881.

10. Van Meter AR, Moreira AL, Youngstrom EA. Meta-analysis of epidemiologic studies of pediatric bipolar disorder. *J Clin Psychiatr.* 2011;72:1250–1256.

11. Kerner B. Genetics of bipolar disorder. *Appl Clin Genet.* 2014;7:33–42.

12. Croarkin PE, Luby JL, Cercy K, et al. Genetic risk score analysis in early-onset bipolar disorder. *J Clin Psychiatr.* 2017. https://doi.org/10.4088/JCP.15m10314. [Epub ahead of print].

13. Nassan M, Croarkin PE, Luby JL, et al. Association of brain-derived neurotrophic factor (BDNF) Val66Met polymorphism with early-onset bipolar disorder. *Bipolar Disord.* 2015;17(6):645–652.

14. Frías Á, Palma C, Farriols N. Comorbidity in pediatric bipolar disorder: prevalence, clinical impact, etiology and treatment. *J Affect Disord.* 2015;174:378–389.

15. Horwitz SM, Storfer-Isser A, Young AS, et al. Development of alcohol and drug use in youth with manic symptoms. *J Am Acad Child Adolesc Psychiatr.* 2017;56(2):149–156.

16. Wilens TE, Biederman J, Martelon M, et al. Further evidence for smoking and substance use disorders in youth with bipolar disorder and comorbid conduct disorder. *J Clin Psychiatr.* 2016;77(10):1420–1427.

17. Sala R, Strober MA, Axelson DA, et al. Effects of comorbid anxiety disorders on the longitudinal course of pediatric bipolar disorders. *J Am Acad Child Adolesc Psychiatr.* 2014;53(1):72–81.

18. Geller B, Luby JL, Joshi P, et al. A randomized controlled trial of risperidone, lithium, or divalproex sodium for initial treatment of bipolar I disorder, manic or mixed phase, in children and adolescents. *Arch Gen Psychiatr.* 2012;69(5):515–528.

19. Tonna M, Amerio A, Odone A, et al. Comorbid bipolar disorder and obsessive-compulsive disorder: state of the art in pediatric patients. *Shanghai Arch Psychiatr.* 2015;27(6):386–387.

20. Elias LR, Miskowiak KW, Vale AM, et al. Cognitive impairment in euthymic pediatric bipolar disorder: a systematic review and meta-analysis. *J Am Acad Child Adolesc Psychiatr.* 2017;56(4):286–296.

21. Dickstein DP, Axelson D, Weissman AB, et al. Cognitive flexibility and performance in children and adolescents with threshold and sub-threshold bipolar disorder. *Eur Child Adolesc Psychiatr.* 2016;25(6):625–638.

22. Hauser M, Galling B, Correll CU. Suicidal ideation and suicide attempts in children and adolescents with bipolar disorder: a systematic review of prevalence and incidence rates, correlates, and targeted interventions. *Bipolar Disord.* 2013;15(5):507–523.

23. Sztein DM, Lane WG. Examination of the comorbidity of mental illness and somatic conditions in hospitalized children in the United States using the kids' inpatient database, 2009. *Hosp Pediatr.* 2016;6(3):126–134.

24. McClellan J, Kowatch R, Findling RL, et al. Practice parameter for the assessment and treatment of children and adolescents with bipolar disorder. *J Am Acad Child Adolesc Psychiatr.* 2007;46(1):107–125.

25. Liu HY, Potter MP, Woodworth KY, et al. Pharmacologic treatments for pediatric bipolar disorder: a review and meta-analysis. *J Am Acad Child Adolesc Psychiatr.* 2011;50(8):749–762.

26. Wagner KD, Redden L, Kowatch RA, et al. A double-blind, randomized, placebo-controlled trial of divalproex extended-release in the treatment of bipolar disorder in children and adolescents. *J Am Acad Child Adolesc Psychiatr.* 2009;48(5):519–532.

27. Wagner KD, Kowatch RA, Emslie GJ, et al. A double-blind, randomized, placebo-controlled trial of oxcarbazepine in the treatment of bipolar disorder in children and adolescents. *Am J Psychiatr.* 2006;163(7):1179–1186.

28. Delbello MP, Findling RL, Kushner S, et al. A pilot controlled trial of topiramate for mania in children and adolescents with bipolar disorder. *J Am Acad Child Adolesc Psychiatr.* 2005;44(6):539–547.

29. Findling RL, Nyilas M, Forbes RA, et al. Acute treatment of pediatric bipolar I disorder, manic or mixed episode, with aripiprazole: a randomized, double-blind, placebo-controlled study. *J Clin Psychiatr.* 2009;70(10):1441–1451.

30. Findling RL, Landbloom RL, Szegedi A, et al. Asenapine for the acute treatment of pediatric manic or mixed episode of bipolar I disorder. *J Am Acad Child Adolesc Psychiatr.* 2015;54(12):1032–1041.

31. DelBello MP, Goldman R, Phillips D et al. Efficacy and safety of lurasidone in children and adolescents with bipolar I depression: a double-blind, placebo-controlled study. *J Am Acad Child Adolesc Psychiatr.* 2017;56(12):1015–1025

32. Tohen M, Kryzhanovskaya L, Carlson G, et al. Olanzapine versus placebo in the treatment of adolescents with bipolar mania. *Am J Psychiatr.* 2007;164(10):1547–1556.

33. Haas M, Delbello MP, Pandina G, et al. Risperidone for the treatment of acute mania in children and adolescents with bipolar disorder: a randomized, double-blind, placebo-controlled study. *Bipolar Disord.* 2009;11(7):687–700.

34. Pathak S, Findling RL, Earley WR, et al. Efficacy and safety of quetiapine in children and adolescents with

mania associated with bipolar I disorder: a 3-week, double-blind, placebo-controlled trial. *J Clin Psychiatr.* 2013;74(1):e100–e109.

35. Findling RL, Cavuş I, Pappadopulos E, et al. Efficacy, long-term safety, and tolerability of ziprasidone in children and adolescents with bipolar disorder. *J Child Adolesc Psychopharmacol.* 2013;23(8):545–557.

36. Findling RL, Kafantaris V, Pavuluri M, et al. Post-acute effectiveness of lithium in pediatric bipolar I disorder. *J Child Adolesc Psychopharmacol.* 2013;23(2):80–90.

37. Joshi G, Wozniak J, Mick E, et al. A prospective open-label trial of extended-release carbamazepine monotherapy in children with bipolar disorder. *J Child Adolesc Psychopharmacol.* 2010;20(1):7–14.

37a. Findling RL, Ginsberg LD. The safety and effectiveness of open-label extended-release carbamazepine in the treatment of children and adolescents with bipolar I disorder suffering from a manic or mixed episode. *Neuropsychiatr Dis Treat.* 2014;10:1589–97.

38. Vitiello B, Riddle MA, Yenokyan G, et al. Treatment moderators and predictors of outcome in the treatment of early age mania (TEAM) study. *J Am Acad Child Adolesc Psychiatr.* 2012;51(9):867–878.

39. Salpekar JA, Joshi PT, Axelson DA, et al. Depression and suicidality outcomes in the treatment of early age mania study. *J Am Acad Child Adolesc Psychiatr.* 2015;54(12):999–1007.

40. Walkup JT, Wagner KD, Miller L, et al. Treatment of early-age mania: outcomes for partial and nonresponders to initial treatment. *J Am Acad Child Adolesc Psychiatr.* 2015;54(12):1008–1019.

41. Findling RL, Frazier JA, Kafantaris V, et al. The collaborative lithium trials (CoLT): specific aims, methods, and implementation. *Child Adolesc Psychiatr Ment Health.* 2008;2(1):21.

42. Findling RL, Landersdorfer CB, Kafantaris V, et al. First-dose pharmacokinetics of lithium carbonate in children and adolescents. *J Clin Psychopharmacol.* 2010;30(4):404–410.

43. Findling RL, Kafantaris V, Pavuluri M, et al. Dosing strategies for lithium monotherapy in children and adolescents with bipolar I disorder. *J Child Adolesc Psychopharmacol.* 2011;21(3):195–205.

44. Findling RL, Robb A, McNamara NK, et al. Lithium in the acute treatment of bipolar I disorder: a double-blind, placebo-controlled study. *Pediatrics.* 2015;136(5):885–894.

45. Detke HC, DelBello MP, Landry J, et al. Olanzapine/Fluoxetine combination in children and adolescents with bipolar I depression: a randomized, double-blind, placebo-controlled trial. *J Am Acad Child Adolesc Psychiatr.* 2015;54(3):217–224.

46. Findling RL, Chang K, Robb A, et al. Adjunctive maintenance lamotrigine for pediatric bipolar I disorder: a placebo-controlled, randomized withdrawal study. *J Am Acad Child Adolesc Psychiatr.* 2015;54(12):1020–1031.

47. Dorfman J, Robb A. Long-term treatment strategies for pediatric bipolar disorder. *Curr Treat Options Psych.* 2016;3:206–220.

48. Findling RL, Landbloom RL, Mackle M, et al. Long-term safety of asenapine in pediatric patients diagnosed with bipolar I disorder: a 50-week open-label, flexible-dose trial. *Paediatr Drugs.* 2016;18(5):367–378.

49. Young AS, Fristad MA. Family-based interventions for childhood mood disorders. *Child Adolesc Psychiatr Clin N Am.* 2015;24(3):517–534.

50. Goldstein TR, Fersch-Podrat RK, Rivera M, et al. Dialectical behavior therapy for adolescents with bipolar disorder: results from a pilot randomized trial. *J Child Adolesc Psychopharmacol.* 2015;25(2):140–149.

51. Miklowitz DJ, Axelson DA, Birmaher B, et al. Family-focused treatment for adolescents with bipolar disorder: results of a 2-year randomized trial. *J Affect Disord.* 2008;82:1053–1061.

52. O'Donnell LA, Axelson DA, Kowatch RA, et al. Enhancing quality of life among adolescents with bipolar disorder: a randomized trial of two psychosocial interventions. *J Affect Disord.* 2017;219:201–208.

53. West AE, Weinstein SM, Peters AT, et al. Child- and family-focused cognitive-behavioral therapy for pediatric bipolar disorder: a randomized clinical trial. *J Am Acad Child Adolesc Psychiatr.* 2014;53(11):1168–1178.

54. MacPherson HA, Weinstein SM, Henry DB, et al. Mediators in the randomized trial of child- and family-focused cognitive-behavioral therapy for pediatric bipolar disorder. *Behav Res Ther.* 2016;85:60–71.

55. Weinstein SM, Henry DB, Katz AC, et al. Treatment moderators of child- and family-focused cognitive-behavioral therapy for pediatric bipolar disorder. *J Am Acad Child Adolesc Psychiatr.* 2015;54(2):116–125.

56. Knutsson J, Bäckström B, Daukantaitė D, et al. Adolescent and family-focused cognitive-behavioural therapy for paediatric bipolar disorders: a case series. *Clin Psychol Psychother.* 2017;24(3):589–617.

CHAPTER 17

Childhood-Onset Schizophrenia

AFSOON ANVARI, BS • FRANCIS LOEB, BS • JUDY RAPOPORT, MD • DAVID I. DRIVER, MD

INTRODUCTION

With symptom onset prior to 13 years of age, Childhood-onset schizophrenia (COS) is an exceptionally rare and devastating psychiatric condition, which clinically and neurobiologically resembles adult-onset schizophrenia (AOS). The etiology of schizophrenia largely remains unknown, but it is widely accepted that it is due to a combination of genetic predisposition and environmental influences.[1-5] Earlier onset cases are more strongly influenced by genetic factors, less so by environmental causes, and are typically more severe in disease manifestation with an overall poorer prognosis.[6,7] Because of the timing of onset and nature of the disease course, COS severely disrupts neurobiologic, cognitive, and social development, causing a significant burden of illness to the patient and the family.

From 1990 to 2017, the National Institute of Mental Health (NIMH) Child Psychiatry Branch (CPB) maintained the largest cohort of COS patients for longitudinal analysis, with inpatient observation available up to 2016. After referral and an extensive prescreen, which included a thorough records review, children and their parents underwent clinical and structural interviews. Ninety percent of prescreened patients were excluded.[8] Patients who met inclusion criteria after screening were admitted to the NIMH inpatient unit where they participated in the inpatient phase of the study. This phase, frequently lasting up to 5 months, included observation, medication washout, diagnosis, and clinical stabilization phases.

Nearly 3500 pediatric patients were referred to the NIMH COS study. Sixty percent of those screened in person ultimately failed to meet criteria for schizophrenia. Of the 217 children admitted to the inpatient phase of the study, only 134 patients ultimately received a diagnosis of COS.[9] Follow-up studies of COS and rule-out patients indicated excellent reliability of both the diagnosis of COS and the alternative diagnoses.[8,10] Trauma, mood, anxiety, developmental, and/or behavioral disorders served as the most frequent alternative diagnoses.

Although COS is commonly associated with auditory hallucinations (94.9% of COS patients),[11] hallucinations are neither necessary nor sufficient for the diagnosis, and diagnosis should not be based on positive symptoms alone. Hallucinations, delusions, and disordered thoughts can be seen in healthy, nonpsychotic children[12] and typically diminish after 7 years of age.[13] Transient visual hallucinations in preschool children are occasionally reported in conjunction with anxiety and stress, and the prognosis is generally benign.[8,11,14] Because the prevalence of COS is so low, there is a very high probability that children presenting with hallucinations and delusions are suffering from something other than COS.

NIMH CPB researchers identified a heterogeneous subgroup of children who presented with transient psychotic symptoms and multiple developmental abnormalities. These children did not fit clearly into any existing DSM category and were ultimately referred to as "multidimensionally impaired" (MDI); the most fitting diagnosis in the *Diagnostic and Statistical Manual of Mental Disorders, Fifth Edition* (*DSM-5*) would be "psychosis not otherwise specified". MDI patients often exhibit stress-related transient episodes of psychosis, emotional instability, impaired interpersonal skills, and information-processing deficits. This diagnostic category can be mistaken as COS and requires a multidisciplinary approach that includes physical therapy, occupational therapy, special education, and antipsychotic treatment.

DEFINITION/SYMPTOM CRITERIA

Schizophrenia, the prototype for psychotic disorders, is defined by delusions, hallucinations, disorganized thought, disorganized behavior, and/or negative symptoms. COS is neither differentiated from schizophrenia in the *DSM-5* (Table 17.1) nor distinguished in previous editions. In an effort to better obtain a homogenous cohort, the NIMH CPB established additional diagnostic criteria for COS to differentiate it from its

TABLE 17.1
DSM-5 Diagnostic Criteria for Schizophrenia 295.90 (F20.9)

A. Symptoms: Two (or more) of the following, each present for a significant portion of time during a 1-month period (or less if successfully treated). At least one of these must be (1), (2), or (3)	1. Delusions. 2. Hallucinations. 3. Disorganized speech (e.g., frequent derailment or incoherence). 4. Grossly disorganized or catatonic behavior. 5. Negative symptoms (i.e., diminished emotional expression or avolition).
B. Interpersonal/occupational dysfunction	For a significant portion of the time since the onset of the disturbance, level of functioning in one or more major areas, such as work, interpersonal relations, or self-care, is markedly below the level achieved before the onset (or when the onset is in childhood or adolescence, there is failure to achieve expected level of interpersonal, academic, or occupational functioning).
C. Duration	Continuous signs of the disturbance persist for at least 6 months. This 6-month period must include at least 1 month of symptoms (or less if successfully treated) that meet Criterion A (i.e., active-phase symptoms) and may include periods of prodromal or residual symptoms. During these prodromal or residual periods, the signs of the disturbance may be manifested by only negative symptoms or by two or more symptoms listed in Criterion A present in an attenuated form (e.g., odd beliefs, unusual perceptual experiences).
D. Exclusion of mood disorder	Schizoaffective disorder and depressive or bipolar disorder with psychotic features have been ruled out because either (1) no major depressive or manic episodes have occurred concurrently with the active-phase symptoms, or (2) if mood episodes have occurred during active-phase symptoms, they have been present for a minority of the total duration of the active and residual periods of the illness.
E. Exclusion of medical condition	The disturbance is not attributable to the physiologic effects of a substance (e.g., a drug of abuse, a medication) or another medical condition.
F. Consideration of autism spectrum disorder or a communication disorder	If there is a history or autism spectrum disorder or a communication disorder of childhood onset, the additional diagnosis of schizophrenia is made only if prominent delusions or hallucinations, in addition to the other required symptoms of schizophrenia, are also present for at least 1 month (or less if successfully treated).

From American Psychiatric Association. Schizophrenia spectrum and other psychotic disorders. In: *Diagnostic and Statistical Manual of Mental Disorders*. 5th ed. Arlington, VA: American Psychiatric Publishing; 2013:87–122, with permission.

later-onset counterparts, adolescent-onset and adult-onset schizophrenia:
1. Onset of psychotic symptoms before 13 years of age
2. Premorbid intelligence quotient (IQ) of 70 or above
3. Absence of significant neurologic problems

The DSM-5 definition of schizophrenia is demonstrated in Table 17.1.[15]

The *DSM-5* did not radically alter the diagnostic criteria seen in the *DSM-IV*. Two changes have been made to Criterion A: (1) at least one of the two required symptoms has to be delusions, hallucinations, or disorganized thinking, and (2) bizarre delusions and special auditory hallucinations (Kurt Schneider's first-rank symptoms in the *DSM-IV*) are no longer given special consideration.[16] Criterion F has also been altered, as pervasive developmental

disorder (PDD) is now considered an autism spectrum disorder (ASD).

For schizophrenia, the majority of the changes between the two editions were seen in the dimensional categorization of symptoms and in the removal of the subtypes of schizophrenia (catatonic, disorganized, paranoid, residual, undifferentiated). Subtypes showed limited diagnostic stability, low reliability, and poor validity.[17] The dimensional categories include delusions, hallucinations, negative symptoms, disorganized speech, cognitive impairment, motor symptoms (includes catatonia), depression, and mania.[15] Dimensions that respond best to atypical antipsychotics are hallucinations, delusions, disorganized speech, and mania.[18]

Despite changes in the new edition, 99.5% of patients in pre-DSM-5 clinical trials meet diagnostic criteria for schizophrenia in the *DSM-5*, suggesting very little impact in the generalizability of previous research as well as in the diagnosis of schizophrenia. Many support omission of the classic subtypes of schizophrenia because of the lack of clinical value and variation in treatment response.[18] Longitudinal studies also support the transition to a dimensional, rather than categoric, approach to psychosis.[19]

EPIDEMIOLOGY

COS is an exceptionally rare psychiatric illness with an estimated incidence of less than 0.04%[8] and a prevalence estimated between 1:30,000[20] and 1:40,000 children.[21] Some studies report a COS prevalence of 1:10,000[22–24] and a prevalence of schizophrenia before the age of 15 years as 1.4:10,000.[25] A nationwide population study in Denmark found a 1.9% prevalence rate of Early Onset Schizophrenia (EOS),[26] higher than estimates in a Finnish study, suggesting that 4.7% of patients with schizophrenia have onset before the age of 19 years.[27] Because of the rare nature of COS, large-scale prevalence studies based on standardized clinical assessments have not been performed. Psychotic symptoms, however, are relatively common in children—both healthy and with other psychiatric conditions—with prevalence reported up to 5%.[28,29]

SCREENING/DIAGNOSIS

An overall lack of systematic, evidence-based diagnostic tools and biologic markers of disease make diagnosing mental health disorders overall particularly challenging. The diagnosis of COS requires an extensive, longitudinal analysis of a patient's clinical presentation and the incorporation of collateral information from family members, caretakers, teachers, and other members of the treatment team. Although developmental impairments are neither diagnostic nor reliable prodromal indicators of disease,[8,30,31] they are frequently present in individuals being considered for a diagnosis of COS,[8] and clinicians must be astute in assessing for them. Surprisingly, developmental abnormalities in language, social, and motor domains appear to be more significant in cases of COS with a later symptom onset.[32–36]

Family dynamics, clinical severity, and the pressure of time to diagnose and treat children with psychotic illness are barriers to obtaining a valid, reliable diagnosis. When considering COS as a diagnosis, clinicians must not be blinded by the presence of hallucinations, as hallucinations are very common in children who are healthy, in those who have behavioral disturbances, and in various other psychiatric disorders.

Differential Diagnoses

Hallucinations are frequently a red herring in the evaluation of a pediatric patient for a primary psychotic disorder. Disorders commonly mistaken for COS include trauma, anxiety, substance induced, mood, and Autism Spectrum Disorders (ASD's). Medical etiologies to consider include epilepsy, chromosomal disorders, anti-NMDA (*N*-methyl-D-aspartate) receptor encephalitis, herpes simplex encephalitis, lysosomal storage diseases, inborn errors of metabolism, neurodegenerative disorders, central nervous system tumors, and progressive organic central nervous system disorders such as sclerosing panencephalitis.

COS is also associated with several chromosomal anomalies. The most clinically relevant chromosomal abnormality seen in COS, with an increased frequency over the general population, is 22q11 deletion, velocardiofacial syndrome (VCF), also known as DiGeorge syndrome. VCF is considered a pleiotropic genetic mutation and is implicated in both schizophrenia and ASD. It is associated with a broad phenotype.[37–40] 22q11.2 deletion syndrome accounts for ~30% of EOS and 1%–2% of AOS.[41]

Given the subgroup of MDI children within the NIMH CPB study, it deserves adequate diagnostic consideration to differentiate between COS and this atypical presentation of psychosis. MDI children feature severe functional impairments, most notably multiple developmental disorders, affective lability, and transient psychotic symptoms that do not meet criteria for a specific DSM-5 diagnosis. MDI is associated with neuropsychologic test abnormalities, eye movement dysfunction, and familial risk factors.[25,33,42,43] Unlike the comorbidities typically seen in COS, attention deficit hyperactivity disorder (ADHD) is highly comorbid within the MDI group.[8] Helpful in differentiating between COS and MDI patients, the following features define the MDI presentation[8]:

1. Transient episodes of psychosis and perceptual disturbance(s), typically presenting as stress-related responses
2. Nearly daily periods of emotional lability disproportionate to precipitants
3. Impaired interpersonal skills despite the desire to initiate peer friendships
4. Cognitive deficits indicated by multiple deficits in information processing
5. No clear thought disorder

EVALUATION AND WORKUP

A thorough evaluation of a child for COS requires a clinician to obtain/review medical records, obtain collateral

TABLE 17.2 Screening and Diagnostic Tools	
Scale for the Assessment of Positive Symptoms (SAPS)	Assessment of positive symptoms of psychosis developed for schizophrenia
Scale for the Assessment of Negative Symptoms (SANS)	Assessment of negative symptoms of psychosis developed for schizophrenia
Brief Psychiatric Rating Scale (BPRS) for Children	21-item clinician-based rating scale to evaluate psychiatric problems in children and adolescents
Social Communication Questionnaire	Screening questionnaire to evaluate communication skills and social functioning in children who may have ASD
Kiddie-Sads-Present and Lifetime Version (K-SADS-PL)	A semistructured diagnostic interview to assess current and past episodes of psychopathology in children and adolescents based on DSM-III-R and DSM-IV criteria. Available supplements include psychotic disorders supplement, affective disorders supplement, anxiety disorders supplement, behavioral disorders supplement, substance abuse and other disorders supplement
Clinical Global Impressions Scale	Assessment of outcome to evaluate treatment efficacy
Children's Global Impressions Scale	An adaptation of the Clinical Global Impression Scale for children
Bunny-Hamburg Global Ratings	Contains two subscales (Psychosis and Depression) that assist in excluding COS as a diagnosis
Abnormal Involuntary Movement Scale	12-item scale administered by clinician to detect and monitor tardive dyskinesia in patients receiving neuroleptic medications
Simpson-Angus Scale	Instrument to assess neuroleptic-induced parkinsonism

ASD, autism spectrum disorder; COS, childhood-onset schizophrenia.

information from all members of the treatment team, carefully observe patient and family interactions over an extended period, and exclude other diagnoses to include organic etiologies of psychosis, comorbid psychiatric disease, and developmental deficits. A thorough medical, physical, and neurologic examination is crucial to exclude organic etiologies. Additionally, given the potential for the use of psychopharmacologic agents to treat the psychotic symptoms, baseline assessments of metabolism, kidney and liver function, vital signs, and abnormal involuntary movements should be obtained as part of the initial evaluation.

Screening and Diagnostic Tools

The screening and diagnosis of COS is based on DSM-5 criteria for schizophrenia, the NIMH criteria for COS, and the longitudinal assessment of a pediatric patient. Rating scales are primarily used as screening tools and to monitor clinical progress (Table 17.2).

The NIMH COS cohort had a 44% false-positive COS diagnosis rate at the initial screening visit[21]; false-positive diagnosis is very likely higher for clinicians who have never or less frequently encountered the disease. Additionally, lengthy, medication-free

observation periods are not feasible in clinical practice. Thus, in an effort to help the clinical community, the NIMH CPB constructed an algorithm for classifying COS. After analyzing multiple variables (e.g., demographics, clinical history measures, IQ, rating scales, and antipsychotic medication), we concluded that COS can be distinguished by greater levels of positive and negative symptoms of psychosis and lower levels of depression.[44] The worksheet developed for child and adolescent patients who had onset of psychosis before 13 years of age uses only the NIMH Global Scale Psychosis Score and the NIMH Global Scale Depression Score to estimate the likelihood of a diagnosis of COS. This two-predictor model has 78.7% sensitivity, 77.6% specificity, 91% positive predictive value, and 55% negative predictive value (see Table 17.3).[44]

Comorbidity

COS is highly correlated with numerous comorbidities, both psychiatric and medical. Medical comorbidities account for almost 60% of premature deaths in adult schizophrenia.[8] Screening children with COS necessitates focused evaluation on growth, language,

TABLE 17.3

National Institute of Mental Health Global Scale: Ratings for Psychosis and Depression[45,46]

Scale	Psychosis	Depression
1–3 Minimal	Ratings of 2–3 may reflect odd or strange manner, apathy, somewhat flat affect, social withdrawal, inattention, or suspiciousness.	Ratings of 2–3 reflect some sadness, gloominess, pessimism, sluggishness, or mildly diminished interests, or diminished sense of competence.
4–6 Mild	Including some distortions of reality, difficulties with logic, instances of inappropriate affect, or inappropriate interpersonal relations. May rarely report hearing voices without responding to them or noninterfering delusions, without elaboration.	More persistent depressive symptoms, which may be directly expressed as sadness and depressive feelings, or as other symptoms such as somatic complaints, some feelings of inability to cope, increased dependency, disinterest in usual activities, or feeling slowed down and less able to function. Ordinarily, such symptoms would be somewhat evident to friends and relatives.
7–9 Moderate	With more evident conceptual disorganization, some reality testing and contact with reality is maintained (e.g., patient will consider staff explanations), but patient could not function for more than a day or two without hospitalization. Symptoms may include hallucinations, throughout the day, interfering delusions, severe thought blocking, loose associations, markedly inappropriate affect.	More pervasive depressive feelings, with helpless and hopelessness, social withdrawal, some psychomotor retardation and/or anxious agitation, and often problems sleeping (e.g., early morning awakening or excess sleep). Symptoms would usually lead to seeking treatment including hospitalization.
10–12 Severe	Major loss of contact with reality. Multiple psychotic symptoms are present including definite thought disorder, pervasive involvement with hallucinations, preoccupation with very bizarre thoughts or ideas, little control over behavior, and inability to function outside a hospital.	Depressive symptoms as described above, but associated with more marked helplessness, a sense of worthlessness, and often preoccupation with death. There may be impaired judgment or loss of insight, noncommunicativeness, and more retardation and/or agitation. Patient is unable to function outside a hospital.
13–15 Very severe	Absence of reality contact, with loss of ego boundaries. Multiple symptoms of psychosis continually present, although the patient will often be sufficiently out of touch that he/she may not verbalize symptoms. Frequently characterized by catatonia, sever agitation or combativeness, smearing, or word salad. Minimal self-care is usually impossible for the patient.	Depressive symptoms as above, but symptoms (e.g., muteness, extreme agitation, or retardation) are more profound and incapacitating. May also include depressive delusions (somatic delusions or delusions of guilt) or regressed behavior. Patents may require close supervision for eating and other basic activities.

From Greenstein D, Kataria R, Gochman P, Dasgupta A. Looking for childhood-onset schizophrenia: diagnostic algorithms for classifying children and adolescents with psychosis. *J Child Adolesc Psychopharm.* 2014;24(7):366–373, with permission.

and overall development. Sixty-seven percent of children with COS have learning disorders and/or show premorbid disturbances in social, motor, and language domains.[8] Adolescent- and adult-onset schizophrenia have similar premorbid impairments, with delays in language, motor development, and social functioning; however, these premorbid impairments tend to be more severe in COS.[32,34,35,47,48]

COS is associated with ASD both genotypically, with shared genetic risk factors,[1] and phenotypically, with social and cognitive disturbances.[49] In the NIMH study

of COS, 20% of children were screened positive for PDD,[8] now considered an ASD in the *DSM-5.* Although studies of adult schizophrenia have not identified ASD in the premorbid history,[50,51] 27% of patients with COS met ASD criteria before onset of psychotic symptoms.[48] COS patients with ASD and other developmental abnormalities have poorer clinical outcome and prognosis, which is correlated to severity of comorbid diagnoses.[52-54] Several studies suggest that developmental deficits could represent a premorbid phenotype in COS.[32,34,35,47,55,56]

The premorbid pathology of COS has been heavily explored. The NIMH cohort of COS patients demonstrated that about 55% of patients had language, motor, and/or social abnormalities several years before onset of psychotic symptoms; 87% of children had premorbid impairments in at least one of 15 domains with an average of 3.89 abnormalities per child.[8,31] Patients with COS often face challenges in the educational school system, with increased rates of poor grades and placement into special education programs.[33,35] Almost half of COS cases demonstrated PDD before onset of psychosis.[48]

Comorbid psychiatric conditions can make diagnosis of COS and management of symptoms more challenging. Beyond ASD and developmental impairments, psychiatric comorbidities include obsessive-compulsive disorder (OCD), ADHD, expressive and receptive language disorders, auditory processing deficits, executive functioning deficits, and mood disorders.[8] Depression was the most frequent comorbid diagnosis seen in 54% of the NIMH screening population, followed by OCD (21%), generalized anxiety disorder (15%), and ADHD (15%).[21] Although stimulants can potentially provoke or worsen psychotic symptoms, a case series demonstrated significant improvement in ADHD inattentive symptoms on stimulants after initial stabilization with an antipsychotic.[57] This small-scale study showed no worsening of psychotic symptoms, reflecting that physicians should continue to treat comorbid conditions. The most appropriate time to incorporate additional pharmacotherapy for comorbid disorders in COS patients is after stabilization with antipsychotics.

Primarily related to antipsychotic treatment side effects, medical comorbidities associated with COS include diabetes, hyperlipidemia, cardiovascular disease, obesity, hyperprolactinemia, and dyskinesia. Typical antipsychotics are more likely to produce hyperprolactinemia and dyskinesia, and atypical antipsychotics are more likely to produce the comorbidities seen in metabolic syndrome.

INTERVENTION

Once a diagnosis is established to a high degree of certainty, it is important not to delay treatment. Although the impact of delayed diagnosis is not well studied in pediatric populations, it is well established that the duration of untreated psychosis in adults is negatively associated with outcome.[58,59] Following the *DSM-5*, recommendation that dimensions be incorporated into clinical practice can facilitate a thorough evaluation, which in turn will inform a well-designed treatment plan.

Nonpharmacologic

Patients with early-onset schizophrenia typically have a more chronic course of illness, greater cognitive impairment, more negative symptoms, more severe social consequences and are typically more treatment refractory than patients with AOS.[60,61] Although psychopharmacologic intervention is foundational, psychotherapeutic and psychosocial interventions must be aggressively pursued to promote psychologic health and functional well-being, particularly during the window of childhood and adolescent brain development.[62] Interventions should be guided by the results of the exploration into comorbidity. The NIMH cohort frequently required speech-language, educational (i.e., treatment of learning disorders), executive functioning, individual therapy, family therapy, physical therapy, occupational therapy, and psychoeducational intervention.

Pharmacologic

Although mood stabilizers, antidepressants, and anxiolytics are often incorporated into the treatment regimen of a COS patient, the mainstay of therapy is antipsychotic medication. Antipsychotic medications are classified as either typical (i.e., first generation) or atypical (i.e., second generation) and differentiated by receptor affinity and associated side effect profiles.

Typical antipsychotics are high-affinity D_2 receptor antagonists. Side effects of antipsychotic therapies are linked to additional dopamine antagonism at unwanted locations of the brain (see Table 17.4). Typical antipsychotics are known for a higher risk of movement-related side effects and extrapyramidal symptoms (EPS) secondary to effects on the nigrostriatal pathway, which contains the vast majority of dopamine receptors in the brain.[63] Nearly all typical antipsychotics have FDA-approval for use in the pediatric population, with the exception of fluphenazine.[62] Chlorpromazine, droperidol, haloperidol, pimozide, thioridazine, and trifluoperazine are approved for use in children, and loxapine, molindone, perphenazine, and thiothixene are approved for use in adolescents.[62]

All antipsychotic agents have the potential of inducing neuroleptic malignant syndrome (NMS), more often seen in typical agents and with no relation to dose.[63] NMS is characterized by rigidity, high fever, autonomic instability, delirium, high creatinine phosphokinase, and elevated liver enzymes; it should be treated promptly with discontinuation of the offending medication, supportive therapy, and/or administration of the

TABLE 17.4
Dopaminergic Antagonism in Antipsychotic Medications

Implicated Pathway	Effects	Comments
Mesolimbic	Reduction in positive symptoms	Site of intended therapeutic effect, due to dopamine overactivity in psychosis
Mesocortical	Potential increase in negative symptoms	Negative symptoms are thought to be secondary to decreased dopamine in the mesocortical pathway

Nigrostriatal	Extrapyramidal symptoms:
	  Dystonia (sustained muscle contraction)
	
	  Parkinsonism (tremor, rigidity, bradykinesia)
	  Akathisia (motor restlessness, anxiety, agitation)
	  Tardive dyskinesia (abnormal involuntary movements, often involve mouth/tongue)
		Treated with:
		  Anticholinergic agent (e.g., benztropine, diphenhydramine)
		  Anticholinergic, antiparkinsonian agent (e.g., trihexyphenidyl, pramipexole)
		  β-blocker (e.g., propranolol), amantadine, benzodiazepine
		  Discontinue medication, switch to clozapine

Tuberoinfundibular	Hyperprolactinemia: amenorrhea, galactorrhea, gynecomastia, diminished libido, impotence	Decrease dose and/or switch medication (especially if on risperidone)

muscle relaxant dantrolene or the dopamine agonist bromocriptine.[63]

Atypical antipsychotics have an affinity for D_2 receptors, D_4 receptors, and 5-HT_{2A} receptors, as well as effects at other neuroreceptors based on specific medication.[64] Central 5-HT_{2A} receptor antagonism is thought to broaden the therapeutic effect while reducing incidence of EPS.[63]

Despite no evidence to demonstrate superior efficacy or tolerability, atypical antipsychotics are the most commonly prescribed form of psychopharmacology for most childhood and adolescent psychiatric disorders requiring treatment with antipsychotic agents, with an increase of 500% in prescriptions seen between 1995 and 2000.[65] The ratio of use for atypical to typical antipsychotics is greater for children (2.7:1) and adolescents (3.8:1) compared with adults (1.6:1),[66] although there has not been defined superiority of atypical use in pediatric patients compared with adults. Atypical agents have been used to treat aggression and oppositional behaviors often seen in ASD[67–71]; they have also shown effectiveness in lowering physical and verbal aggression scores in schizophrenia.[72]

Randomized-controlled trials against placebo have demonstrated efficacy of risperidone, olanzapine, quetiapine, aripiprazole, and paliperidone in adolescent schizophrenia, with no significant response differences between antipsychotic therapy.[73–77] In pediatric cases of schizophrenia, clozapine is the only antipsychotic that has demonstrated superior efficacy in clinical outcome.[77–79]

Although clozapine is a third-line medication, epidemiologic studies demonstrate that its use occurs later than recommended by current clinical guidelines.[26,80] In a study of clozapine use in COS and EOS using Danish medical registries, researchers found that 17.6% of patients had tried clozapine with an average of three antipsychotic medication trials before initiation of clozapine with an 88.8% favorable clinical response.[26] Significant predictors of clozapine use included older age at diagnosis, family history of schizophrenia, and attempted suicide,[26] possibly reflecting demographic characteristics that prompt a clinician to more readily prescribe a third-line agent.

Clozapine is associated with significant clinical improvement and low rates of discontinuation in EOS, with common adverse events, including sedation, hypersalivation, enuresis, and constipation.[81] Weight gain and metabolic changes are common (8%–22%) with infrequent macrovascular complications; although neutropenia is concerning, it occurs in 6%–15% of patients and is usually transient with <0.1% of patients experiencing agranulocytosis.[81] Rates of neutropenia in children and adolescents treated with clozapine are considerably higher than the adult population; despite this, neutropenia is largely benign with the vast majority of patients able to tolerate continued clozapine therapy.[82] Risk factors associated with neutropenia include younger age, African-American ethnicity, and male gender.[82]

The American Academy of Child and Adolescent Psychiatry recommends that atypical antipsychotic medications be used as a substitute rather than as an adjunct to the currently prescribed antipsychotic; polypharmacy should be avoided whenever possible.[83] Dosing should begin small and be increased based on the patient's response; an adequate medication trial is one at optimal dose for 6–8 weeks.[84] Although atypical agents are more frequently prescribed for the pediatric population, they have less FDA-approval than typical agents and few are approved for use in children. Aripiprazole and risperidone have been approved for treatment of aggression and irritability in pediatric ASD.[84] Aripiprazole, asenapine, olanzapine, paliperidone, quetiapine, and risperidone are FDA-approved medications for use in adolescents for schizophrenia and/or bipolar I disorder.[62,84]

Side effect profiles of atypical drugs are typically more variable than typical antipsychotics; in general, they exhibit lower rates of EPS and hyperprolactinemia. Aripiprazole and quetiapine are preferred therapies for patients sensitive to EPS or hyperprolactinemia, although aripiprazole is known for QT prolongation among the atypical antipsychotic medications.[63] Short-term cardiovascular side effects seen across atypicals, although infrequent, include prolongation of the QT interval, tachycardia, orthostatic hypotension, and pericarditis.[63,76,78,85] Atypical antipsychotics, most notably olanzapine and clozapine, are more likely to produce metabolic syndrome, a side effect to which children and adolescents appear more vulnerable than adults; aripiprazole, lurasidone, ziprasidone, paliperidone, and asenapine are considered more weight-neutral options.[63,76,77,84] The atypical antipsychotics show varying levels of glucose, cholesterol, and triglyceride elevation, and the FDA issued a boxed warning based on an increased risk of diabetes while on these medications.[84]

The American Psychiatric Association recommends monitoring to include personal and family history at baseline, body mass index every 4 weeks, waist circumference at baseline and annually, blood pressure every 12 weeks, fasting plasma glucose every 12 weeks, and fasting lipid profile every 12 weeks.[86]

IMPLICATIONS FOR CLINICAL PRACTICE

COS remains a devastating, multifactorial disease with numerous genetic and environmental factors implicated. Unfortunately, there is no known effective intervention to prevent psychosis. The gold standard clinical approach remains rooted in early identification, thorough evaluation, aggressive treatment, and close monitoring.

The evaluation of a patient for COS involves a multidisciplinary evaluation with a particular focus on comorbidities as they are highly prevalent in both the COS and rule-out populations. Proper treatment planning includes a multidisciplinary team engaging the patient in various therapies and nonpharmacologic interventions with antipsychotic medication as a foundation.

Clozapine is the only antipsychotic medication found to be clinically superior in treatment-refractory patients with both COS and its adult counterpart, and its use should not be delayed when it is indicated.

All antipsychotic medications are associated with adverse side effects, and although in varying degrees, EPS and metabolic side effects are common to both the typical and atypical antipsychotics medication. Adherence to the established guidelines for antipsychotic monitoring is imperative.

Even child and adolescent psychiatrists, who are best equipped to treat COS, often struggle in diagnosis and management of this disease. Clinicians should be astute and patient in their approach, heavily involve the family, and seek consult from a multidisciplinary team to achieve the greatest degree of clinical functioning.

REFERENCES

1. Asarnow RF, Forsyth JK. Genetics of childhood-onset schizophrenia. *Child Adolesc Psychiatr Clin N Am*. 2013;22:675–687.
2. Ahn K, An SS, Shugart YY, Rapoport JL. Common polygenic variation and risk for childhood-onset schizophrenia. *Mol Psychiatry*. 2016;21:94–96.
3. Rapoport JL, Addington AM, Frangou S, et al. The neurodevelopmental model of schizophrenia: update 2005. *Mol Psychiatry*. 2005;10:434–449.
4. Sullivan PF, Kendler KS, Neale MC. Schizophrenia as a complex trait: evidence from a meta-analysis of twin studies. *Arch Gen Psychiatry*. 2003;60(12):1187–1192.
5. Moran P, Stokes J, Marr J, et al. Gene x environment interactions in schizophrenia: evidence from genetic mouse models. *Neural Plast*. 2016;2016:2173748. https://doi.org/10.1155/2016/2173748.
6. Childs B, Scriver CR. Age at onset and causes of disease. *Perspect Biol Med*. 1986;29(3 Pt 1):437–460.
7. Clemmensen L, Vemal DL, Steinhausen H. A systematic review of the long-term outcome of early onset schizophrenia. *BMC Psychiatry*. 2012;12(150):1–16.
8. Driver DI, Gogtay N, Rapoport JL. Childhood onset schizophrenia and early onset schizophrenia spectrum disorders. *Child Adolesc Psychiatr Clin N Am*. 2013;22(4):539–555. https://doi.org/10.1016/j.chc.2013.04.001.
9. Craddock K, David CN, Driver DI, et al. Early-onset schizophrenia and psychotic illnesses. *Clin Man Child Adolesc Psychopharmacol*. 2017;3:439–501.

10. Calderoni D, Wudarsky M, Bhangoo R, et al. Differentiating childhood-onset schizophrenia from psychotic mood disorders. *J Am Acad Child Adolesc Psychiatry.* 2001;40(10):1190–1196.

11. David CN, Greenstein D, Clasen L, et al. Childhood onset schizophrenia: high rate of visual hallucinations. *J Am Acad Child Adolesc Psychiatry.* 2011;50(7):681–686.

12. Lukianowicz N. Hallucinations in non-psychotic children. *Psychiatr Clin (Basel).* 1969;2(6):321–337.

13. Caplan R. Thought disorder in childhood. *J Am Acad Child Adolesc Psychiatry.* 1994;33(5):605–615.

14. Polanczyk G, Moffitt TE, Arseneault L, et al. Etiological and clinical features of childhood psychotic symptoms: results from a birth cohort. *Arch Gen Psychiatry.* 2010;67:328–338.

15. American Psychiatric Association. Schizophrenia spectrum and other psychotic disorders. In: *Diagnostic and Statistical Manual of Mental Disorders.* 5th ed. Arlington, VA: American Psychiatric Publishing; 2013:87–122.

16. Hans-Jurgen M, Bandelow B, Bauer M, et al. DSM-5 reviewed from different angles: goal attainment, rationality, use of evidence, consequences-part 2: bipolar disorders, schizophrenia spectrum disorders, anxiety disorders, obsessive-compulsive disorders, trauma- and stressor-related disorders, personality disorders, substance-related and addictive disorders, neurocognitive disorders. *Eur Arch Psychiatry Clin Neurosci.* 2015;265:87–106.

17. Kuroki T, Ishitobi M, Kamio Y, et al. Current viewpoints on DSM-5 in Japan. *Psychiatry Clin Neurosci.* 2016;70(9):371–393.

18. Mattila T, Koeter M, Wohlfarth T, et al. Impact of DSM-5 changes on the diagnosis and acute treatment of schizophrenia. *Schizophr Bull.* 2015;41(3):637–643.

19. Rapoport JL, Giedd JN, Gogtay N. Neurodevelopmental model of schizophrenia: update 2012. *Mol Psychiatry.* 2012;17(12):1228–1238.

20. Mattai AK, Jill JL, Lenroot RK. Treatment of early-onset schizophrenia. *Curr Opin Psychiatry.* 2010;23:304–310.

21. Gochman P, Miller R, Rapoport JL. Childhood-onset schizophrenia: the challenge of diagnosis. *Curr Psychiatry Rep.* 2011;13(5):321–322.

22. Burd L, Kerbeshian J. A North Dakota prevalence study of schizophrenia presenting in childhood. *J Am Acad Child Adolesc Psychiatry.* 1987;26:347–350.

23. Remschmidt HE, Schulz E, Martin M, et al. Childhood-onset schizophrenia: history of the concept and recent studies. *Schizophr Bull.* 1994;20(4):727–745.

24. Gonthier M, Lyon MA. Childhood-onset schizophrenia: an overview. *Psychol Sch.* 2004;41:803–811.

25. McKenna K, Gordon CT, Lanane M, et al. Looking for childhood-onset schizophrenia: the first 71 cases screened. *J Am Acad Child Adolesc Psychiatry.* 1994;33(6):636–644.

26. Schneider C, Papachristou E, Wimberley T, et al. Clozapine use in childhood and adolescent schizophrenia: a nationwide population-based study. *Eur Neuropsychopharmacol.* 2015;25:857–863.

27. Cannon M, Jones P, Juttunen MO, et al. School performance in Finnish children and later development of schizophrenia: a population-based longitudinal study. *Arch Gen Psychiatry.* 1999;56:457–463.

28. Kelleher I, Cannon M. Psychotic-like experiences in the general population: characterizing a high-risk group for psychosis. *Psychol Med.* 2011;41(1):1–6.

29. Kelleher I, Connor D, Clarke MC, et al. Prevalence of psychotic symptoms in childhood and adolescence: a systematic review and meta-analysis of population-based studies. *Psychol Med.* 2012;42(9):1857–1863.

30. Payá B, Rodríguez-Sánchez JM, Otero S, et al. Premorbid impairments in early-onset psychosis: differences between patients with schizophrenia and bipolar disorder. *Schizophr Res.* 2013;146:103–110.

31. Driver DI, Greenstein D, Farmer M, et al. Poster #T66 Premorbid impairments in childhood-onset schizophrenia. *Schizophr Res.* 2014;153:S312.

32. Alaghband-Rad J, McKenna K, Gordon CT, et al. Childhood-onset schizophrenia: the severity of premorbid course. *J Am Acad Child Adolesc Psychiatry.* 1995;34(10):1273–1283.

33. Nicolson R, Rapoport JL. Childhood-onset schizophrenia: rare but worth studying. *Biol Psychiatry.* 1999;46(10):1418–1428.

34. Hollis C. Child and adolescent (juvenile onset) schizophrenia. A case control study of premorbid developmental impairments. *Br J Psychiatry.* 1995;166(4):489–495.

35. Nicolson R, Lenane M, Singaracharlu S, et al. Premorbid speech and language impairments in childhood-onset schizophrenia: association with risk factors. *Am J Psychiatry.* 2000;157(5):794–800.

36. Green WH, Padron-Gayol M, Hardesty AS, et al. Schizophrenia with childhood onset: a phenomenological study of 38 cases. *J Am Acad Child Adolesc Psychiatry.* 1992;31(5):968–976.

37. Squarcione C, Torti MC, Di Fabio F, Biondi M. 22q11 deletion syndrome: a review of the neuropsychiatric features and their neurobiological basis. *Neuropsychiatr Dis Treat.* 2013;9:1873–1884.

38. Yuen T, Chow EWC, Silversides CK, Bassett AS. Premorbid adjustment and schizophrenia in individuals with 22q11.2 deletion syndrome. *Schizophr Res.* 2013;151:221–225.

39. Fiksinski AM, Breetvelt EJ, Duijff SN, et al. Autism Spectrum and psychosis risk in the 22q11.2 deletion syndrome. Findings from a prospective longitudinal study. *Schizophr Res.* 2017;188. [Epub].

40. Demily C, Franck N. Cognitive behavioral therapy in 22q11.2 microdeletion with psychotic symptoms: what do we learn from schizophrenia? *Eur J Med Gen.* 2016;59:596–603.

41. Monks S, Niarchou M, Davies AR, et al. Further evidence for high rates of schizophrenia in 22q11.2 deletion syndrome. *Schizophr Res.* 2014;(153):231–236.

42. Kumra S, Jacobsen LK, Lenane M, et al. "Multidimensionally impaired disorder": is it a variant of very early-onset schizophrenia? *J Am Acad Child Adolesc Psychiatry.* 1998;37(1):91–99.

43. Towbin KE, Dykens EM, Pearson GS, et al. Conceptualizing "borderline syndrome of childhood" and "childhood schizophrenia" as a developmental disorder. *J Am Acad Child Adolesc Psychiatry.* 1993;32(4):775–782.

44. Greenstein D, Kataria R, Gochman P, Dasgupta A. Looking for childhood-onset schizophrenia: diagnostic algorithms for classifying children and adolescents with psychosis. *J Child Adolesc Psychopharmacol.* 2014;24(7):366–373.

45. Murphy DL, Pickar D, Alterman IS. Methods for the quantitative assessment of depressive and manic behavior. In: Burdock EL, Sudilovsky A, Gershon S, eds. *The Behavior of Psychiatric Patients.* New York: Marcel Dekker; 1982:355–392.

46. Sunderland T, Alterman IS, Yount D, et al. A new scale for the assessment of depressed mood in demented patients. *Am J Psychiatry.* 1988;145(8):955–959.

47. Russell A, Bott L, Sammons C. The phenomena of schizophrenia occurring in childhood. *J Am Acad Child Adolesc Psychiatry.* 1989;28:399–407.

48. Rapoport J, Chavez A, Greenstein D, et al. Autism spectrum disorders and childhood-onset schizophrenia: clinical and biological contributions to a relation revisited. *J Am Acad Child Adolesc Psychiatry.* 2009;48(1):10–18.

49. Canitano R, Pallagrosi M. Autism spectrum disorders and schizophrenia spectrum disorders: excitation/inhibition imbalance and developmental trajectories. *Front Psychiatry.* 2017;8(69):1–7.

50. Done DJ, Crow TJ, Johnstone EC, et al. Childhood antecedents of schizophrenia and affective illness: social adjustment at ages 7 and 11. *BMJ.* 1994;309(6956):699–703.

51. Jones P, Rodgers B, Murray R, et al. Child development risk factors for adult schizophrenia in the British 1946 birth cohort. *Lancet.* 1994;344(8934):1398–1402.

52. Gupta S, Rajaprabhakaran R, Arndt S, et al. Premorbid adjustment as a predictor of phenomenological and neurobiological indices in schizophrenia. *Schizophr Res.* 1995;16(3):189–197.

53. Gupta S, Andreasen NC, Arndt S, et al. Neurological soft signs in neuroleptic-naive and neuroleptic-treated schizophrenic patients and in normal comparison subjects. *Am J Psychiatry.* 1995;152(2):191–196.

54. Gupta SK, Kunka RL, Metz A, et al. Effect of alosetron (a new 5-HT3 receptor antagonist) on the pharmacokinetics of haloperidol in schizophrenic patients. *J Clin Pharmacol.* 1995;35(2):202–207.

55. Asarnow JR, Ben-Meir S. Children with schizophrenia spectrum and depressive disorders: a comparative study of premorbid adjustment, onset pattern and severity of impairment. *J Child Psychol Psychiatry.* 1988;29(4):477–488.

56. Watkins JM, Asarnow RF, Tanguay PE. Symptom development in childhood onset schizophrenia. *J Child Psychol Psychiatry.* 1988;29(6):865–878.

57. Tossell JW, Greenstein DK, Davidson AL, et al. Stimulant drug treatment in childhood-onset schizophrenia with comorbid ADHD: an open-label case series. *J Child Adolesc Psychopharmacol.* 2004;14:448–454.

58. Singh SP. Outcome measures in early psychosis; relevance of duration of untreated psychosis. *Br J Psychiatry Suppl.* 2007;50:s58–s63.

59. Black K, Peters L, Rui Q, et al. Duration of untreated psychosis predicts treatment outcome in an early psychosis program. *Schizophr Res.* 2001;47(2–3):215–222.

60. Hassan GA, Taha GR. Long term functioning in early onset psychosis: two years prospective follow-up study. *Behav Brain Funct.* 2011;7(28):1–10.

61. Correll CU. Symptomatic presentation and initial treatment for schizophrenia in children and adolescents. *J Clin Psychiatry.* 2010;71(29).

62. Chan V. Schizophrenia and psychosis: diagnosis, current research trends, and model treatment approaches with implications for transitional age youth. *Child Adolesc Psychiatr Clin N Am.* 2017;26:341–366.

63. Black DW, Andreasen NC. Psychopharmacology and electroconvulsive therapy. In: *Introductory Textbook of Psychiatry.* 6th ed. Arlington, VA: American Psychiatric Publishing; 2014:541–590.

64. Burstein ES, Ma J, Wong S, et al. Intrinsic efficacy of antipsychotics at human D2, D3, and D4 dopamine receptors: identification of the clozapine metabolite N-desmethyl-clozapine as a D2/D3 partial agonist. *J Pharmacol Exp Ther.* 2005;315:1278–1287.

65. Patel NC, Sanchez RJ, Johnsrud MT, et al. Trends in antipsychotic use in a Texas Medicaid population of children and adolescents: 1996 to 2000. *J Child Adolesc Psychopharmacol.* 2002;12:221–229.

66. Sikich L, Hamer RM, Bashford RA, et al. A pilot study of risperidone, olanzapine, and haloperidol in psychotic youth: a double-blind, randomized, 8-week trial. *Neuropsychopharmacology.* 2004;29:133–145.

67. Pappadopulos E, Macintyre II JC, Crismon ML, et al. Treatment recommendations for the use of antipsychotics for aggressive youth (TRAAY). Part II. *J Am Acad Child Adolesc Psychiatry.* 2003;42:145–161.

68. DelBello M, Grcevich S. Phenomenology and epidemiology of childhood psychiatric disorders that may necessitate treatment with atypical antipsychotics. *J Clin Psychiatry.* 2004;65(suppl 6):12–19.

69. Burcu M, Zito JM, Ibe A, et al. Atypical antipsychotic use among Medicaid-insured children and adolescents: duration, safety, and monitoring implications. *J Child Adolesc Psychopharmacol.* 2014;24:112–119.

70. Aman MG, Bukstein OG, Gadow KD, et al. What does risperidone add to parent training and stimulant for severe aggression in child attention-deficit/hyperactivity disorder? *J Am Acad Child Adolesc Psychiatry.* 2014;53(41):47–60.

71. Gadow KD, Arnold LE, Molina BS, et al. Risperidone added to parent training and stimulant medication: effects on attention-deficit/hyperactivity disorder, oppositional defiant disorder, conduct disorder, and peer aggression. *J Am Acad Child Adolesc Psychiatry.* 2014;53:948–959.

72. Fond G, Boyer L, Favez M, et al. Medication and aggressiveness in real-world schizophrenia. Results from the FACE-SZ dataset. *Psychopharmacology.* 2016;223:571–578.

73. Kumra A, Datta SS, Wright SD, et al. Atypical antipsychotics for psychosis in adolescents. *Cochrane Database Syst Rev.* 2013;10:CD009582.
74. Sikich L, Frazier JA, McClellan J, et al. Double-blind comparison of first- and second-generation antipsychotics in early-onset schizophrenia and schizo-affective disorder: findings from the Treatment of Early-Onset Schizophrenia Spectrum Disorders (TEOSS) study. *Am J Psychiatry.* 2008;165:1420–1431.
75. Findling RL, Johnson JL, McClellan J, et al. Double-blind maintenance safety and effectiveness findings from the Treatment of Early-Onset Schizophrenia Spectrum (TEOSS) study. *J Am Acad Child Adolesc Psychiatry.* 2010;49:583–594.
76. McClellan J, Stock S, American Academy of Child and Adolescent Psychiatry (AACAP) Committee on Quality Issues (CQI). Practice parameter for the assessment and treatment of children and adolescents with schizophrenia. *J Am Acad Child Adolesc Psychiatry.* 2013;52:976–990.
77. Correll CU, Kratochvil CJ, March JS. Developments in pediatric psychopharmacology: focus on stimulants, antidepressants, and antipsychotics. *J Clin Psychiatry.* 2011;72:655–670.
78. Kumra S, Oberstar JV, Sikich L, et al. Efficacy and tolerability of second-generation antipsychotics in children and adolescents with schizophrenia. *Schizophr Bull.* 2008;34:60–71.
79. Sporn AL, Vermani A, Greenstein DK, et al. Clozapine treatment of childhood-onset schizophrenia: evaluation of effectiveness, adverse effects, and long-term outcome. *J Am Acad Child Adolesc Psychiatry.* 2007;46(10):1349–1356.
80. Vera I, Rezende L, Molina V, et al. Clozapine as treatment of first choice in first psychotic episodes. What do we know? *Actas Esp Psiquiatr.* 2012;40(5):281–289.
81. Schneider C, Corrigall R, Hayes D, et al. Systematic review of the efficacy and tolerability of clozapine in the treatment of youth with early onset schizophrenia. *Eur Psychiatry.* 2014;29(1):1–10.
82. Maher KN, Tan M, Tossell JW, et al. Risk factors for neutropenia in clozapine-treated children and adolescents with childhood-onset schizophrenia. *J Child Adolesc Psychopharmacol.* 2013;23:110–116.
83. American Academy of Child and Adolescent Psychiatry. Practice parameter on the use of psychotropic medication in children and adolescents. *J Am Acad Child Adolesc Psychiatry.* 2009;48:961–973.
84. Giles LL, Martini R. Challenges and promises of pediatric psychopharmacology. *Acad Pediatr.* 2016;16:508–518.
85. Jensen KG, Juul K, Fink-Jensen A, et al. Corrected QT changes during antipsychotic treatment of children and adolescents: a systematic review and meta-analysis of clinical trials. *J Am Acad Child Adolesc Psychiatry.* 2015;54:225–236.
86. American Diabetes Association, American Psychiatric Association, American Association of Clinical Endocrinologists, North American Association for the Study of Obesity. Consensus development conference on antipsychotic drugs and obesity and diabetes. *Diabetes Care.* 2004;27:596–601.

FURTHER READING

1. Ahn K, Gogtay N, Andersen TM, et al. High rate of disease-related copy number variations in childhood onset schizophrenia. *Mol Psychiatry.* 2014;19:568–572.
2. Nicolson R, Giedd JN, Lenane M, et al. Clinical and neurobiological correlates of cytogenetic abnormalities in childhood-onset schizophrenia. *Am J Psychiatry.* 1999;156(10):1575–1579.
3. Rapoport JL, Gogtay N. Childhood onset schizophrenia: support for a progressive neurodevelopmental disorder. *Int J Dev Neurosci.* 2011;29(3):251–258.
4. Gordon CT, Frazier JA, McKenna K, et al. Childhood-onset schizophrenia: an NIMH study in progress. *Schizophr Bull.* 1994;20(4):697–712.
5. Volkmar FR. Childhood and adolescent psychosis: a review of the past 10 years. *J Am Acad Child Adolesc Psychiatry.* 1996;35:843–851.
6. Kolvin I. Studies in the childhood psychoses. I. Diagnostic criteria and classification. *Br J Psychiatry.* 1971;118(545):381–384.
7. Poulton R, Caspi A, Moffitt TE, et al. Children's self-reported psychotic symptoms and adult schizophreniform disorder: a 15-year longitudinal study. *Arch Gen Psychiatry.* 2000;57:1053–1058.
8. Jablensky A. Schizophrenia in DSM-5: assets and liabilities. *Schizophr Res.* 2013;150:36–37.
9. Nemeroff CB, Weinberger D, Rutter M, et al. DSM-5: a collection of psychiatrist views on the changes, controversies, and future directions. *BMC Med.* 2013;11(202):1–19.
10. Ross CA. Problems with autism, catatonia, and schizophrenia in DSM-5. *Schizophr Res.* 2014;158:264–265.
11. Dahl EK, Cohen DJ, Provence S. Clinical and multivariate approaches to the nosology of pervasive developmental disorders. *J Am Acad Child Psychiatry.* 1986;25(2):170–180.
12. Petti TA, Vela RM. Borderline disorders of childhood: an overview. *J Am Acad Child Adolesc Psychiatry.* 1990;29(3):327–337.
13. Van der Gaag RJ, Buitelaar J, Van den Ban E, et al. A controlled multivariate chart review of multiple complex developmental disorder. *J Am Acad Child Adolesc Psychiatry.* 1995;34(8):1096–1106.
14. Cohen DJ, Paul R, Volkmar FR. Issues in the classification of pervasive and other developmental disorders: toward DSM-IV. *J Am Acad Child Psychiatry.* 1986;25(2):213–220.
15. Ad-Dab'bagh Y, Greenfield B. Multiple complex developmental disorder: the "multiple and complex" evolution of the "childhood borderline syndrome" construct. *J Am Acad Child Adolesc Psychiatry.* 2001;40(8):954–964.
16. Nicolson R, Lenane M, Brookner F, et al. Children and adolescents with psychotic disorder not otherwise specified: a 2- to 8-year follow-up study. *Compr Psychiatry.* 2001;42(4):319–325.
17. Gogtay N, Ordonez A, Herman DH, et al. Dynamic mapping of cortical development before and after the onset of pediatric bipolar illness. *J Child Psychol Psychiatry.* 2007;48(9):852–862.

18. Lawrie SM, Abukmeil SS. Brain abnormality in schizophrenia. A systematic and quantitative review of volumetric magnetic resonance imaging studies. *Br J Psychiatry*. 1998;172:110–120.

19. Wright IC, Rabe-Hesketh S, Woodruff PW, et al. Meta-analysis of regional brain volumes in schizophrenia. *Am J Psychiatry*. 2000;157(1):16–25.

20. Shenton ME, Dickey CC, Frumin M, et al. A review of MRI findings in schizophrenia. *Schizophr Res*. 2001;49(1-2): 1–52.

21. Pantelis C, Yucel M, Wood SJ, et al. Structural brain imaging evidence for multiple pathological processes at different stages of brain development in schizophrenia. *Schizophr Bull*. 2005;31(3):672–696.

22. Mathalon DH, Sullivan EV, Lim KO, et al. Progressive brain volume changes and the clinical course of schizophrenia in men: a longitudinal magnetic resonance imaging study. *Arch Gen Psychiatry*. 2001;58(2):148–157.

23. Gur RE, Cowell P, Turetsky BI, et al. A follow-up magnetic resonance imaging study of schizophrenia. Relationship of neuroanatomical changes to clinical and neurobehavioral measures. *Arch Gen Psychiatry*. 1998;55(2):145–152.

24. Anvari AA, Friedman LA, Greenstein D, et al. Hippocampal volume change relates to clinical outcome in childhood-onset schizophrenia. *Psychol Med*. 2015;45(12):2667–2674.

25. Lieberman J, Chakos M, Wu H, et al. Longitudinal study of brain morphology in first episode schizophrenia. *Biol Psychiatry*. 2001;49(6):487–499.

26. DeLisi LE. Regional brain volume change over the life-time course of schizophrenia. *J Psychiatr Res*. 1999;33(6):535–541.

27. Gogtay N. Cortical brain development in schizophrenia: insights from neuroimaging studies in childhood-onset schizophrenia. *Schizophr Bull*. 2008;34(1):30–36.

28. Gogtay N, Weisinger B, Bakalar JL, et al. Psychotic symptoms and gray matter deficits in clinical pediatric populations. *Schizophr Res*. 2012;140(1-3):149–154.

29. Sporn AL, Greenstein DK, Gogtay N, et al. Progressive brain volume loss during adolescence in childhood-onset schizophrenia. *Am J Psychiatry*. 2003;160(12):2181–2189.

30. Gogtay N, Sporn A, Clasen LS, et al. Structural brain MRI abnormalities in healthy siblings of patients with childhood-onset schizophrenia. *Am J Psychiatry*. 2003;160(3):569–571.

31. Gogtay N, Sporn A, Clasen LS, et al. Comparison of progressive cortical gray matter loss in childhood-onset schizophrenia with that in childhood-onset atypical psychoses. *Arch Gen Psychiatry*. 2004;61(1):17–22.

32. Hollis C. Adult outcomes of child- and adolescent-onset schizophrenia: diagnostic stability and predictive validity. *Am J Psychiatry*. 2000;157:1652–1659.

33. Eggers C, Bunk D. The long-term course of childhood-onset schizophrenia: a 42-year follow-up. *Schizophr Bull*. 1997;23:105–117.

34. Ienciu M, Romosan F, Bredicean C, et al. First episode psychosis and treatment delay–causes and consequences. *Psychiatr Danub*. 2010;22(4):540–543.

35. Franz L, Carter T, Leiner AS, et al. Stigma and treatment delay in first-episode psychosis: a grounded theory study. *Early Interv Psychiatry*. 2010;4(1):47–56.

36. Norman RM, Mallal AK, Manchanda R, et al. Does treatment delay predict occupational functioning in first-episode psychosis? *Schizophr Res*. 2007;91(1-3):259–262.

37. Compton MT, Esterberg ML. Treatment delay in first-episode nonaffective psychosis: a pilot study with African American family members and the theory of planned behavior. *Compr Psychiatry*. 2005;46(4):291–295.

38. Harrigan SM, McGorry PD, Krstev H. Does treatment delay in first-episode psychosis really matter? *Psychol Med*. 2003;33(1):97–110.

39. Khandaker GM, Stochl J, Zammit S, et al. A population-based longitudinal study of childhood neurodevelopmental disorders, IQ and subsequent risk of psychotic experiences in adolescent. *Psychol Med*. 2014;44:3229–3238.

40. Moran LV, Masters GA, Pingali S, et al. Prescription stimulant use is associated with earlier onset of psychosis. *J Psychiatr Res*. 2015;71:41–47.

41. Andrianarisoa M, Boyer L, Godin O, et al. Childhood trauma, depression and negative symptoms are independently associated with impaired quality of life in schizophrenia. Results from the national FACE-SZ cohort. *Schizophr Res*. 2017;185:173–181.

42. Kilian S, Burns JK, Seedat S, et al. Factors moderating the relationship between childhood trauma and premorbid adjustment in first-episode schizophrenia. *PLoS One*. 2017;12(1):1–14.

43. Scherr M, Hamann M, Schwerthoffer D, et al. Environmental risk factors and their impact on the age of onset of schizophrenia: comparing familial to non-familial schizophrenia. *Nord J Psychiatry*. 2012;66(2):107–114.

44. Barker V, Bois C, Neilson E, et al. Childhood adversity and hippocampal and amygdala volumes in a population at familial high risk of schizophrenia. *Schizophr Res*. 2016;175:42–47.

45. Botellero VL, Skranes J, Bjuland KJ, et al. A longitudinal study of associations between psychiatric symptoms and disorders and cerebral gray matter volumes in adolescents born very preterm. *BMC Pediatr*. 2017;17(45):1–17.

46. Knuesel I, Chicha L, Britschgi M, et al. Maternal immune activation and abnormal brain development across CNS disorders. *Nat Rev Neurol*. 2014;10(11):643–660.

47. McGrath JJ, Petersen L, Agerbo E, et al. A comprehensive assessment of parental age and psychiatric disorders. *JAMA Psychiatry*. 2014;71(3):301–309.

48. Limosin F. Neurodevelopmental and environmental hypotheses of negative symptoms of schizophrenia. *BMC Psychiatry*. 2014;14(88):1–6.

49. Husted JA, Ahmed R, Chow EWC, et al. Early environmental exposures influence schizophrenia expression even in the presence of strong genetic predisposition. *Schizophr Res*. 2012;137:166–168.

50. Howes OD, McCutcheon R, Owen MJ, Murray RM. The role of genes, stress, and dopamine in the development of schizophrenia. *Biol Psychiatry*. 2017;81:9–20.

51. Davis J, Eyre H, Jacka FN, et al. A review of vulnerability and risks for schizophrenia: beyond the two hit hypothesis. *Neurosci Biobehav Rev.* 2016;65:185–194.

52. Gogos JA, Gerber DJ. Schizophrenia susceptibility genes: emergence of positional candidates and future directions. *Trends Pharmacol Sci.* 2006;27(4):226–233.

53. Weinberger DR. Implications of normal brain development for the pathogenesis of schizophrenia. *Arch Gen Psychiatry.* 1987;44(7):660–669.

54. Feinberg I. Schizophrenia: caused by a fault in programmed synaptic elimination during adolescence? *J Psychiatr Res.* 1982;17(4):319–334.

55. Miyamoto S, LaMantia AS, Duncan GE, et al. Recent advances in the neurobiology of schizophrenia. *Mol Interv.* 2003;3(1):27–39.

56. Weinberger DR. The biological basis of schizophrenia: new directions. *J Clin Psychiatry.* 1997;58(suppl 10):22–27.

57. Marin O. Interneuron dysfunction in psychiatric disorders. *Nat Rev Neurosci.* 2012;13(2):107–120.

58. Henn FA. Dopamine: a marker of psychosis and final common driver of schizophrenia psychosis. *Am J Psychiatry.* 2011;168(12):1239–1240.

59. Lewis DA, Gonzalez-Burgos G. Neuroplasticity of neocortical circuits in schizophrenia. *Neuropsychopharmacology.* 2008;33(1):141–165.

60. Beneyto M, Lewis DA. Insights into the neurodevelopmental origin of schizophrenia from postmortem studies of prefrontal cortical circuitry. *Int J Dev Neurosci.* 2011;29(3):295–304.

61. Howes OD, Bose SK, Turkheimer F, et al. Dopamine synthesis capacity before onset of psychosis: a prospective [18F]-DOPA PET imaging study. *Am J Psychiatry.* 2011;168(12):1311–1317.

62. Howes OD, Kapur S. The dopamine hypothesis of schizophrenia: version III–the final common pathway. *Schizophr Bull.* 2009;35(3):549–562.

63. Addington AM, Rapoport JL. The genetics of childhood-onset schizophrenia: when madness strikes the prepubescent. *Curr Psychiatry Rep.* 2009;11:156–161.

64. Ordonez AE, Luscher ZI, Gogtay N. Neuroimaging findings from childhood onset schizophrenia patients and their non-psychotic siblings. *Schizophr Res.* 2016;173:124–131.

65. Gogtay N, Giedd JN, Lusk L, et al. Dynamic mapping of human cortical development during childhood through early adulthood. *Proc Natl Acad Sci USA.* 2004;101(21):8174–8179.

66. Gogtay N, Greenstein D, Lenane M, et al. Cortical brain development in nonpsychotic siblings of patients with childhood-onset schizophrenia. *Arch Gen Psychiatry.* 2007;64(7):772–780.

67. Greenstein D, Lerch J, Shaw P, et al. Childhood onset schizophrenia: cortical brain abnormalities as young adults. *J Child Psychol Psychiatry.* 2006;47(10):1003–1012.

68. Greenstein D, Lenroot R, Clausen L, et al. Cerebellar development in childhood onset schizophrenia and nonpsychotic siblings. *Psychiatry Res Neuroimaging.* 2011;193: 131–137.

69. Waltman D, Knowlton BJ, Cohen JR, et al. DTI microstructural abnormalities in adolescent siblings of patients with childhood-onset schizophrenia. *Psychiatry Res Neuroimaging.* 2016;258:23–29.

70. Mattai AA, Weisinger B, Greenstein D, et al. Normalization of cortical gray matter deficits in nonpsychotic siblings of patients with childhood-onset schizophrenia. *J Am Acad Child Adolesc Psychiatry.* 2011;50(7):697–704.

71. Chakravarty MM, Rapoport JL, Giedd JN, et al. Striatal shape abnormalities as novel neurodevelopmental endophenotypes in schizophrenia: a longitudinal study. *Hum Brain Mapp.* 2015;36:1458–1469.

72. Wagshal D, Knowlton BJ, Cohen JR, et al. Cognitive correlates of gray matter abnormalities in adolescent siblings of patients with childhood-onset schizophrenia. *Schizophr Res.* 2015;161:345–350.

73. Zalesky A, Pantelis C, Cropley V, et al. Delayed development of brain connectivity in adolescents with schizophrenia and their unaffected siblings. *JAMA Psychiatry.* 2015;72(9):900–908.

74. Watsky RE, Ludovici Pollard K, Greenstein D, et al. Severity of cortical thinning correlates with schizophrenia spectrum symptoms. *J Am Acad Child Adolesc Psychiatry.* 2016;55(2):130–136.

75. Sawa A, Snyder SH. Schizophrenia: diverse approaches to a complex disease. *Science.* 2002;296(5568):692–695.

76. Kleinman JE, Law AJ, Lipska BK, et al. Genetic neuropathology of schizophrenia: new approaches to an old question and new uses for postmortem human brains. *Biol Psychiatry.* 2011;69(2):140–145.

77. Brennand KJ, Simone A, Jou J, et al. Modelling schizophrenia using human induced pluripotent stem cells. *Nature.* 2011;493:221–225.

78. Tandon R, Keshavan MS, Nasrallah HA. Schizophrenia, "just the facts" what we know in 2008. Part 2. Epidemiology and etiology. *Schizophr Res.* 2008;102(1–3): 1–18.

79. Keshavan MS, Tandon R, Boutros NN, et al. Schizophrenia, "just the facts": what we know in 2008. Part 3: neurobiology. *Schizophr Res.* 2008;106(2–3):89–107.

80. Tsuang MT, Faraone SV. The case for heterogeneity in the etiology of schizophrenia. *Schizophr Res.* 1995;17(2):161–175.

Clinical Pearls Appendix

Chapters	Clinical Pearls
1. Gender Dysphoria in Childhood and Adolescence	• Gender dysphoria is a term created by the Diagnostic and Statistical Manual of Mental Disorders, Fifth Edition (DSM-5) to describe the distress that might be present in the context of incongruence between sex assigned at birth and gender identity. • Individuals who experience incongruence between biologic sex and gender identity are forced to face intense minority stress, overtly and covertly, and it is unsurprising that transgender adolescents often have alarmingly high rates of mental health issues, including increased suicidal ideation and suicide attempts. • Between ages of 5–7 years, children begin to understand *gender constancy*, the concept that everyone's gender is stable. For some children, this period where gender constancy solidifies is when we begin to see an increase in gender dysphoria because there is less fluidity in gender cognitively at this period. • Social transition has been identified as a protective factor for many transgender and gender nonconforming youth. • Most children and teens who meet criteria for gender dysphoria do not have a cooccurring mental health issue.
2. School Refusal	• School refusal is conceptualized based on the functionality of the school refusal behaviors, which fall into one of the four major categories. These categories are divided into students who refuse school to (1) avoid school-related stimuli that provoke a general sense of negative affectivity (i.e., anxiety and depression); (2) escape school-related aversive social and/or evaluative situations; (3) gain attention from significant others (e.g., parents); and/or (4) pursue tangible reinforcement outside of school. • Being bullied has been linked to higher rates of absenteeism. • With regard to diagnostic evaluation, it is important to consider a broad range of disorders as well as the **absence of a diagnosable mental disorder**. • School-refusing children often report a range of somatic complaints. • As school refusal is a complicated behavior that involves the interaction of individual, family, and school variables, effective treatment will need to be comprehensive. Four specific treatment components have been identified: (1) individual exposure-based cognitive behavioral therapy, (2) group therapy for youth exhibiting school refusal behavior, (3) parent management training, and (4) school consultation and collaboration.
3. Attention Deficit Hyperactivity Disorder and Anxiety	• Comorbid anxiety disorders are reported to occur in 30%–40% in clinical psychiatric samples of children with attention deficit hyperactivity disorder (ADHD) as well as pediatric samples. • Parents are more reliable informants for externalizing disorders such as ADHD, and children and adolescents are more reliable informants for internalizing disorders such as anxiety. • The Vanderbilt ADHD Teacher (VADTRS) and Parent rating scales (VADPRS) are straightforward instruments that follow DSM-IV criteria for ADHD and include 12 criteria for conduct disorder and 7 criteria from the Pediatric Behavior Scale, which screen for anxiety and depression in children aged 6–12 years. Both versions of the Vanderbilt ADHD Rating Scale have been validated and shown to be statistically significant instruments. The VADTRS and VADPRS are in the public domain and available widely free-of-charge. • Assessing sleep is very important. • Stimulant treatment significantly decreased risk of anxiety when compared with placebo. Therefore comorbid anxiety is not a contraindication for stimulant treatment.

Chapters	Clinical Pearls
4. Tourette Syndrome	• Tourette syndrome is not a functional disorder; however, tics are often exacerbated by stress, disappear (for the most part) in sleep, and are usually suppressible (at least for brief periods). • Tics peak at approximately 10 years and have a tendency to improve during adolescence. • Age of onset or initial complexity does not predict prognosis. • There is no evidence that ADHD medications directly cause tics; however, the mechanism of action of stimulants can sometimes bring out or exacerbate tics in the genetically primed individual. • Medications are appropriate for many moderately to seriously affected individuals, but the majority will not require drug treatment if tics are mild and do not interfere with the child's ability to function at home or in school.
5. Management of ADHD in Youth With Comorbid Epilepsy	• The presence of epilepsy predisposes children to a much higher likelihood of being diagnosed with psychiatric illnesses such as depression, anxiety, ADHD, conduct disorder, developmental delay, or autistic spectrum disorder. • Children with epilepsy are much more likely to have ADHD. Children with ADHD are much more likely to have abnormal epileptiform discharges on an EEG and eventually develop a seizure disorder than those without ADHD. As many as 40% or more of children with epilepsy will also have ADHD. • Many clinicians undertreat ADHD in this population, leading to additional morbidity. • The significant overlap of the common finding of inattention in both, patients with ADHD and patients with epilepsy, makes it imperative to establish whether the ADHD symptoms were present before the onset of seizures. • Patients with epilepsy controlled well on one antiepileptic medication were, in general, able to be started on methylphenidate without any new seizure onset or complication.
6. Evolution From Feeding Disorders to Avoidant-Restrictive Food Intake Disorder	• Eating disorders in young children and infants are generally referred to as "feeding disorders," to emphasize the relationship between caregiver and child that may be strained or dysregulated in these conditions. • Many times, parents are blamed for their children's low appetite or selectivity, creating more shame and isolation in those parents, which leads to more anxiety and perpetuates the dysfunctional cycle of negative parent-child interactions. • The DSM-5 differentiates avoidant-restrictive food intake disorder (ARFID) from more common feeding difficulties by requiring at least one of the following: (1) significant weight loss (or failure to achieve expected weight gain or faltering growth in children), (2) significant nutritional deficiency, (3) dependence on enteral feeding or oral nutritional supplements, and (4) marked interference with psychosocial functioning. • The DSM-5 describes three main types of ARFID: (1) those with an apparent lack of interest in food and eating, (2) those with sensory aversions to specific food characteristics, and (3) those with a conditioned negative association and fear of eating due to or in anticipation of an aversive experience. • Regular meal and bedtimes are very important for these children.
7. Eating Disorders	• In the DSM-5 criteria for anorexia nervosa, the amenorrhea criterion was removed, and there is no longer a weight criterion. Instead, the degree of being underweight is determined via age, gender, and developmental trajectory. • Almost one-third of adolescents with anorexia nervosa reported suicidal ideation. • To meet criteria for binge eating disorder, individuals must have recurrent episodes of binge eating (as defined in bulimia) but do not engage in compensatory behaviors. • In a majority of cases, there is no need for medication. • Treatment should focus on increasing weight to a developmentally appropriate level and then reevaluating for comorbid conditions.

8. Childhood Stress and Trauma	<ul><li>The most common reasons that children and adolescents are referred to treatment are disruptive behaviors and ADHD; in both cases it is highly likely that the problematic behaviors have been caused or exacerbated by chronic stress and traumatic experiences.</li><li>Disorders related to chronic stress and traumatic experiences manifest not only as posttraumatic stress disorder (PTSD) but also as diagnoses consistent with disruptive behaviors (e.g., disruptive mood dysregulation disorder [DMDD], ADHD, and oppositional defiant disorder), mood issues (e.g., depression and anxiety), learning disorders, and other common childhood psychiatric disorders.</li><li>Chronic stress and traumatic experiences leading to psychopathology or a single incident event leading to PTSD are caused by injury to neurophysiology such as hypothalamic-pituitary-adrenal axis dysregulation, genes via epigenetic mechanisms (e.g., methylation/demethylation, telomeric shortening,) and to brain structure through multiple pathways.</li><li>Any diagnostic assessment should include an assessment of TRAUMA and a comprehensive developmental history, including a psychosocial evaluation of stress and trauma exposure.</li><li>Core components to evidence-based trauma treatments include (1) engagement, (2) psychoeducation, (3) emotional regulation, (4) promotion of positive adjustment, (5) parenting skills, (6) trauma narrative, (7) promotion of safety, (8) attachment and strengthening relationships, (9) attention to social context, and (10) posttrauma growth.</li></ul>
9. Factitious Disorder Imposed on Another	<ul><li>Munchausen by proxy, which has never been a formal International Statistical Classification of Diseases and Related Health Problems (ICD) or DSM diagnosis, remains the most commonly used term to describe abusive illness or condition falsification due to Factitious Disorder Imposed on Another (FDIA).</li><li>This disorder always includes a caretaker knowingly giving or producing false information. The DSM-5 characterizes the types of actions constituting illness falsification as the exaggeration, fabrication, simulation, or induction of physical or psychologic impairments.</li><li>A thorough and comprehensive record review and chronologic summary, along with an analysis of the suspected abusers' behaviors, is the foundation on which assessment of suspected pediatric condition falsification and FDIA rests.</li><li>Underlying medical or psychiatric disorders in the child that are congruent with the symptoms being reported **do not need to be ruled out** for a conclusion of abusive condition falsification or neglect to be made.</li><li>The abuser(s) should be required to engage in a medical monitoring plan designed to rapidly identify the recurrence of medical setting behaviors associated with pediatric condition falsification. All care must be directed through a single pediatrician and his or her predetermined backup provider to avoid doctor shopping and confusion about the treatment plan.</li></ul>
10. Pediatric Sleep Disorders	<ul><li>A sleepy toddler or preschooler exhibits paradoxical hyperactivity, irritability, and impulsivity, whereas sleepy older children exhibit signs and symptoms similar to that of adults with chronic sleep disruption such as low energy and drowsiness.</li><li>The peak age of occurrence of obstructive sleep apnea is between 2 and 6 years, which is usually a period when adenotonsillar hypertrophy and lymphoid hyperplasia are common. There is a second peak of obstructive sleep apnea in adolescence because of other risk factors such as obesity.</li><li>Diagnosis of obstructive sleep apnea is confirmed by a polysomnogram.</li><li>Insufficient sleep is the most common cause of sleepiness in adolescents.</li><li>Improving sleep hygiene is critical in treating children and adolescents with insomnia.</li></ul>
11. Concussion in Children and Adolescents	<ul><li>Concussions are considered a mild traumatic brain injury and can occur with contact to the head or with acceleration/deceleration forces.</li><li>Concussion may or may not involve loss of consciousness. In fact, most sports-related concussions are not associated with loss of consciousness.</li><li>The vast majority of patients with concussion will have a normal head CT and experience typical postconcussion symptoms, permitting observation in the outpatient setting.</li><li>Standard concussion treatment entails resting until all symptoms fully resolve followed by a graded program of exertion before medical clearance and return to play.</li><li>With conservative management that includes both physical and cognitive rest, many patients return to baseline within a few days.</li></ul>

12. Pediatric Delirium

- Pediatric delirium is a medical emergency that requires immediate management; however, in the hospital and outpatient settings, it often goes underdiagnosed.
- Pediatric delirium may present with three motoric subtypes: these include hyperactive, hypoactive, and mixed delirium. Hypoactive delirium is more likely to be overlooked by care providers or misdiagnosed as depression.
- A wider array of screening tools for delirium in pediatric patients is now available.
- To decrease the risk of delirium in ventilated patients, α-2 agonists, such as dexmedetomidine and clonidine, have been gaining favor as sedatives in this population.
- Psychologic distress is common after delirium, including symptoms of posttraumatic stress, anxiety, and depression.

13. Pediatric Catatonia

- Catatonia is frequently not recognized in the medical and psychiatric pediatric settings.
- In children, the catatonia symptoms may be mistaken for oppositional behaviors.
- There are no pathognomonic findings on imaging for catatonia.
- The first-line medications for catatonia are the benzodiazepines. There are no established guidelines for dosing or dose titration.
- In the treatment of catatonia, it is essential to identify and treat the underlying medical or neuropsychiatric condition.

14. Pediatric Inflammatory Brain Disease

- Symptoms of inflammatory brain disease vary greatly depending on the underlying etiology.
- Determining if the primary disease is due to CNS vasculitis versus an autoimmune encephalopathy is a helpful starting point.
- The hallmark of Pediatric Inflammatory Brain Disease (PIBD) is the *involvement of multiple domains*, including neurologic, cognitive, and psychiatric findings.
- Patients with inflammatory brain disorder appear to be very sensitive to adverse effects of psychotropic medications.
- Beyond the acute phase of illness, children can suffer from emotional, cognitive, and physical symptoms. Although some children's obsessive-compulsive disorder, tics, anxiety, mood disorder symptoms, attentional problems resolve, others do not. Some are left with ongoing emotional, processing, attentional, and fine motor difficulties. Some are left with ongoing pain and poor muscle tone.

15. Disruptive Mood Dysregulation Disorder

- Although irritability is a symptom of several psychiatric disorders, chronic irritability has been shown to have unique neurobiologic correlates and confers unique risk for functional impairment as compared with the comorbid disorders often seen with DMDD.
- Irritability causes significant functional impairment and has been shown to be a risk factor for significant morbidity.
- Irritability can be measured, and there are validated scales, which are reasonable tools for clinical settings.
- DMDD increases risk for anxiety and depression.
- There are nonpharmacologic interventions, which have been shown to change the psychologic underpinnings of DMDD and alter brain circuitry.

16. Pediatric Bipolar Disorder

- The prevalence of bipolar I disorder in the general population is approximately 1%, and when one expands to the bipolar spectrum (bipolar II and cyclothymia), the rate increases to 4%–6% of the population.
- In the DSM-5, to meet criteria for bipolar disorder, one must have met criteria for **at least one manic episode.** This includes an elevated, expansive, or irritable mood for most of the day, nearly every day, for at least a week or for any duration if hospitalized.
- Five cardinal symptoms that help distinguish pediatric bipolar disorder from ADHD are elations, grandiosity, flight of ideas/racing thoughts, decreased need for sleep, and hypersexuality.
- Up to half of those with bipolar disorder have a lifetime suicide attempt. Suicide in bipolar should be a focus of treatment, and early diagnosis, treatment, and intervention may help mitigate the long-term suicide risk.
- Pharmacotherapy is the cornerstone of the treatment of pediatric bipolar disorder.

17. Childhood-Onset
    Schizophrenia

- Hallucinations are neither necessary nor sufficient for a diagnosis of schizophrenia.
- The vast majority of patients with multidimensional impairments do not develop schizophrenia in adolescence or adulthood.
- Always evaluate for caregiver illness and impairment.
- Clozapine is a third-line medication that has demonstrated superior efficacy in individuals with schizophrenia who have failed at least two previous antipsychotic trials.
- Judicious monitoring for antipsychotic side effects is imperative, irrespective of the type used.

Index

Note: Page numbers followed by "t" indicate tables and "b" indicate boxes.

Printed in the United States
By Bookmasters